Modern Diagnostics: Emerging Electromagnetic Technologies

Modern Diagnostics: Emerging Electromagnetic Technologies

Editor: Shemeka Hoover

AMERICAN
MEDICAL PUBLISHERS
www.americanmedicalpublishers.com

AMERICAN
MEDICAL PUBLISHERS
www.americanmedicalpublishers.com

Cataloging-in-Publication Data

Modern diagnostics : emerging electromagnetic technologies / edited by Shemeka Hoover.
p. cm.
Includes bibliographical references and index.
ISBN 978-1-63927-730-8
1. Diagnostic imaging. 2. Diagnostic imaging--Technological innovations.
3. Electromagnetism in medicine. 4. Electromagnetism--Therapeutic use.
5. Electromagnetism--Physiological effect. 6. Electromagnetism--Technological innovations.
I. Hoover, Shemeka.
RC78.7.D53 M63 2023

American Medical Publishers,
41 Flatbush Avenue,
1st Floor, New York,
NY 11217, USA

ISBN 978-1-63927-730-8 (Hardback)

Contents

Preface

Over the recent decade, advancements and applications have progressed exponentially. This has led to the increased interest in this field and projects are being conducted to enhance knowledge. The main objective of this book is to present some of the critical challenges and provide insights into possible solutions. This book will answer the varied questions that arise in the field and also provide an increased scope for furthering studies.

Electromagnetism refers to the force of electric and magnetic fields which is frequently used in various technologies. Electromagnetic technologies are also used in medical imaging and diagnostics. The advancements in electromagnetic engineering such as computational methods, imaging theory and algorithms, measurement techniques, etc. have led to the development of this technology. Such advancements have led to development of low-cost, portable, and accurate microwave sensing/imaging systems which can help in overcoming various challenges existing in medical diagnostics. Currently, the electromagnetism research is focused on the use of microwave technologies in medical imaging and diagnostics. Microwave medical imaging makes use of the prominent dielectric contrast between healthy and disease-affected tissues to detect a pathological condition. The objective of microwave sensing technology is to monitor physiological parameters such as heart-rate, or disease-related biomarkers in the blood. A new medical application named microwave tomography is emerging as an effective means to monitor thermal ablation. In this book, various advancements in electromagnetic technology having applications in medical diagnostics have been looked at in detail. Medical researchers, scientists and students actively engaged in this field will find it full of crucial and unexplored concepts.

I hope that this book, with its visionary approach, will be a valuable addition and will promote interest among readers. Each of the authors has provided their extraordinary competence in their specific fields by providing different perspectives as they come from diverse nations and regions. I thank them for their contributions.

Editor

1

Application of Linear Gradient Magnetic Field in Arterial Profile Scanning Imaging

Yanjun Liu [1,2], Guoqiang Liu [2,3,*], Dan Yang [1,4,5,*] and Bin Xu [6]

1 College of Information Science and Engineering, Northeastern University, Shenyang 110819, China; 1800720@stu.neu.edu.cn
2 Institute of Electrical Engineering Chinese Academy of Sciences, Beijing 100190, China
3 School of Electronics, Electrical and Communication Engineering, University of Chinese Academy of Sciences, Beijing 100190, China
4 Key Laboratory of Data Analytics and Optimization for Smart Industry MOE, Northeastern University, Shenyang 110819, China
5 Liaoning Province Key Laboratory of Infrared Optoelectric Materials and Micro-Nano Devices, Northeastern University, Shenyang 110819, China
6 College of Computer Science and Engineering, Northeastern University, Shenyang 110819, China; xubin@mail.neu.edu.cn
* Correspondence: gqliu@mail.iee.ac.cn (G.L.); yangdan@mail.neu.edu.cn (D.Y.)

Abstract: *Background and Objectives*: Cardiovascular and cerebrovascular diseases caused by arterial stenosis and sclerosis are the main causes of human death. Although there are mature diagnostic techniques in clinical practice, they are not suitable for early disease prediction and monitoring due to their high cost and complex operation. The purpose of this paper is to study the coupling effect of arterial blood flow and linear gradient magnetic field, and to propose a method for the reconstruction of the arterial profile, which will lay a theoretical foundation for new electromagnetic artery scanning imaging technology. *Methods and Models*: A combination coil composed of gradient coils and drive coils is applied as a magnetic field excitation source. By controlling the excitation current, a linearly gradient magnetic field with a line-shaped zero magnetic field is generated, and the zero magnetic field is driven to scan in a specific direction. According to the magnetoelectric effect of blood flow, under the action of the external magnetic field, the voltage signals on the body surface can be detected by measuring electrodes. The location of the artery center line can be determined by the time–space relationship between voltage signals and zero magnetic field scanning. In addition, based on the reciprocity theorem integral equation, a numerical model between the amplitude of the voltage signal and the arterial radius is derived to reconstruct the arterial radius. The above physical process was simulated in the finite element analysis software COMSOL, and the voltage signals obtained from the simulation verified the arterial profile reconstruction. *Results*: Through finite element simulation verification, the imaging method based on a linear gradient magnetic field has a numerical accuracy of 90% and a spatial resolution of 1 mm. Moreover, under 100 Hz low-frequency alternating current excitation, the single scanning time is 0.005 s, which is far shorter than the arterial blood flow change cycle, meeting the requirements of real-time imaging. The results demonstrate the effectiveness and high theoretical feasibility of the proposed method in real-time arterial imaging. *Conclusions:* This study indicates the potential application of linear gradient magnetic fields in arterial profile imaging. Compared with traditional electromagnetic imaging methods, the proposed method has the advantages of fast imaging speed and high resolution, showing the certain application value in early real-time imaging of arterial disease. However, further studies are necessary to confirm its effectiveness in clinical practice by more medical data and real cases.

Keywords: electromagnetic sensor; linear gradient magnetic field; artery stenosis; finite element; magnetoelectric effects of blood flow; reciprocal theory

---

1. Introduction

According to investigation [1], cardiovascular and cerebrovascular diseases are the main causes of human death, and the main cause of cardiovascular and cerebrovascular diseases such as coronary heart disease and angina is atherosclerosis, which leads to arterial stenosis and affects the normal circulation of blood. At present, the commonly used diagnostic techniques for arterial stenosis include digital subtraction angiography (DSA), CT angiography (CTA), magnetic resonance angiography (MRA), and medical ultrasound examination. DSA is the gold standard of angiography, but because of its high trauma, it is generally used for preoperative examination [2,3]. CTA has the advantages of fast imaging and low trauma, but it still needs to inject a contrast agent, and X-ray has some potential harm to human body [4,5]. MRA is currently considered non-invasive and safe, but its diagnosis is costly and therefore not suitable for routine medical examinations [6,7]. Medical ultrasound examination technology has relatively low cost, high resolution, and can be used for real-time imaging. However, its disadvantages lie in the poor penetration of ultrasound to bone, extremely limited brain imaging, and the operator's manipulation is very important [8,9]. Superb skills and rich experience are necessary for obtaining high-quality images and making accurate diagnosis. Therefore, it is still expected to develop a non-invasive, low-cost, fast imaging, high-resolution, and easy to operate angiography technology, which can be applied to the early diagnosis of diseases in the future, even using portable, home-based diagnostic equipment.

In recent years, electromagnetic imaging technology for medical diagnosis has made great progress, and many novel imaging technologies have emerged, such as electrical impedance tomography, magnetic acoustic tomography, magneto-acousto-electrical tomography, magnetic induction tomography, thermoacoustic tomography, and so on [10–15]. Dr. Ruben Specogna and Dr. Antonio Affanni et al. effectively fused optical and impedance data and proposed novel biosensor and inversion technology for monitoring and predicting thrombosis characteristics, which provided a new idea for electromagnetic arterial blood flow imaging [16,17]. In 2016, Dr. Ali of The University of Huddersfield verified the linear relationship between electrode potential difference signal and blood flow under a uniform magnetic field through numerical simulation and experiment [18], which greatly promoted the research progress of the electromagnetic non-invasive blood flow measurement method.

In addition, 3D reconstruction technology has made significant progress in vascular diagnosis and treatment in recent years. Dr. Andrzej Polanczyk et al. proposed a method to reconstruct the 3D geometry of blood vessels using computational fluid dynamics and medical data to predict the outcome after surgery, and the comparison with real postoperative data shows that the reconstruction method has a high accuracy [19]. In fact, 3D reconstruction technology can not only be applied in clinical diagnosis and treatment, it can also be used as an important tool in the research of cutting-edge medical imaging technology. For example, it could combine digital twinning technology to build more realistic vascular simulation models, which would greatly facilitate non-medical researchers and promote the development of interdisciplinary research between medicine and engineering. It should be noted that this study focuses on the arterial imaging method based on the magnetoelectric effect of blood flow, so the finite element vascular model with electromagnetic parameters and flow velocity parameters is adopted. The influence of more hydrodynamic parameters will be considered in future studies.

In our previous work [20,21], based on the reciprocity theorem, we derived the integral equation of the surface potential signal and arterial blood flow velocity in detail and realized arterial imaging by inverting blood flow velocity distribution. However, this imaging method itself is an underdetermined and ill-conditioned problem. The higher resolution depends on more electrodes to obtain more surface potential data, and a large number of operations are required in the inversion process, resulting in the slow imaging speed, which is also one of the common problems of inversion imaging technology. Therefore, an arterial profile scanning imaging method based on a linear gradient magnetic field is proposed in this paper. A linear gradient magnetic field has been widely used in magnetic particle imaging [22], but the application of arterial flow imaging has not been studied so far. The advantage of this method is that the imaging speed is fast and does not require a lot of inversion calculation. Moreover, there is no need to generate a uniform magnetic field in the measurement area, so the volume of the excitation coil is saved, which is conducive to the miniaturization of the detection system.

The purpose of this paper is to study the coupling effect of arterial blood flow and a linear gradient magnetic field, and to propose a method for reconstruction of the arterial profile, which will lay a theoretical foundation for new electromagnetic artery scanning imaging technology. The organizational structure and main contributions of this paper are as follows. A combined coil structure that can drive rapid scanning of the zero magnetic field region is introduced in Section 2.2, a numerical model between the amplitude of the surface potential signal and the artery radius is derived in Section 2.3, and the algorithm process of arterial profile scanning imaging is introduced in Section 2.4. The finite element simulation results and the final imaging results are analyzed in Section 3. Finally, in Section 4, the general conclusions are summarized, and the future research direction is prospected.

2. Methods and Models

2.1. Basic Electromagnetic Theory

2.1.1. Magnetoelectric Effects of Blood Flow

Arterial blood flow has both fluidity and electrical conductivity. When the direction of the external magnetic field is perpendicular to the direction of blood flow, according to Faraday's law, the blood flow velocity will be coupled with the magnetic field to form a current source $\boldsymbol{J}_e$:

$$\boldsymbol{J}_e = \sigma \boldsymbol{v} \times \boldsymbol{B} \tag{1}$$

where σ is blood conductivity, $\boldsymbol{v}$ is blood flow velocity, and $\boldsymbol{B}$ is magnetic flux density. From Ohm's law vector equation and current continuity theorem, it can be further deduced that:

$$\nabla \cdot (\sigma \nabla u) = \nabla \cdot (\sigma \boldsymbol{v} \times \boldsymbol{B}) \tag{2}$$

where u is a scalar potential. From the above equation, it can be seen that the interaction between arterial blood flow velocity and external magnetic field will form an induced potential field within a certain range of human body, which is the magnetoelectric effect of blood flow. At this time, the potential signal caused by blood flow can be obtained through the measuring electrode on the skin surface.

2.1.2. Reciprocity Theorem Integral Equation

Rayleigh–Carson reciprocity theorem is often used to describe the relationship between two independent groups of sources and fields [23,24]. In the previous work [20], we derived the integral Equation (3) based on the reciprocity theorem, which was used to describe the relationship between the surface potential signal $u(\boldsymbol{r})$, blood flow velocity $\boldsymbol{v}(\boldsymbol{r})$, and magnetic flux density $\boldsymbol{B}(\boldsymbol{r})$:

$$u(\boldsymbol{r}) = \int_V \boldsymbol{J}_r(\boldsymbol{r}) \cdot (\boldsymbol{v}(\boldsymbol{r}) \times \boldsymbol{B}(\boldsymbol{r})) \mathrm{d}V \tag{3}$$

where $\boldsymbol{r}$ is the spatial position vector of the arterial blood flow area and $\mathrm{d}V$ is the volume of the arterial blood flow area. $\boldsymbol{J}_r(\boldsymbol{r})$ is the reciprocal current density; its physical meaning is the current density field generated by injecting 1 A DC current at the location of the measuring electrode when there is no external magnetic field. The closer $\boldsymbol{r}$ is to the electrode, the larger $\boldsymbol{J}_r(\boldsymbol{r})$ is. Therefore, when the position of the measuring electrode is determined, $J_r(r)$ is also determined. Some relevant studies also consider $J_r(r)$ as the contribution ability or weight value of flow velocity at different positions to the surface potential signal [18,25].

According to Equation (3), when the magnetic field and flow velocity are not correlated with time, the surface potential signal can be regarded as a function related to space, and the location of arterial blood flow can be reconstructed by using potential data and an image reconstruction algorithm. However, this imaging method is a typical underdetermined and ill-conditioned problem. The higher resolution depends on more electrodes to obtain more surface potential data, and a large number of operations are required in the inversion process, resulting in the slow imaging speed, which is not conducive to real-time imaging. In order to improve the related problems, an arterial profile scanning imaging method based on a linear gradient magnetic field is proposed in this paper.

2.2. *Combined Coil for Arterial Profile Imaging*

According to Equation (3), a surface potential signal is generated by the mutual coupling of blood flow velocity and the magnetic field, which means that when there is no magnetic field in the artery blood flow area or there is an equal and opposite magnetic field on both sides of the center line of the artery blood flow area, the surface potential signal will greatly attenuate or even disappear. According to this difference, a combined coil that can generate a linear gradient magnetic field with a zero magnetic field region is designed, an alternating magnetic field is applied to drive the zero magnetic field area to scan the measuring body parts, and the location of the artery is located by establishing a time–space relationship. This section mainly introduces the structure of the combined coil and the current excitation mode. The implementation of linear gradient magnetic field and zero magnetic field region scanning will be shown in Section 3.

2.2.1. Combined Coil Structure

The structure of the combined coil for the arterial profile scanning imaging is shown in Figure 1. It is an open measurement structure, consisting of four gradient coils (GC_1, GC_2, GC_3, and GC_4) with the same size and two driving coils (DC_1 and DC_2) with the same size. The central air area is the measured area, and the measured objects can be entered from the side.

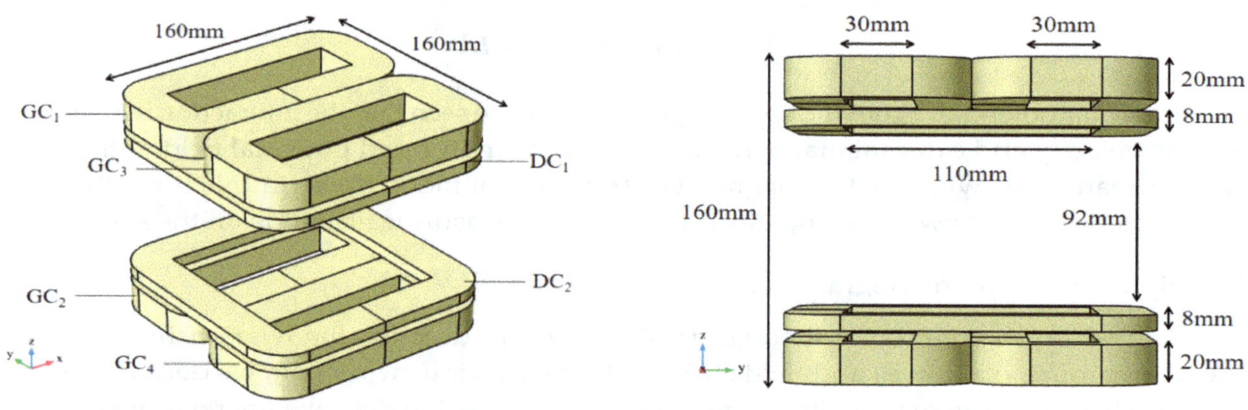

Figure 1. Schematic diagram of combined coil structure. (**a**) 3D view; (**b**) y-z view.

First of all, the same direct current is injected into the coaxial gradient coil, and a direct current of the same magnitude but opposite direction is injected into the gradient coil of different axes, namely $I_{GC_1} = I_{GC_2} = -I_{GC_3} = -I_{GC_4}$. The combined coil is established in the Cartesian coordinate system, as shown in Figure 1. The origin of coordinates is located in the center of the air gap area between the upper and lower coils, and the axial direction of the combined coil is in the direction of the z-axis.

Due to symmetry and superposition of the magnetic field, a linear region with a magnetic field strength of 0 will be generated near the x-axis (y = z = 0). The magnetic fields on both sides of the zero magnetic field region have opposite directions and the same intensity. On the whole, it is a linear gradient magnetic field along the y-axis. Compared with the circular coil of the same size, the rectangular coil will generate a more uniform zero magnetic field region and a larger linear range, which is conducive to scanning imaging.

In addition, in order to make the zero magnetic field region scan the measured region, two methods can be considered: mechanical control and electrical scanning. The mechanical control method is to drive the gradient coils to move in parallel along the y-axis through the mechanical and electrical devices, so that the zero magnetic field region can scan the measured region. However, this method may cause some uncertain errors in the scanning process and slow down the scanning speed. Therefore, the electrical scanning method is adopted in this paper to realize the fast scanning. The realization method is to apply the same low-frequency AC current to the driving coil DC_1 and DC_2 at the same time. Then, an alternating magnetic field will be generated in the measured region, and the position of the zero magnetic field region will be changed. The excitation alternating current I_{drive} adopted in this paper is in the following form:

$$I_{drive} = A\cos(2\pi f t) \tag{4}$$

where A is the amplitude of the ac current, which determines the maximum displacement of zero magnetic field region scanning, and f is the alternating frequency. The time required for the zero magnetic field to scan the whole measured region is a half cycle of the alternating magnetic field, that is, the time required for I_{drive} to change from A to $-A$. Therefore, the relationship between the scanning cycle T_S and f is as follows:

$$T_S = \frac{1}{2f} \tag{5}$$

Therefore, in the final scanning process, the magnetic field $\boldsymbol{B}$ in the measured region is the superposition of linear gradient magnetic field $\boldsymbol{B}_G$ and alternating magnetic field $\boldsymbol{B}_D$:

$$\boldsymbol{B}(\boldsymbol{r},t) = \boldsymbol{B}_G(\boldsymbol{r}) + \boldsymbol{B}_D(\boldsymbol{r},t) \tag{6}$$

2.2.2. Time–Space Relationship

According to the combined coil and excitation mode in Section 2.2.1, the continuous scanning of the zero magnetic field on the measured region can be realized; thus, a set of continuous time-varying potential signals can be obtained, and the potential signal at each time point can reflect the spatial position of the zero magnetic field. Therefore, the signal acquisition step size δ_{TR} and the imaging spatial resolution δ_{SR} have the following time–space relationship:

$$\frac{\delta_{TR}}{T_S} = \frac{\delta_{SR}}{W} \tag{7}$$

where W is the total length of the scanning path, and the length scanned by the zero magnetic field within δ_{TR} is δ_{SR}. Therefore, a set of time–space sequences will be obtained:

$$\mathbf{T} = \begin{bmatrix} t_1 \\ t_2 \\ \vdots \\ t_N \end{bmatrix}; \mathbf{Y} = \begin{bmatrix} y_1 \\ y_2 \\ \vdots \\ y_N \end{bmatrix}; N = \frac{W}{\delta_{SR}} + 1 = \frac{T_S}{\delta_{TR}} + 1 \tag{8}$$

where $\mathbf{T}$ represents time sequences, $\mathbf{Y}$ represents space sequences, and N is the number of sequences. Since the zero magnetic field is scanned along the y-axis, the x-axis coordinate does not change, so the

y-axis coordinate y_i is used to represent the space position. Thus, when a time point t_i is given, we can directly determine its corresponding space position y_i.

2.3. Relationship between Surface Potential Signal and Arterial Radius

For convenience, the human non-arterial tissue and the artery were respectively equivalent to two cylinders with different radii, as shown in Figure 2, in which the cylinder with a relatively small radius was the area of arterial blood flow, while the cylinder with a relatively large radius was the non-arterial tissue. A pair of measuring electrodes were placed on the surface of the body to detect the surface potential signal. The direction of arterial flow velocity set in the model was the positive direction of the x-axis. The magnetic field generated by the combined coil was mainly in the direction of the z-axis. The zero magnetic field region in the shape of a line is in the direction of the x-axis and the scanning direction is in the direction of the y-axis. The profile to be imaged in this study is the x-y plane, as shown in Figure 2b.

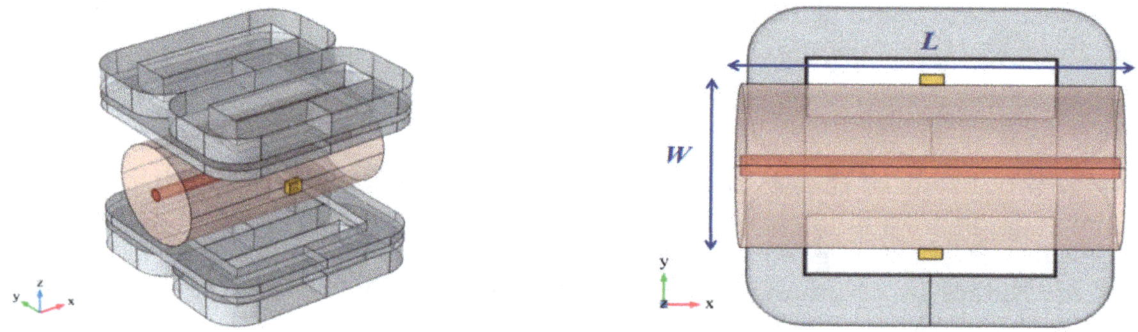

(a) (b)

Figure 2. Schematic diagram of surface potential signal simulation measurement in an artery model. (**a**) 3-D view; (**b**) x-y view.

According to the magnetoelectric effect of blood flow, the coupling of external magnetic field and arterial blood flow velocity will form an induced electric potential field. At this time, the potential signal can be detected through the measuring electrode on the skin surface. When the external magnetic field is related to time, the generated potential signal is also related to time. Therefore, the reciprocity theorem integral Equation (3) should be extended to the following form:

$$u(\boldsymbol{r},t) = \int_V \boldsymbol{J}_r(\boldsymbol{r}) \cdot (\boldsymbol{v}(\boldsymbol{r}) \times \boldsymbol{B}(\boldsymbol{r},t))\mathrm{d}V \tag{9}$$

According to Equation (9), when the magnetic field in the artery blood flow area is zero at t_0, the potential signal $u(\boldsymbol{r}, t_0)$ is also zero, so the position of the artery center line can be inferred from the moment of zero potential. Since the change of magnetic field is linear and continuous, the generated potential signal is also approximately linear and continuous, which cannot directly reflect the boundary information of the arterial blood flow area. However, in the actual diagnosis of arterial stenosis, it is necessary to observe the radius of the arterial blood flow area. According to Equation (9), it can be preliminarily determined that the amplitude of the potential signal is related to the volume of the integral region. Therefore, the mathematical relationship between the amplitude of the potential signal and the radius of the artery can be considered to solve the problem.

In addition, it should be noted that the arterial blood flow velocity $\boldsymbol{v}$ actually changes periodically, but the zero magnetic field scanning cycle T_S in this study is far less than the blood flow change cycle. Taking the vertebral artery as an example, the fitting function curve of blood flow velocity $\boldsymbol{v}$ in a cardiac cycle is given in reference [26,27], as shown in Figure 3, where the parameters of the fitting function are determined by a large number of experiments. As can be seen from Figure 3, the cycle time of blood flow change is about 0.8 s, while when the alternating frequency of excitation current is 100 Hz, the scanning cycle T_S is only 5×10^{-3} s. Therefore, for a study within a scanning cycle, v can be regarded as a constant.

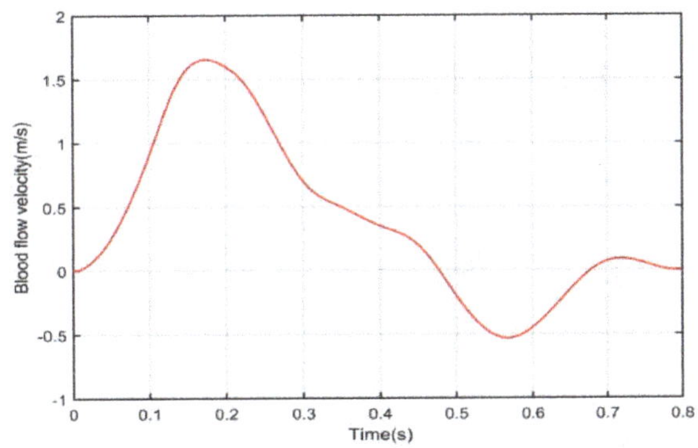

Figure 3. Changes in arterial blood velocity over time during a cardiac cycle [26,27].

In Figure 2, the direction of the blood flow is along the x-axis and the direction of the magnetic field is along the z-axis, and they are perpendicular to each other. According to the vector calculation rules, only the y component plays a role in $\boldsymbol{J}_r$. Therefore, we can convert the vector parameters in Equation (9) into the form of scalar parameter multiplication:

$$u(y_c,t) = \pi r^2 L J_r(y_c) v B(y_c,t) \tag{10}$$

where,

$$J_r(y_c) = \frac{1}{L}\int_{-\frac{L}{2}}^{\frac{L}{2}} J_r(x,y_c)\mathrm{d}x \tag{11}$$

$$B(y_c,t) = \frac{1}{L}\int_{-\frac{L}{2}}^{\frac{L}{2}} B(x,y_c,t)\mathrm{d}x \tag{12}$$

where r is the radius of the artery, L is the length of the measured region as shown in Figure 2, and it is also the length of the zero magnetic field region in the shape of a line. y_c is the y-axis coordinate corresponding to the center line of the artery. Since the radius of the artery is relatively small, the change of each parameter value in the radial direction of the artery is not significant, so we consider replacing the value of each point in the radial direction with the value of the center line of the artery. $J_r(y_c)$ is the average of the y component of the reciprocal current density $\boldsymbol{J}_r$ on the line $y = y_c$, and $B(y_c,t)$ is the average of the z component of the magnetic flux density $\boldsymbol{B}$ on the line $y = y_c$. In Figure 2, the origin point of the coordinate system is just at the intersection of the connecting line between two electrodes position and the center line of the artery. Therefore, the integral range of Equations (10) and (11) is from $-L/2$ to $L/2$.

In fact, $[LJ_r(y_c)]$ in Equation (10) can also be equivalent to the average current density J of a cylinder with a unit axial length. Figure 4 shows the distribution of the equivalent current density J, where the left electrode position is injected with 1 A DC current and the right electrode is grounded. The yellow arrow in Figure 4a is the current flow direction, and the green curve is the isoline of current density. As can be seen from Figure 4b, the values of the reciprocal current density are distributed symmetrically with y = 0 as the center line, the values near the electrode are very large, and the farther from the electrode, the smaller the value. This also indicates that the distance between the arterial blood flow and the electrode is negatively correlated with the contribution of the blood flow to the electrode surface potential signal.

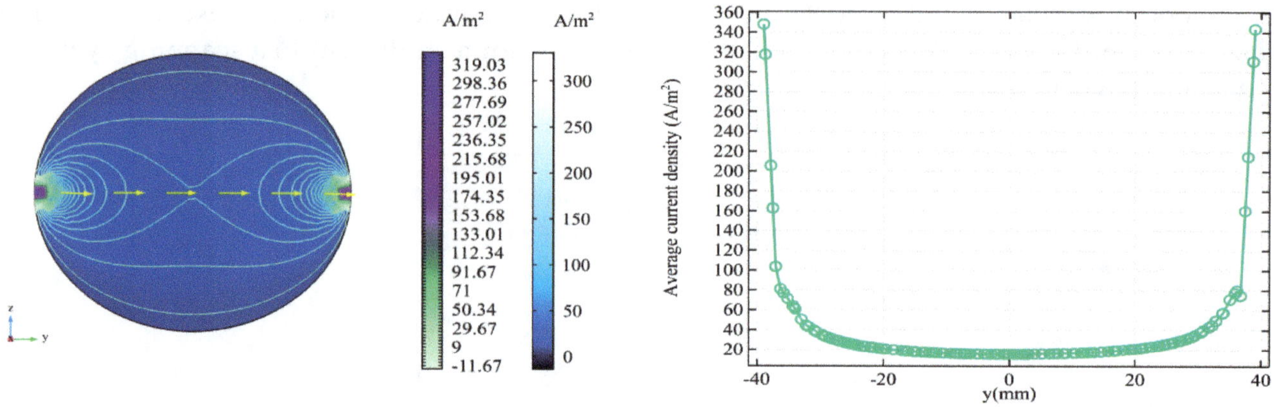

(a) (b)

Figure 4. The reciprocal current density distribution on the cross-section. (**a**) y–z views; (**b**) The current density distribution on the connection line of the two electrodes (z = 0).

Therefore, Equation (10) can be further simplified as follows:

$$u(y_c, t) = \pi r^2 J(y_c) v B(y_c, t) \tag{13}$$

The derivative of the time term in the equation is as follows:

$$\frac{\partial u(y_c, t)}{\partial t} = \pi r^2 J(y_c) v \frac{\partial B(y_c, t)}{\partial t} \tag{14}$$

$\partial u/\partial t$ represents the slope of the time-varying potential signal curve. $\partial B/\partial t$ is constant when the magnetic field at y_c linearly changes, and v and $J(y_c)$ are also constant. Therefore, the slope of the potential signal curve is mainly related to the radius of the artery. The larger the radius, the higher the slope of the potential signal curve, leading to the greater peak value of the potential signal. According to the excitation current mode in Equation (4), the magnetic field is the largest at the beginning time t_s and the end time t_e of a scanning cycle, so the amplitude of the potential signal is the largest at the time t_s and t_e. Since the actual position of the artery is not always at the center of the measured region, the potential amplitude at the two moments is not always the same. However, when the scanning cycle has been determined, $|u(y_c, t_s) - u(y_c, t_e)|$ remains unchanged. Therefore, $|u(y_c, t_s) - u(y_c, t_e)|$ and r satisfy the following relation:

$$|u(y_c, t_s) - u(y_c, t_e)| = K_{se}(y_c) r^2 \tag{15}$$

where the proportionality coefficient K_{se} satisfies:

$$K_{se}(y_c) = |K(y_c, t_s) - K(y_c, t_e)| = \pi J(y_c) v |B(y_c, t_s) - B(y_c, t_e)| \tag{16}$$

In Equation (16), J and B are determined by the structure of the measuring electrode and combined coil structure and the mode of the excitation current, which are called inherent parameters of the system and independent of the measured object. Thus, a linear relationship between the amplitude of surface potential signal and the square of the arterial radius can be established. After the proportional coefficient K_{se} is calculated according to prior knowledge, the radius of the arterial blood flow area can be solved.

2.4. Principle of Arterial Profile Scanning Imaging

Arterial profile scanning imaging based on a linear gradient magnetic field mainly includes location imaging and a radius reconstruction of the arterial, and its basic process is shown in Figure 5.

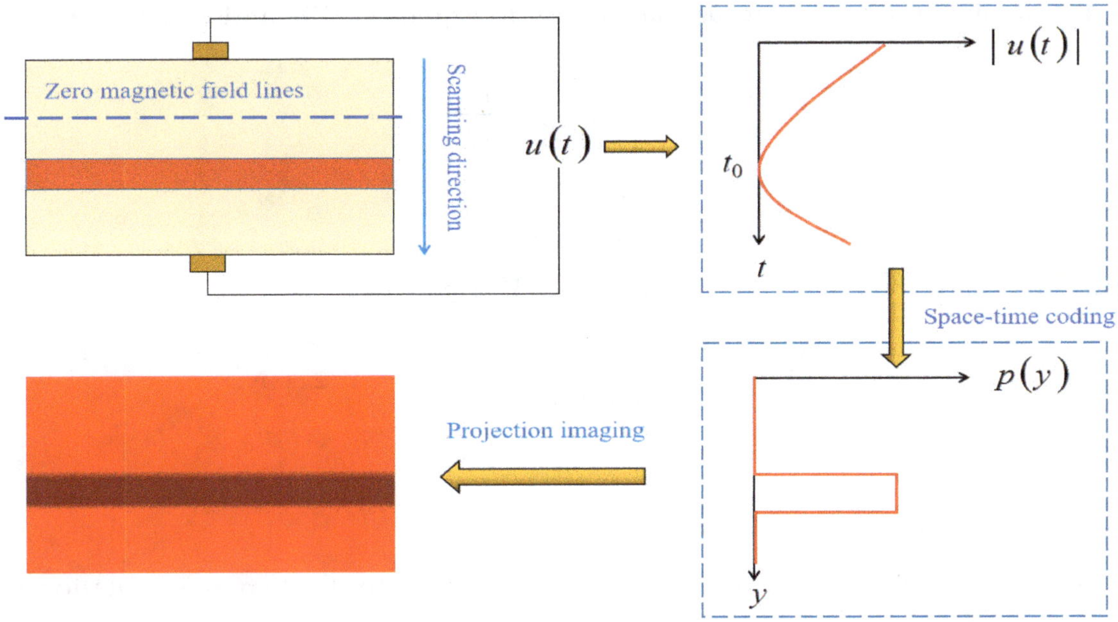

Figure 5. Schematic diagram of arterial profile scanning imaging based on a linear gradient magnetic field.

Firstly, the gradient coils are used to generate the linear gradient magnetic field with a zero magnetic field region, and at the same time, the driving coils are used to generate an alternating magnetic field to drive the zero magnetic field region to scan along the y-axis, so as to establish the time–space relationship. Then, a time-varying potential signal $u(t)$ is obtained by using measuring electrodes, and the center line position of the arterial is determined by the time characteristic of $u(t)$. Then, the arterial radius is solved by Equation (15), and then the one-dimensional projection sequence $p(y)$ is obtained. Finally, $p(y)$ is projected onto a two-dimensional plane in-line projection to obtain the arterial profile. The implementation steps of transforming potential signals into projection sequences are as follows:

Step 1: The surface potential signal sequence is obtained by measurement:

$$\mathbf{U} = \begin{bmatrix} u_1 \\ u_2 \\ \vdots \\ u_N \end{bmatrix}; N = \frac{W}{\delta_{SR}} + 1 = \frac{T_S}{\delta_{TR}} + 1 \tag{17}$$

where u_1 is the potential value at the first time point of the scanning cycle, and u_N is the potential value at the last time point of the scanning cycle.

Step 2: Find the time t_0 corresponding to zero potential, and calculate the scanning distance w of the zero magnetic field region; then, determine the center line coordinate y_c of the artery through the time–space relationship (7):

$$w = \frac{\delta_{TR}}{\delta_{SR}} t_0 \tag{18}$$

$$y_c = -\frac{W}{2} + w \tag{19}$$

Step 3: Calculate the proportional coefficient K_{se} according to Equation (16).

Step 4: Calculate the artery radius r according to Equation (15), and determine the boundary coordinates y_{b1} and y_{b2}:

$$r = \sqrt{\frac{|u_1 - u_N|}{K_{se}(y_c)}} \tag{20}$$

$$\begin{aligned} y_{b1} &= y_c - r \\ y_{b2} &= y_c + r \end{aligned} \tag{21}$$

Step 5: Determine the final projection sequence $\mathbf{P} = [p_1 \cdots p_N]^T$:

$$p_i = \begin{cases} |u_1 - u_N| & y_{b1} \le y_i \le y_{b2} \\ 0 & y_i < y_{b1}, y_i > y_{b2} \end{cases}, i = 1, 2 \cdots N. \tag{22}$$

3. Results

3.1. Finite Element Modeling

First, according to the structure of Figures 1 and 2, a 3D finite element simulation model was constructed in COMSOL, including the combined coil model and the single artery equivalent model. The geometric dimensions of the artery model refer to the dimensions of the common carotid artery in reference [27]. The mesh generation structure of the model is shown in Figure 6.

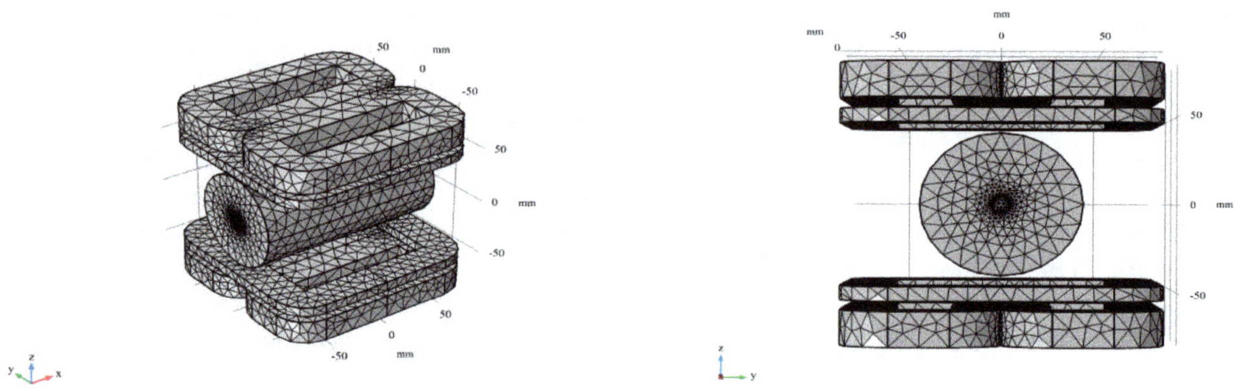

(a) (b)

Figure 6. 3D finite element simulation model. (**a**) 3D view; (**b**) y-z view.

In the study, the arterial model is the area we're interested in, so we set the arterial model mesh to "Extra fine" in "Predefined" and the combined coil model to "Normal". The finite element model contains 23,786 mesh vertices and 141,253 tetrahedra. These settings ensure a balance between CPU time and numerical accuracy.

In addition, some necessary parameter settings include the following. The blood flow velocity was set at 0.7 m/s and the electrical conductivity of the artery model was set to 1.09 S/m of the conductivity of the blood (the typical conductivity value) [28]. The material of the combined coil model was set to copper, and its conductivity is 5.998×10^7 S/m. The relative permeability of the whole model was set as 1. The four gradient coils have the same specifications with 500 turns, and the two drive coils have the same specifications with 200 turns. The current applied to the gradient coil group was 10 A, and the amplitude and frequency of the alternating current of the drive coil group were 13 A and 100 Hz, respectively. Therefore, the scanning cycle T_S of the zero magnetic field line is 5×10^{-3} s, the length W of the scanning path of the zero magnetic field line is 80 mm, and when the expected spatial resolution δ_{SR} is 1 mm, according to Equation (7), the signal acquisition step size δ_{TR} should be 6.25×10^{-5} s.

3.2. Magnetic Field Analysis

3.2.1. Linear Gradient Magnetic Field

When only the gradient coils (GC_1, GC_2, GC_3, and GC_4) was given 10 A current, the linear gradient magnetic field generated was shown in Figure 7. In order to observe the overall magnetic field distribution in the measured region more clearly, a cuboid air field with a size of 200 mm × 200 mm × 80 mm was added. It can be clearly seen in Figure 7b that the zero magnetic field region in the shape of a line was generated near y = 0, which is caused by the different excitation current directions of coils with different axes. The magnetic flux density modulus on both sides of the zero magnetic field is basically same, but the magnetic field direction is opposite. The x–y plane shown in Figure 7 is the plane to be imaged. When an alternating magnetic field is applied, the zero magnetic field will move along the y-axis for scanning.

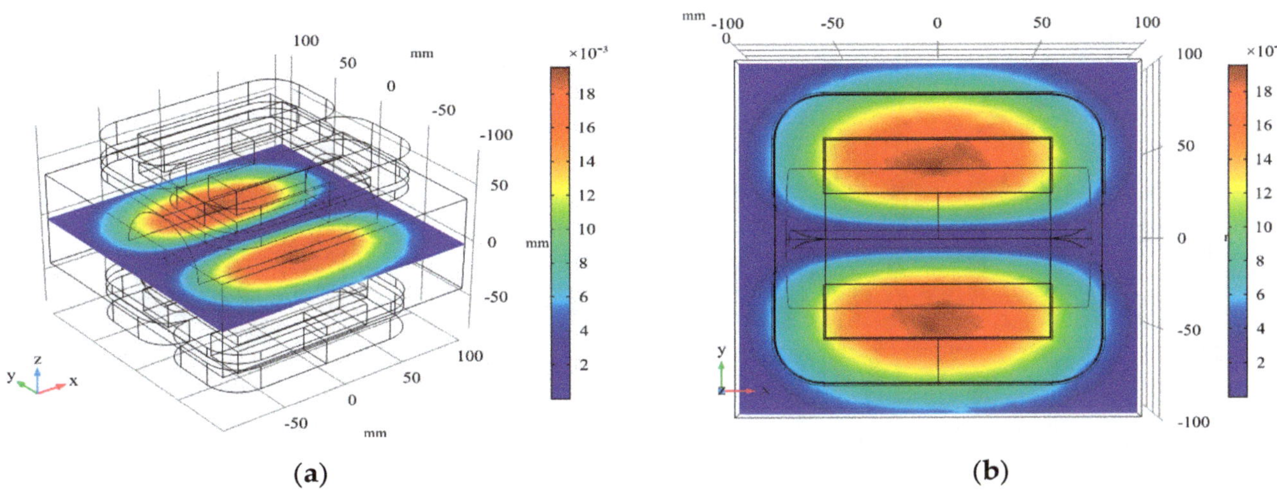

Figure 7. The magnetic flux density modulus distribution of the linear gradient field generated by the gradient coils. (**a**) 3D view; (**b**) x–y view.

The relationship between the excitation current I_G of the gradient coils and the generated magnetic field B_G is shown in Figure 8. Figure 8a,b are the magnetic field distribution on the line between points (0, −100, 0) and (0, 100, 0). Figure 8c,d are the magnetic field distribution on the line between points (0, −40, 0) and (0, 40, 0), namely the artery model range.

As can be seen from Figure 8a, the magnetic field within the scope of action of the combined coil is a sinusoidal wave distribution, reaching its peak value near the central axis of the gradient coil, and the excitation current and magnetic field peak value show a linear relationship. When I_G is 10 A, 20 A, 30 A, 40 A, and 50 A, the peak value of the gradient magnetic field B_G generated is 0.019 T, 0.038 T, 0.057 T, 0.076 T and 0.095 T, respectively. The linear region between the positive and negative peaks is the linear gradient magnetic field we need, as shown in Figure 8c. The measured object will be placed within this range, and this linearity ensures that the magnetic field at each point in the scanning process of the zero magnetic field can also change linearly with time. Figure 8b,d show good numerical symmetry of the magnetic field on both sides of the zero magnetic field.

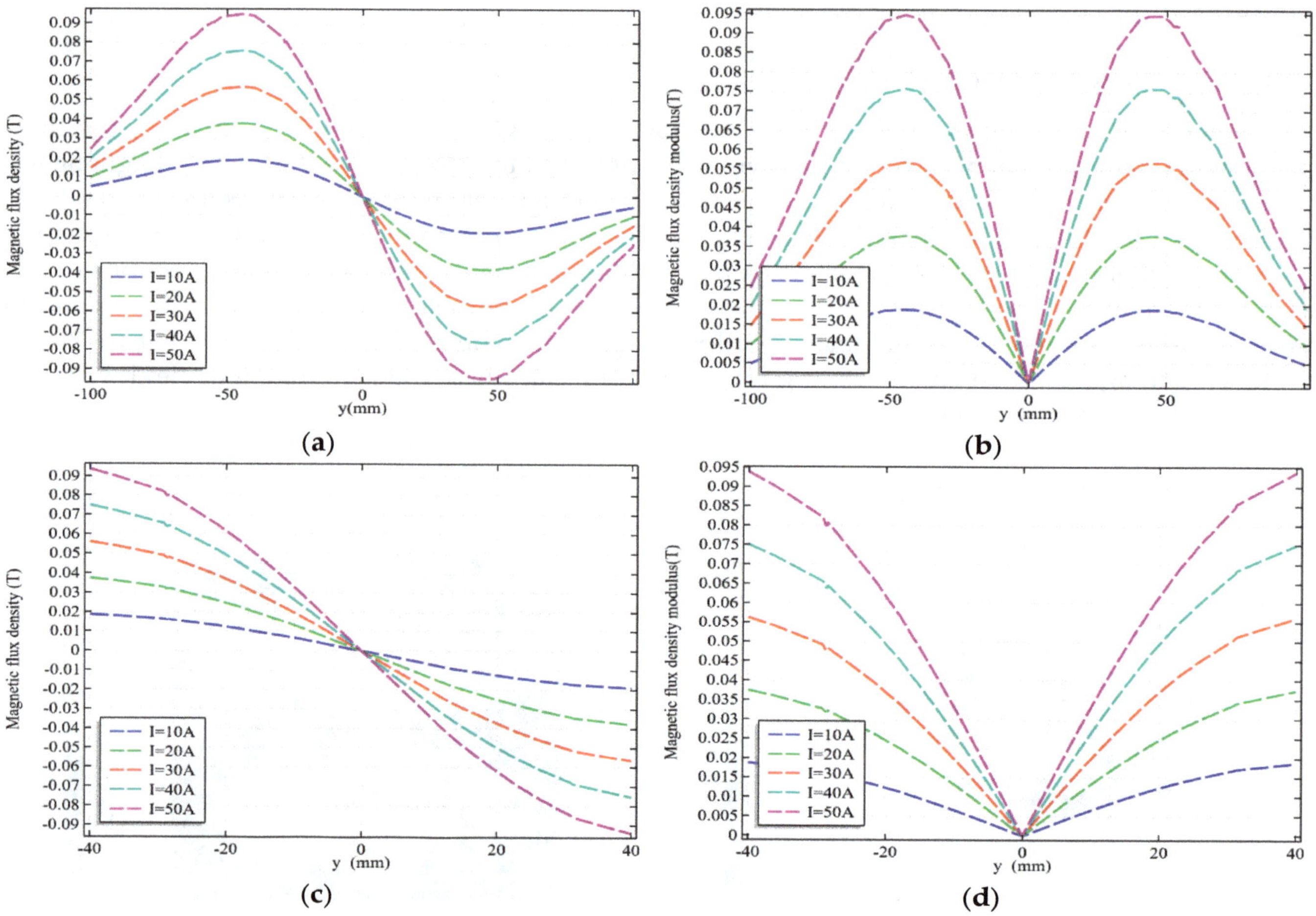

Figure 8. The linear gradient magnetic fields with different excitation currents near x = 0. (**a**) The magnetic flux density of the entire observed region; (**b**) The magnetic flux density modulus of the entire observed region; (**c**) The magnetic flux density within the radial range of the artery model; (**d**) The magnetic flux density modulus values within the radial range of the model.

3.2.2. Zero Magnetic Field Scanning

After the linear gradient magnetic field and zero magnetic field region are generated from the gradient coil group, an alternating current is injected into the driving coils (DC_1 and DC_2) to generate the alternating magnetic field, and zero magnetic field scanning can be realized through the superposition of the magnetic field. The scanning process is shown in Figure 9. Figure 9a shows the positions of the zero magnetic field region when currents with different amplitude are applied to the drive coils, respectively. The color bar is adjusted to highlight the positions of the zero magnetic field region. It can be clearly seen that the zero magnetic field region moves from y = −50 to y = 50 as the excitation current goes from 15 A to −15 A. Figure 9b shows the magnetic field distribution on the *y*-axis corresponding to Figure 9a, showing the details of the superposition of magnetic fields with different driving currents. Therefore, when the cosine excitation method as shown in Equation (4) is adopted for the driving coils, the zero magnetic field region will complete a quick scan on the measured plane within half a cosine cycle. Since the radial range of the artery model was [−40, 40], the excitation current amplitude we chose was 13 A.

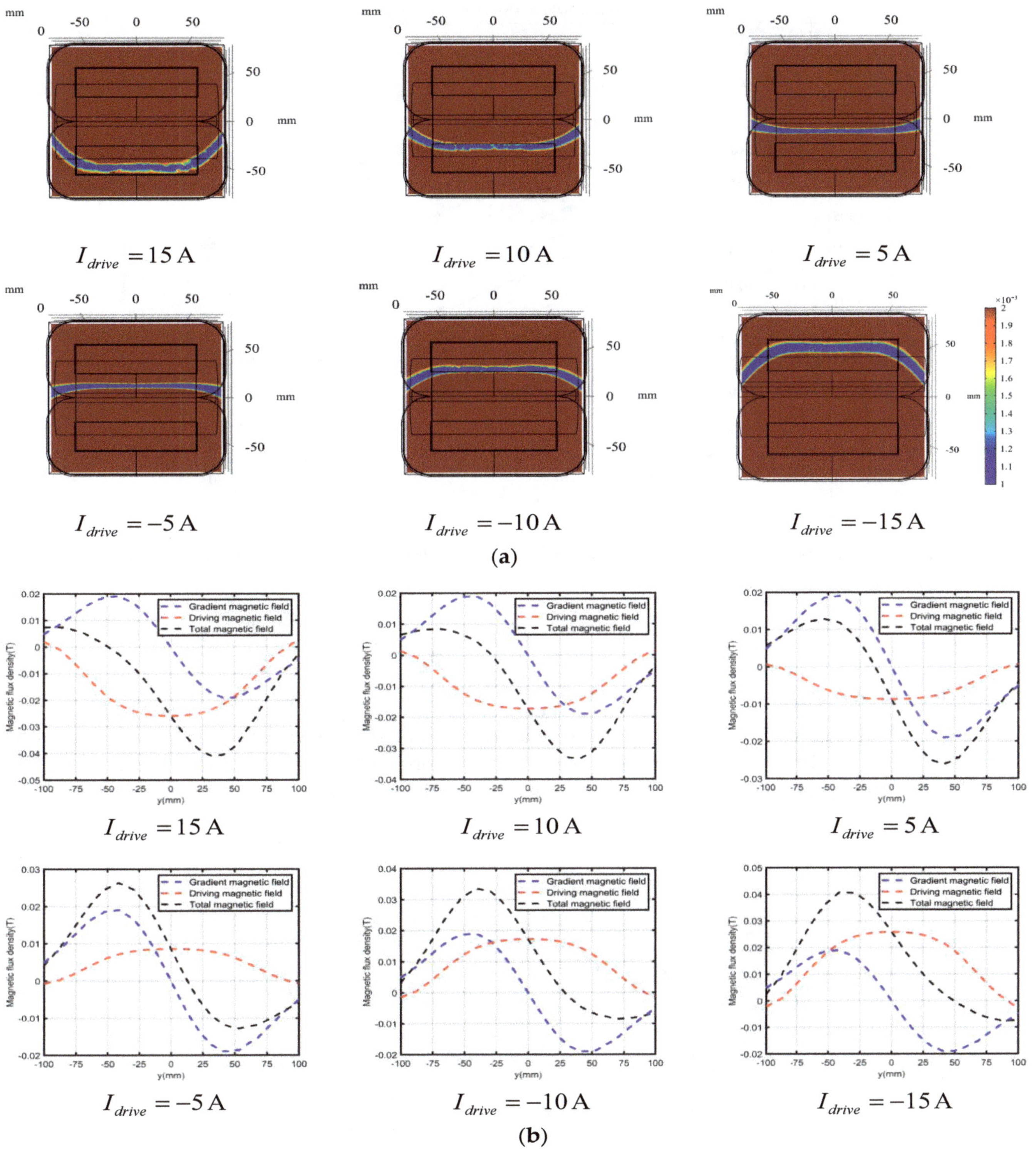

Figure 9. Distribution of magnetic fields with different driving currents. (**a**) position of zero magnetic field region; (**b**) Superposition of linearly gradient magnetic fields with different driving magnetic fields.

The magnetic field distribution in the radial direction (along the y-axis) of the artery model, namely within the scanning imaging region, is shown in Figure 10. The zero magnetic field moves from $y = -40$ to $y = 40$ over time, and the closer to the center, the more uniform the change. The magnetic field of each point changes linearly with time, that is, the rate of change of magnetic field $\partial B/\partial t$ is approximately constant.

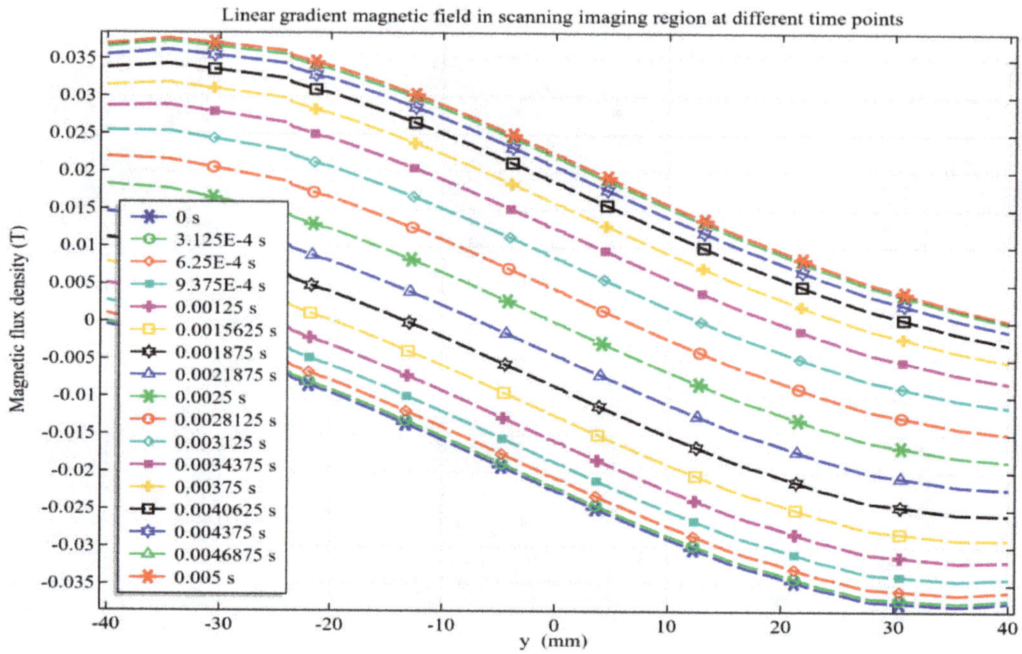

Figure 10. Linear gradient magnetic field distribution at different time points within the range of the artery model.

3.3. *Scanning Imaging Results*

3.3.1. Arterial Position Imaging

As shown in Figure 11, in order to test the sensitivity of the proposed scanning imaging method to the arterial position, different d values were set for simulation, and the radius of the artery was set as 5 mm. The electrode potential signals in a scanning cycle with different d values are shown in Figure 12.

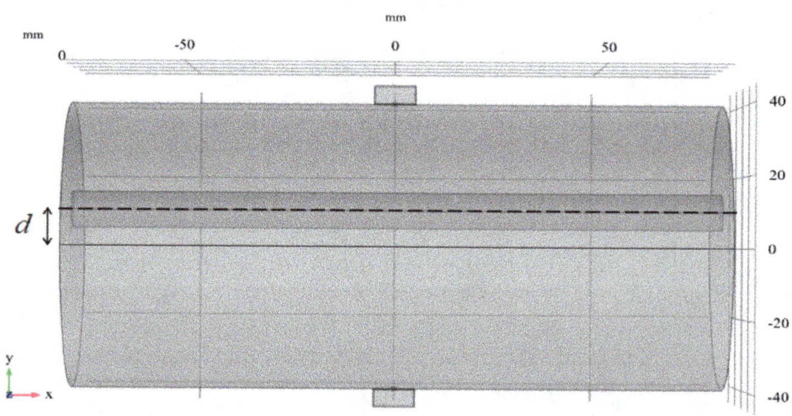

Figure 11. d represents the distance from the center of the artery to y = 0.

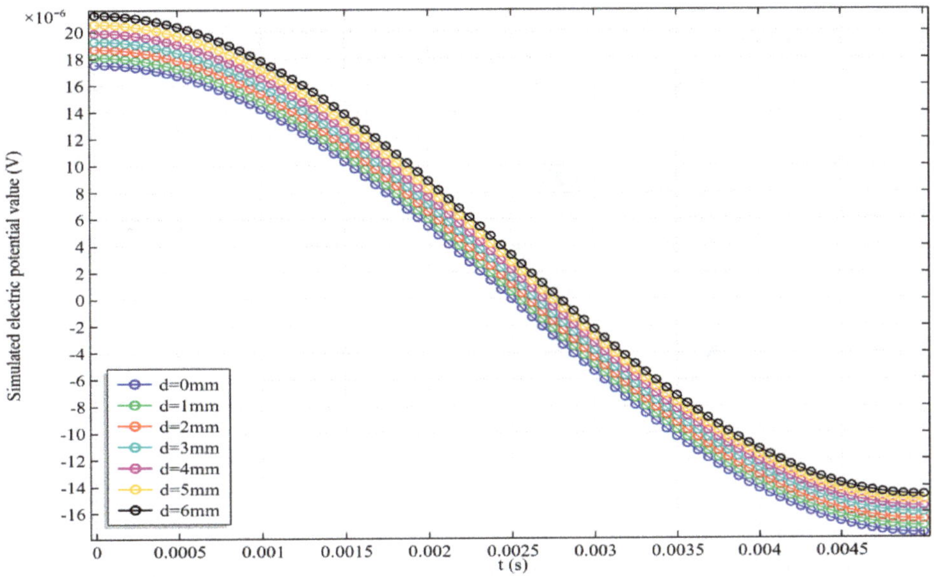

Figure 12. The electrode potential signal during a scanning cycle with different d values.

$d = 0$ mm in Figure 12 indicates that the center line of the artery is at y = 0. According to the excitation mode, when t = 0.0025 s, the alternating magnetic field is 0; then, the zero magnetic field is at y = 0, so at this moment, the electrode potential decreases to zero. According to the magnetic field analysis in Section 3.2, the scanning direction of the zero magnetic field is from y = −40 to y = 40. Therefore, when d gradually increases, the artery gradually moves to the positive y-axis, and the time corresponding to the zero potential also increases, which is in line with expectations. According to the imaging steps in Section 2.4, the arterial radius r and projection sequence $\mathbf{P}$ can be calculated for imaging. The imaging results are shown in Figure 13, and the error analysis between the reconstructed value and the real value of the radius is shown in Figure 14. In order to clearly observe the difference in the position of reconstructed arteries, four images with d values of 0 mm, 2 mm, 4 mm, and 6 mm were presented.

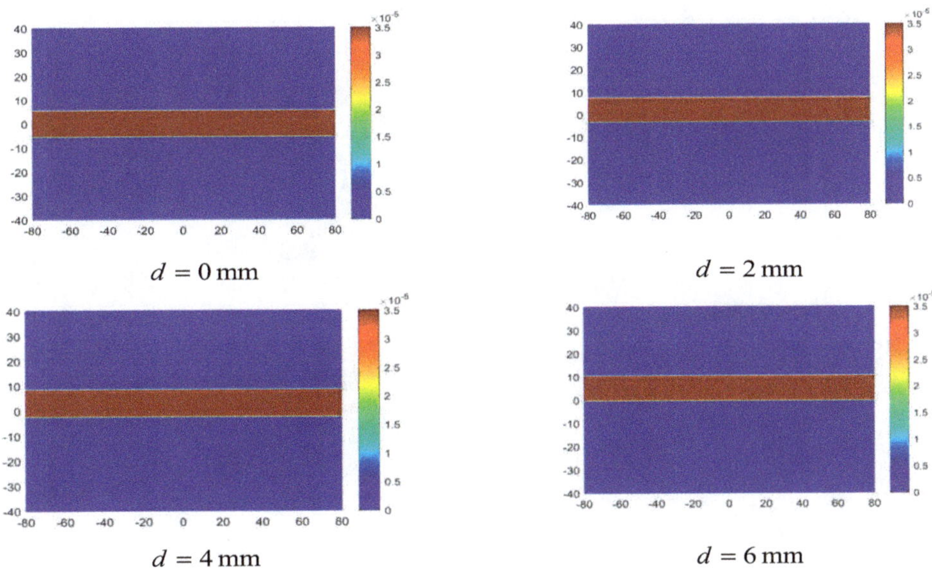

Figure 13. Imaging results of arterial blood flow profile with different d values.

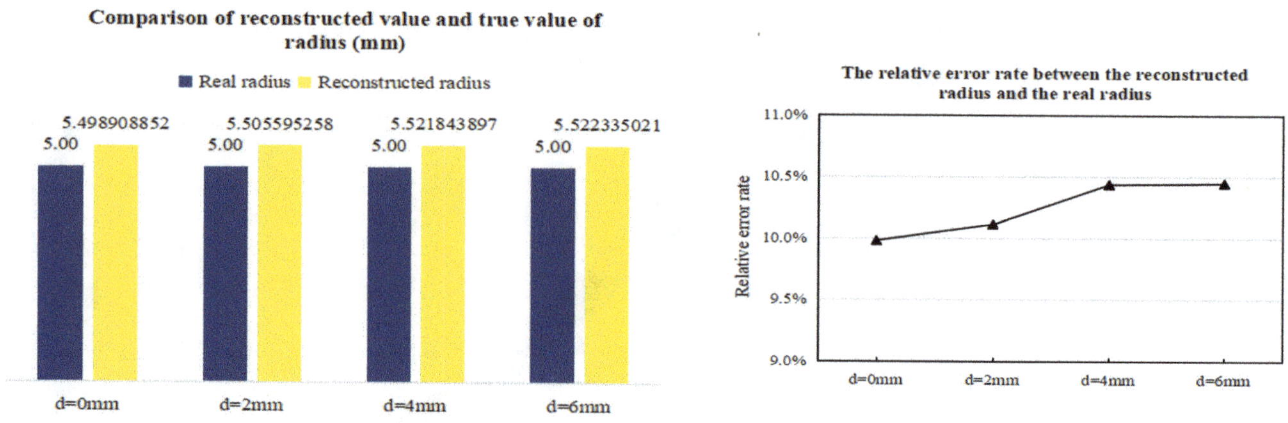

(**a**) (**b**)

Figure 14. Error of reconstructed value and true value of artery radius with different *d* values. (**a**) The comparison of the reconstructed radius value with the true value. (**b**) The relative error between the reconstructed radius value and the true value.

It can be seen from Figure 13 that the reconstructed radius is highly consistent with the true radius, and the reconstruction accuracy is about 90%. Although the reconstruction error increases slightly with the increase of *d* value, the dispersion degree between the four groups of errors is very low, with the relative error rate between 10% and 10.5%, which indicates that the scanning imaging method proposed in this paper has no specificity for arterial location. In addition, since the absolute error of the four groups of results is around 0.5 mm, it can be speculated that the error may be due to the approximate calculation of K_{se}. To verify this hypothesis, arterial models with different *r* values were set for imaging.

3.3.2. Imaging Results of Arterial Profile with Different Radii

Four groups of artery models with different radius *r* were set, in which *r* was 1 mm, 2 mm, 3 mm, and 4 mm respectively, and the center line of the four groups of arteries was y = 0. The electrode potential signal is shown in Figure 15.

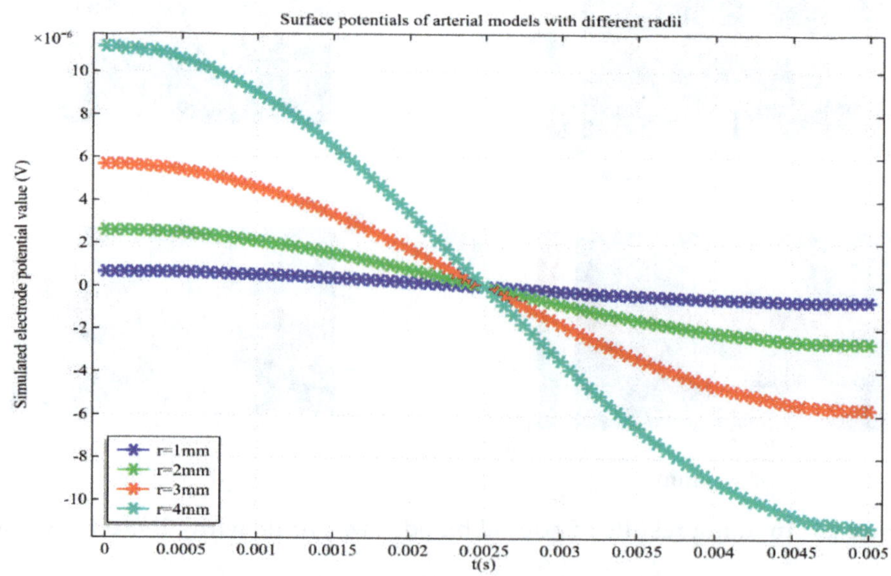

Figure 15. The electrode potential signal during a scanning cycle with different *r*.

In Figure 15, the zero potential at half of the scanning cycle indicates that the center line of the artery is at y = 0, and with the decrease of r, the slope and amplitude of the potential signal gradually decrease, which is consistent with the analysis in Equation (14). The comparison between the reconstructed value of radius and the true value is shown in Figure 16, and the imaging results of the arterial profile are shown in Figure 17.

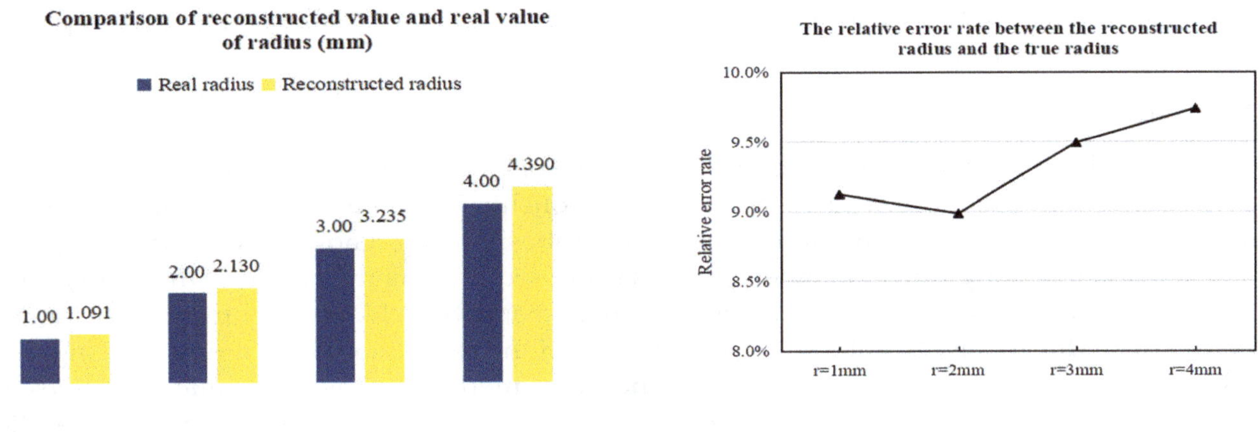

(a) (b)

Figure 16. Error of reconstructed value and true value of artery radius with different r values. (**a**) The comparison of the reconstructed radius value with the true value. (**b**) The relative error between the reconstructed radius value and the true value.

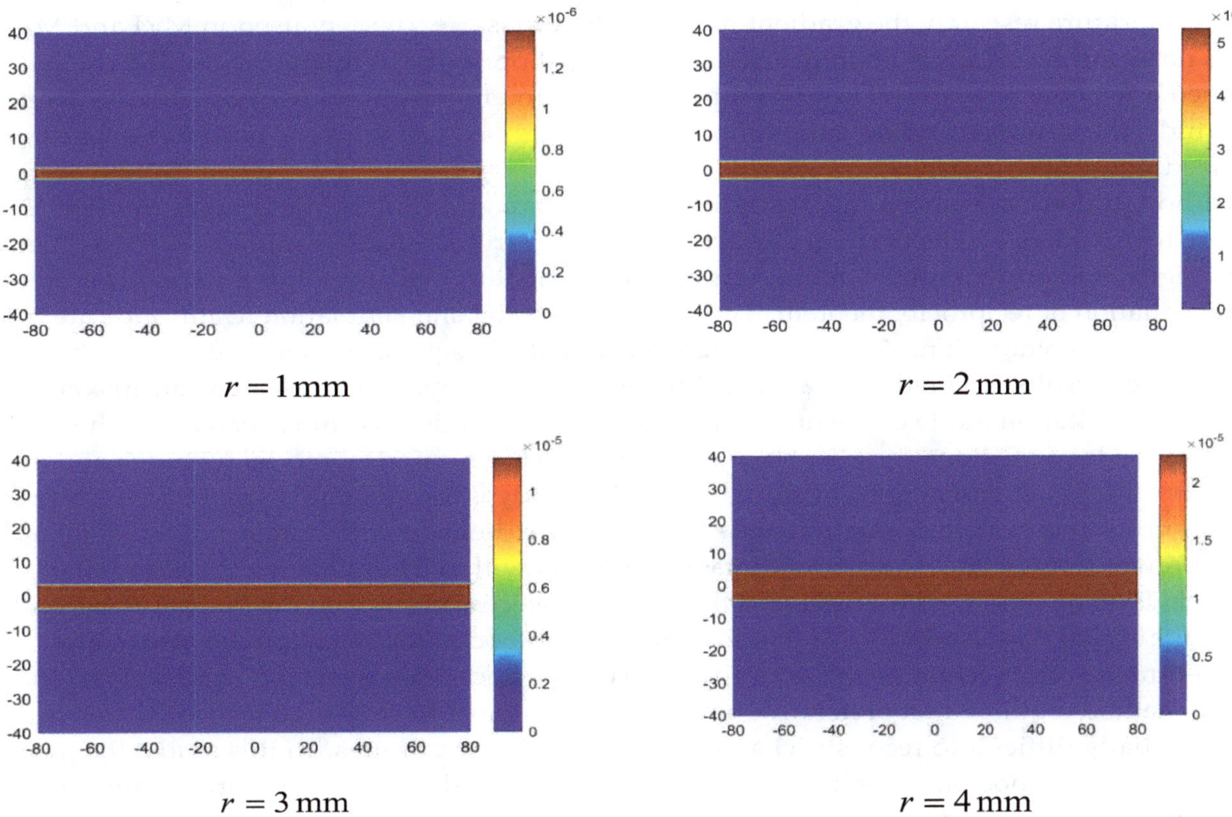

Figure 17. Imaging results of arterial blood flow profile with different r values.

It can be seen from Figure 16 that the reconstruction results of the artery model with different radius all have an error of about 9.5%, which further proves that this is an approximate error generated by calculating the K_{se}. This error can be improved by adding a correction factor greater than 1 to K_{se}.

On the other hand, the approximate error decreases with the decrease of the radius. The reason for this phenomenon is that the value of the artery center line is used to replace the value of each point in the radial direction in the imaging process. Therefore, the smaller the radius, the more accurate the approximation. When r = 1 mm, the error increases slightly, because the zero magnetic field region is not a standard line shape, so when the arterial blood flow area is too narrow, the error will increase. In general, the accuracy of radius reconstruction results of each group of models is above 90%, and the spatial resolution is 1 mm, indicating that the scanning imaging method proposed in this paper has high theoretical feasibility.

4. Discussion

In this study, firstly, the magnetoelectric effect of arterial blood flow is analyzed, and the reciprocity theorem integral equation used to describe the relationship between detecting voltage signal and arterial blood flow velocity is introduced. Based on the above theory, a novel arterial scanning imaging approach using a linear gradient magnetic field is proposed. The main content of this study includes three parts: generation and scanning of a linear gradient magnetic field, establishment of the numerical model between the voltage signal and artery radius, and the realization of scanning imaging.

Tobias Knopp et al. earlier studied the generation method of free magnetic field lines along a specific direction, proposed a combined coil structure consisting of two mutually perpendicular Maxwell coil pairs [29], and applied it to magnetic particle imaging (MPI) to improve the magnetic field scanning efficiency [30]. Can Barıs Top et al. studied a combined coil similar to this study, mainly analyzing the scanning trajectories of free magnetic field lines in MPI [22]. Koray Ertan et al. studied the coupling effects among gradient coil arrays and proposed a circuit model and analytical formula for driving mutually coupled gradient coil arrays in magnetic resonance imaging (MRI) [31]. According to previous literature research, the gradient magnetic field has been widely used in MRI and MPI, but there is no report on its application in arterial imaging at present. Compared with MRI and MPI, the combined coil in this study is relatively simple and easy to implement. However, with the deepening of the study, the structure and excitation mode of the combined coil may still need to be continuously optimized in further studies.

Although there have been many studies on electromagnetic blood flow measurement [32–34], there are few studies on electromagnetic artery imaging. In this study, a numerical model between voltage signal and artery radius under linear gradient magnetic field scanning is derived based on the integral equation of reciprocity theorem. The numerical model and simulation results indicate that the amplitude of the voltage signal is approximately linear with the square of artery radius, which is similar to the research results of Maythem [18]. The difference is that Maythem' s research conclusion is based on the static excitation mode of the uniform magnetic field, while this study focuses on the scanning excitation mode of the linear gradient magnetic field, so the numerical model includes not only the space term but also the time term. In other words, this study is a supplement and improvement to the existing knowledge system of electromagnetic artery measurement and imaging.

In previous study [20,21], an artery imaging method with uniform magnetic field excitation was proposed. The voltage signal was detected through a 16-electrode array on the body surface, and then the voltage signal was used to solve the distribution of blood velocity inside the artery, after which the two-dimensional section of the artery was reconstructed. However, the results show that this imaging method requires a lot of iterative operations in order to achieve high reconstruction accuracy, and it is usually difficult to reconstruct an image within a few minutes. In this study, the proposed arterial imaging method based on linear gradient magnetic field scanning excitation adopts scanning projection imaging instead of iterative operation. Therefore, the imaging speed is greatly improved, and the research results indicate that the imaging speed is positively correlated with the amplitude and frequency of the alternating current. In theory, hundreds of images can be obtained within 1 s, showing high application potential for the early diagnosis of arteriosclerosis and monitoring arterial expansion and contraction.

Although the arterial imaging method based on a linear gradient magnetic field shows good application potential, this study still has some limitations. First of all, the finite element simulation model constructed in this study only considers the electromagnetic parameters and flow velocity of blood, without considering the influence of fluid dynamics. In fact, the distribution of blood flow velocity in blood vessels is not completely uniform due to the stress of the blood vessel wall and blood. Meanwhile, due to the complexity of the arterial vascular structure, it may require multiple scans to accurately reconstruct the arterial profile. These factors may influence the imaging results and need to be considered in further studies. In addition, in order to verify the clinical validity of the proposed method, more medical data from real patients are needed.

5. Conclusions

Through finite element simulation verification, the combined coil proposed in this study can generate a linear gradient magnetic field with a line-shaped zero magnetic field, and it can drive the zero magnetic field to scan in a specific direction under the excitation of the cosine alternating current. The simulation results show that the scanning speed is positively correlated with the amplitude and frequency of the alternating current. When the low-frequency excitation of 100 Hz is applied, the single scanning cycle is 0.005 s, which is far shorter than the arterial blood flow change cycle, meeting the requirements of real-time imaging. Furthermore, the voltage data obtained from each scan can be directly used for projection imaging, without a large amount of inversion calculation, which shows the potential advantage of the proposed method in the real-time imaging of arteries.

In addition, the numerical models (15) and (16) were established between the voltage signal and the artery radius in this study. Combined with the numerical models and the simulated voltage signals, the artery radius can be calculated, and then the arterial profile image can be reconstructed according to the time-space projection imaging method in Section 2.4. The simulation results of the artery models with different radii show that the slope of the voltage signal is proportional to the square of the artery radius in a scanning period, which is consistent with the numerical models and proves the rationality of the numerical models. The imaging results show that the accuracy of reconstruction radius is about 90% and the spatial resolution is 1 mm. Compared with traditional electromagnetic imaging methods, the proposed method has the advantages of fast imaging speed and high resolution, showing the certain application value in early real-time imaging of arterial disease. However, further studies are necessary to confirm its effectiveness in clinical practice by more medical data and real cases

Author Contributions: Conceptualization, Y.L. and G.L.; methodology, D.Y.; software, Y.L.; validation, G.L., D.Y. and B.X.; investigation, Y.L.; writing—original draft preparation, Y.L.; writing—review and editing, G.L. and D.Y.; visualization, B.X.; supervision, D.Y.; funding acquisition, D.Y. All authors have read and agreed to the published version of the manuscript.

References

1. World Health Organization. Available online: http://www.who.int/mediacentre/factsheets/fs310/en/ (accessed on 22 June 2020).
2. Anxionnat, R.; Bracard, S.; Ducrocq, X.; Trousset, Y.; Launay, L.; Kerrien, E.; Braun, M.; Vaillant, R.; Scomazzoni, F.; Lebedinsky, A.; et al. Intracranial Aneurysms: Clinical Value of 3D Digital Subtraction Angiography in the Therapeutic Decision and Endovascular Treatment1. *Radiology* **2001**, *218*, 799–808. [CrossRef] [PubMed]
3. Nakayama, A.; Imamura, H.; Matsuyama, Y.; Kitamura, H.; Miwa, S.; Kobayashi, A.; Miyagawa, S.; Kawasaki, S. Value of Lipiodol Computed Tomography and Digital Subtraction Angiography in the Era

of Helical Biphasic Computed Tomography as Preoperative Assessment of Hepatocellular Carcinoma. *Ann. Surg.* **2001**, *234*, 56–62. [CrossRef] [PubMed]

4. Sun, Z.; Choo, G.H.; Ng, K.H. Coronary CT angiography: Current status and continuing challenges. *Br. J. Radiol.* **2012**, *85*, 495–510. [CrossRef] [PubMed]
5. Husmann, L.; Valenta, I.; Gaemperli, O.; Adda, O.; Treyer, V.; Wyss, C.A.; Veit-Haibach, P.; Tatsugami, F.; von Schulthess, G.K.; Kaufmann, P.A. Feasibility of low-dose coronary CT angiography: First experience with prospective ECG-gating. *Eur. Heart J.* **2007**, *29*, 191–197. [CrossRef]
6. Uchino, A.; Kato, A.; Takase, Y.; Kudo, S. Middle cerebral artery variations detected by magnetic resonance angiography. *Eur. Radiol.* **2000**, *10*, 560–563. [CrossRef]
7. Hundley, W.G.; Clarke, G.D.; Landau, C.; Lange, R.A.; Willard, J.E.; Hillis, L.D.; Peshock, R.M. Noninvasive determination of infarct artery patency by cine magnetic resonance angiography. *Circulation* **1995**, *91*, 1347. [CrossRef] [PubMed]
8. Ritchie, C.J.; Edwards, W.S.; Mack, L.A.; Cyr, D.R.; Kim, Y. Three-dimensional ultrasonic angiography using power-mode Doppler. *Ultrasound Med. Biol.* **1996**, *22*, 277–286. [CrossRef]
9. Nagai, S.; Abe, S.; Sato, T.; Hozawa, K.; Yuki, K.; Hanashima, K.; Tomoike, H. Ultrasonic assessment of vascular complications in coronary angiography and angioplasty after transradial approach. *Am. J. Cardiol.* **1999**, *83*, 180–186. [CrossRef]
10. Wang, H.; Xu, G.; Zhang, S.; Geng, D.; Yang, Q.; Yan, W. Implementation of Generalized Back Projection Algorithm in 3-D EIT. *IEEE Trans. Magn.* **2011**, *47*, 1466–1469. [CrossRef]
11. Griffiths, H.; Stewart, W.R.; Gough, W. Magnetic Induction Tomography: A Measuring System for Biological Tissues. *Ann. N. Y. Acad. Sci.* **1999**, *873*, 335–345. [CrossRef]
12. Wang, J.; Wang, X. Application of particle filtering algorithm in image reconstruction of EMT. *Meas. Sci. Technol.* **2015**, *26*, 7. [CrossRef]
13. Li, X.; Xu, Y.; He, B. Imaging Electrical Impedance From Acoustic Measurements by Means of Magnetoacoustic Tomography With Magnetic Induction (MAT-MI). *IEEE Trans. Biomed. Eng.* **2007**, *54*, 323–330. [CrossRef] [PubMed]
14. Guo, L.; Liu, G.; Xia, H. Magneto-Acousto-Electrical Tomography with Magnetic Induction for Conductivity Reconstruction. *IEEE Trans. Biomed. Eng.* **2015**, *62*, 2114–2124. [CrossRef]
15. Li, Y.; Liu, G.; Xia, H.; Xia, Z.; Yang, Y. Conductivity Reconstruction and Numerical Simulation for Magnetically Mediated Thermoacoustic Imaging. *IEEE Trans. Magn.* **2017**, *53*, 1–4. [CrossRef]
16. Zanet, D.D.; Battiston, M.; Lombardi, E.; Specogna, R.; Trevisan, F.; Marco, L.D.; Affanni, A.; Mazzucato, M. Impedance biosensor for real-time monitoring and prediction of thrombotic individual profile in flowing blood. *PLoS ONE* **2017**, *12*, e0184941. [CrossRef] [PubMed]
17. Affanni, A.; Chiorboli, G.; Codecasa, L.; Cozzi, M.; Marco, L.D.; Mazzucato, M.; Morandi, C.; Specogna, R.; Tartagni, M.; Trevisan, F. A novel inversion technique for imaging thrombus volume in microchannels fusing optical and impedance data. *IEEE Trans. Magn.* **2014**, *50*, 1021–1024. [CrossRef]
18. Maythem, A. Development of an Electromagnetic Induction Method for NonInvasive Blood Flow Measurement. Ph.D. Thesis, University of Huddersfield, Queensgate, Huddersfield, UK, 2016.
19. Andrzej, P.; Michal, P.; Tomasz, W.; Stefanczyk, L.; Strzelecki, M. Computational Fluid Dynamics as an Engineering Tool for the Reconstruction of Hemodynamics after Carotid Artery Stenosis Operation: A Case Study. *Medicina* **2018**, *54*, 42. [CrossRef]
20. Liu, Y.; Yang, D.; Liu, G.; Wang, W.; Xu, B. Numerical model and finite element simulation of arterial blood flow profile reconstruction in a uniform magnetic field. *J. Phys. D Appl. Phys.* **2020**, *53*, 11. [CrossRef]
21. Yang, D.; Liu, Y.-J.; Xu, B.; Duo, Y.-H. A Blood Flow Volume Linear Inversion Model Based on Electromagnetic Sensor for Predicting the Rate of Arterial Stenosis. *Sensors* **2019**, *19*, 3006. [CrossRef]
22. Top, C.B.; Güngör, A.; Ilbey, S.; Guven, H.E. Trajectory Analysis for Field Free Line Magnetic Particle Imaging. *Med. Phys.* **2019**, *46*, 1592–1607. [CrossRef]
23. Carson, J.R. A generalization of the reciprocal theorem. *Bell Syst. Tech. J.* **1924**, *3*, 393–399. [CrossRef]
24. Rau, U. Reciprocity relation between photovoltaic quantum efficiency and electroluminescent emission of solar cells. *Phys. Rev. B Condens. Matter* **2007**, *76*, 85303. [CrossRef]

25. Bevir, M.K. The theory of induced voltage electromagnetic flowmeters. *J. Fluid Mech.* **2006**, *43*, 577–590. [CrossRef]
26. Jozwik, K.; Obidowski, D. Numerical simulations of the blood flow through vertebral arteries. *J. Biomech.* **2010**, *43*, 177–185. [CrossRef] [PubMed]
27. Viedma, A.; Jiménez-Ortiz, C.; Marco, V. Extended Willis circle model to explain clinical observations in periorbital arterial flow. *J. Biomech.* **1997**, *30*, 265. [CrossRef]
28. Abdalla, S.; Al-Ameer, S.S.; Al-Magaishi, S.H. Electrical properties with relaxation through human blood. *Biomicrofluidics* **2010**, *4*, 34101. [CrossRef]
29. Knopp, T.; Erbe, M.; Sattel, T.F.; Biederer, S.; Buzug, T.M. Generation of a static magnetic field-free line using two Maxwell coil pairs. *Appl. Phys. Lett.* **2010**, *97*, 092505. [CrossRef]
30. Knopp, T.; Erbe, M.; Sattel, T.F.; Biederer, S.; Buzug, T.M. A Fourier slice theorem for magnetic particle imaging using a field-free line. *Inverse. Probl.* **2011**, *27*, 095004. [CrossRef]
31. Ertan, K.; Soheil, T.; Atalar, E. Driving mutually coupled gradient array coils in magnetic resonance imaging. *Magn. Reson. Med.* **2019**, *82*, 1187–1198. [CrossRef]
32. Szwast, M.; Piatkiewicz, W. Hall Effect in Electrolyte Flow Measurements: Introduction to Blood Flow Measurements. *Artif. Organs* **2012**, *36*, 551–555. [CrossRef]
33. Kanai, H.; Yamano, E.; Nakayama, K.; Kawamura, N.; Furuhata, H. Transcutaneous Blood Flow Measurement by Electromagnetic Induction. *IEEE Trans. Biomed. Eng.* **2007**, *BME-21*, 144–151. [CrossRef] [PubMed]
34. Guldvog, I.; Kjaernes, M.; Thoresen, M.; Walloe, L. Blood flow in arteries determined transcutaneously by an ultrasonic doppler velocitymeter as compared to electromagnetic measurements on the exposed vesels. *Acta Physiol.* **2010**, *109*, 211–216. [CrossRef] [PubMed]

2

Breast Cancer Detection—A Synopsis of Conventional Modalities and the Potential Role of Microwave Imaging

Brian M. Moloney [1,2,*], Declan O'Loughlin [3], Sami Abd Elwahab [2] and Michael J. Kerin [2]

1 Department of Diagnostic Radiology, Galway University Hospitals, Galway H91 YR71, Ireland
2 Discipline of Surgery, Lambe Institute for Translational Research, School of Medicine, National University of Ireland Galway, Galway H91 YR71, Ireland
3 Electrical and Electronic Engineering, National University of Ireland Galway, Galway H91 CF50, Ireland
* Correspondence: b.moloney1@nuigalway.ie

Abstract: Global statistics have demonstrated that breast cancer is the most frequently diagnosed invasive cancer and the leading cause of cancer death among female patients. Survival following a diagnosis of breast cancer is grossly determined by the stage of the disease at the time of initial diagnosis, highlighting the importance of early detection. Improving early diagnosis will require a multi-faceted approach to optimizing the use of currently available imaging modalities and investigating new methods of detection. The application of microwave technologies in medical diagnostics is an emerging field of research, with breast cancer detection seeing the most significant progress in the last twenty years. In this review, the application of current conventional imaging modalities is discussed, and recurrent shortcomings highlighted. Microwave imaging is rapid and inexpensive. If the preliminary results of its diagnostic capacity are substantiated, microwave technology may offer a non-ionizing, non-invasive, and painless adjunct or stand-alone modality that could possibly be implemented in routine diagnostic breast care.

Keywords: breast imaging; breast cancer; microwave breast imaging; multimodal imaging

---

1. Introduction

Breast cancer is the most commonly diagnosed female malignancy and is the fifth leading cause of cancer death. Annually, approximately 1.67 million cases of invasive breast cancer are diagnosed worldwide, and it is the cause of approximately 522,000 deaths [1]. The lifetime risk of developing breast cancer stands at one in eight females [2]. The incidence of breast cancer in developed countries continues to rise; however, the rate of mortality has undergone a substantial decline [3]. This is attributable to both improved methods of treatment, and implementation of screening programs and improved imaging techniques [4]. Critically, early detection ensures the best outcome for the patient, with survival grossly determined by the stage of the disease at the time of initial diagnosis [5]. In this era of a rising incidence of breast cancer, ensuring diagnosis at the earliest possible stage requires further improvement in the capabilities of current diagnostic modalities and the development of novel imaging systems. Here current conventional imaging applications are reviewed, such as mammography, digital breast tomosynthesis, ultrasonography, and magnetic resonance imaging. These modalities exploit a variety of properties of biological tissues to form an image:

- Mammography and digital breast tomosynthesis exploit the attenuation of x-rays as they pass through breast tissue measured by the attenuation coefficient of the tissue;

- Magnetic resonance imaging uses radio waves, magnetic field gradients, and contrast agents to excite and measure the location of hydrogen atoms;
- Ultrasound exploits differences in acoustic impedance between tissue types as sound waves propagate in the breast.

The potential of microwave breast imaging, a non-ionizing imaging modality that represents a promising method of breast cancer detection, is then discussed. Microwave breast imaging exploits the dielectric properties of biological tissues to form images, potentially providing complementary information to conventional modalities. While it is not expected that the acoustic, x-ray attenuation and dielectric properties are completely independent (all of the x-ray attenuation, acoustic impedance, and dielectric properties are influenced by water content), it is still expected that the dielectric properties would be influenced by other factors such as fractions of bound water and ion concentrations, suggesting that microwave breast imaging may be a useful adjunct imaging modality.

2. Mammography

Although the use of radiography to differentiate benign from cancerous specimen tissue was recorded as far back as 1913 [6], its use to clinically evaluate the symptomatic patient was delayed until the 1930's, when Stafford Warren, who is credited with the invention of the mammogram, pioneered a stereoscopic technique for mammography [7]. To this day, mammography remains the gold standard investigation of symptomatic women aged 40 and over and for the whole population breast cancer screening. While it offers a cost-effective method of investigating breast cancer, its effectiveness is severely hindered by several limitations. For most women, breast compression is an uncomfortable experience. In a study of 954 patients, Keemers-Gels et al. [8] reported that as many as 79% of patients undergoing breast cancer screening found mammography to be mild to severely painful. Additionally, this study established that the pain associated with breast compression during mammography was the main deterrent for women who indicated that they would not attend for further screening. Mammography is also limited in identifying tumors that present without a characteristic mass (as is frequently the case with invasive lobular breast cancer), without calcification (as can occur in entities like non-calcified ductal carcinoma), and in breasts of higher density [9]. The sensitivity of screening mammography, which aims to detect pre-clinical breast cancer in asymptomatic women, is estimated to be between 68 and 90%, with the lower margin of this range applicable to mammographically dense breasts, as is common in younger aged women. Even in women with lower breast density (> 75 years), the sensitivity for screening mammography is 88.4%. With diagnostic mammography, which involves the evaluation of patients with symptoms and signs suggestive of breast cancer, the sensitivity is slightly higher, at 93% [10].

2.1. *Screening Mammography*

Uninterrupted controversy continues to surround screening mammography and the true impact it has on breast cancer. While early breast cancer detection is undoubtedly beneficial for the patient, the benefits of screening appear to be less than as first thought. On the one hand, the use of this modality in organized screening programs remains the only screening test proven to reduce breast cancer mortality supported by randomized trials and subsequent meta-analyses [11,12]. In the randomized control trials (RCTs) and meta-analysis (Table 1) conducted on screening mammography deemed to be of sound methodologic quality, there was a reduction in breast cancer mortality between 20% to 45% in female participants aged 40 to 70 years. Modern mammography screening cites a similar reduction in breast cancer mortality of 28% [13].

Table 1. Randomized trials in mammography screening.

Trial	Country
Greater New York Health Insurance Plan (HIP) [14]	United States
Two-County Trial (TCT) [15]	Sweden
Malmo Mammography Screening Trial (MMST) [16]	Sweden
18-year follow-up meta-analysis of Swedish RCTs [17]	Sweden
Goteborg trial [18]	Sweden
National Breast Screening Study-1 (NBSS-1) [19]	Canada
National Breast Screening Study-2 (NBSS-2) [20]	Canada
Trial on women 40 years old at entry [21]	United Kingdom

However, these RCTs have been subject to criticism, with concerns raised that they are irrelevant to the modern era of breast cancer management as they were conducted prior to the introduction of taxane adjuvant therapy and the standardized acceptance of adjuvant hormone treatment for estrogen receptor-positive disease [22]. This has led some authors to doubt that the benefits of screening mammography would persist under present conditions.

In a seminal publication in 2012, Bleyer et al. [23] interrogated the US Surveillance, Epidemiology, and End Results data to examine trends of early- and late-stage breast cancer among women 40 years of age or older over a 30-year period. In this study, the group demonstrated that screening mammography resulted in a doubling in the annual incidence of early-stage breast cancer that is detected. However, it was calculated that breast cancer was overdiagnosed in up to 31% of all cases, accounting for 1.3 million women over the past 30-year study period. Furthermore, this group demonstrated that screening mammography only marginally reduced the rate of incidence of late-stage breast cancer and concluded that screening was having a minor impact on breast cancer mortality overall.

In a 2012 Cochrane review, Gøtzsche et al. [24] extracted data from eight RCTs, comprising 600,000 women (39–74 years) comparing mammographic screening with no mammographic screening. It was demonstrated that in trials with adequate randomization, screening did not impact breast cancer mortality after a 10 year follow up (Relative Risk 1.02, 95% CI 0.95 to 1.10). In 2013, the Swiss Medical Board (SMB) estimated the benefits, harms, and cost-effectiveness of organized breast screening. This report highlighted the difficulty in demonstrating that the benefits of mammography screening outweighed the harms. Accepting that screening offers a relative risk reduction of breast-cancer mortality of 20%, it was stressed that this came at the cost of a substantial diagnostic cascade. Contrary to public perception, for every female breast-cancer death prevented over a 10-year course of annual screening (initiated at 50 years), as many as 670 patients are likely to have a false-positive outcome with repeat mammography; as many as 100 will have an unnecessary biopsy, and up to 14 will have an overdiagnosed breast cancer that would never have presented clinically [25]. A conclusion was drawn that screening mammography was not cost-effective, and the group recommended that national screening be abolished [26]. To add to the murkiness of international opinion, a 2015 review funded by the Swiss cancer league was published that identified that the SMB report was fundamentally flawed in several aspects expected in appropriate cost-effectiveness analysis [27].

In the UK, following the introduction of the NHS Breast Cancer Screening Program in 1988, women aged 50 to 70 are invited to participate in breast screening every three years, with women over 70 able to self-refer. In 2012, an independent review was convened to reach conclusions about the benefits and harms of breast screening on the currently available literature. Focusing on the UK setting, the panel concluded that 20% was a reasonable estimate of the relative risk reduction of breast cancer mortality and that breast screening saves one life for every 2,000 women screened, or up to 1,300 lives per year in the UK [28].

In the US, a review of five Breast Cancer Surveillance Consortium breast imaging registries, consisting of over 400,000 patients aged 40–90, with linkages to pathology and tumor registries was published in February 2016 [29]. The rates of false-positive (a patient recalled for further investigation, with no underlying breast cancer) and false negative (a patient-reported as normal, despite underlying breast cancer) results and risk factors for recommendations for further imaging and biopsies were analyzed. Rates of false-positives were highest in women aged 40–49 (121.2 per 1000) and decreased with increasing age (50–59 (93.2 per 1000), 60–69 (80.8 per 1000)). This study highlighted that false-positive mammography results are more common in younger women and fortifies opinions that breast screening may be better suited for patients over the age of 50 years. This judgment was supported by the United States Preventive Services Task Force (USPSTF), who reviewed the evidence of breast cancer screening in reducing breast cancer-specific mortality, as well as treatment-related morbidity and harms of breast screening [30]. The USPSTF recommended biennial screening mammography for women between the ages of 50 and 74 years and recommended against routine screening mammography in women aged 40 to 49 years.

The Republic of Ireland National Breast Screening Program, BreastCheck, commenced in February 2000. The service offered a free digitalized screening mammography service to women aged 50 to 64 every two years in eleven of the 26 counties. The program was expanded to include a further three counties in 2004, and finally, to include all 26 counties in December 2007. The program is currently in the process of extending the age-range on a phased basis, with the intention that by 2021, all women aged 50–69 will be invited for screening [31]. Since its initiation, the target population invitation acceptance rate has remained somewhat constant over time ranging from 68% to 76% of those invited [31]. Two standard mammographic view are obtained, craniocaudal (CC) and mediolateral-oblique (MLO). The compression plane for CC is transaxial, while the MLO image plane is approximately 45 to 60 degrees from the axial plane, paralleling the course of the pectoralis muscle heading into the axilla. Each image is independently assessed by two consultant breast radiologists. Each breast radiologists must read at least 5,000 screening cases per year and have specific training in mammography. Patients who have suspicious abnormalities identified on their initial mammograms are recalled to a dedicated assessment clinic for further investigations, such as additional view mammography, ultrasound, or biopsy, as detailed in Figure 1. All cases requiring biopsy are discussed at a tertiary breast center multidisciplinary meeting [32].

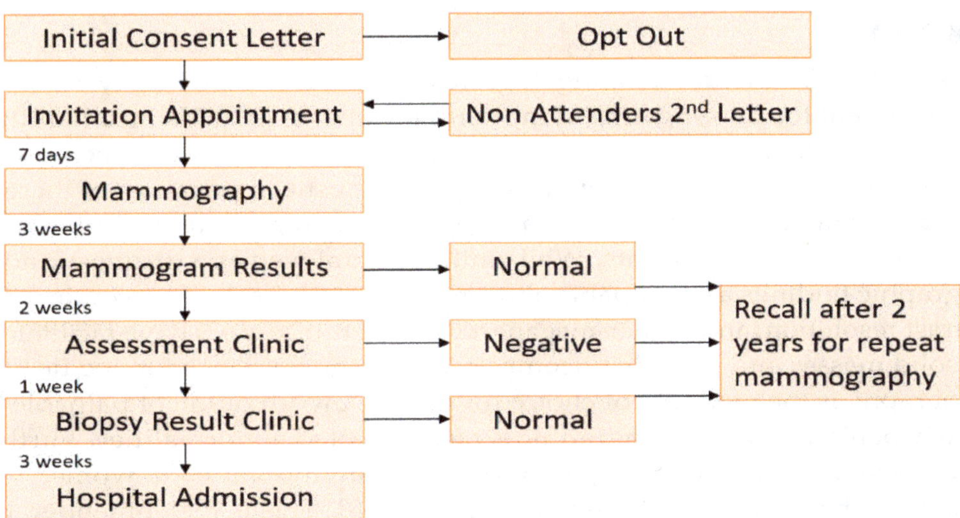

Figure 1. Screening process flow sheet and timescales for the BreastCheck screening program.

2.2. *Symptomatic Breast Mammography*

Diagnostic mammography is indicated for women over the age of 35 years, presenting with a palpable lump. If a benign correlate for a palpable lump (i.e., fibroadenoma, lipoma, hamartoma, or benign lymph node) is distinguished on mammography, no further imaging or biopsy is required, and clinical follow-up is adequate. If no abnormality can be seen with mammography or a finding is distinguished that is not clearly benign, further imaging is usually deemed appropriate, with targeted breast sonography employed. In Ireland, National Quality Assurance Standards ensure that urgent referrals are seen within two weeks. These include (1) Patients over 35 years of age with a discrete lump (2) Patients with suspicious signs, including; ulceration, skin tethering, unilateral nipple eczema, recent nipple inversion retraction or distortion, or (3) Individuals that the General Practitioner deems to have a significant probability of breast cancer at any age, and finally (4) Patients who develop an acute breast abscess. Further referral pathways exist for routine referrals to be evaluated within 12 weeks [33].

3. Digital Breast Tomosynthesis (DBT)

Tomosynthesis (3-Dimensional mammography) is a modification of digital mammography that uses a moving x-ray tube and digital detector to create a series of low dose exposures that are acquired from consecutive exposures along a limited arc angle while the breast is compressed. Individually, these low dose radiographs are only a fraction of the total dose used during conventional digital mammography. If a breast is imaged from 15 projections around a 45-degree arc, a radiograph will be generated every 3 degrees. These two-dimensional exposures are then used to reconstruct three-dimensional images of the breasts using algorithms to generate multiple, thin (usually 1 mm) slices in the same plane as the mammogram [34].

The addition of DBT to conventional digital mammography has been shown to increase rates of cancer detection. In a randomized clinical trial of women aged 45 to 75 years, cancer detection for patients screened with mammography and DBT was higher (n = 9777, 8.6 per 1000) than patients who underwent mammography alone (n = 9783, 4.5 per 1000, RR 1.9) [35]. This is counterbalanced by increased radiation dose, increased cost, and increased radiologist interpretation time [35]. Overall, the procedure is well-tolerated by patients, and its use is becoming increasingly widespread, usually at the discretion of the radiologist.

4. Breast Sonography

Breast sonography offers a non-ionizing, high resolution, low cost, highly sensitive (81.7%) and specific (88%) instrument for investigating symptomatic patients [36]. Using a handheld transducer, breast sonography has a definitive role in establishing the relationships between glandular, fat, and fibrous components of breast tissue based on the different acoustic impedances of these tissues. This is difficult to elucidate by mammography alone, as the fibrous and glandular components of the breast have similar X-ray attenuation coefficients. While initially employed as a diagnostic adjunct to further assess mammographic findings and palpable abnormalities, technical advances, including improved spatial and contrast resolution, and higher-megahertz (MHz) transducers have facilitated the use of US to characterize solid masses and provide uncomplicated image guidance for needle biopsy [37].

Breast sonography is the modality of choice for further investigation of palpable breast findings that are not clearly benign and mammographic screen-detected abnormalities. Furthermore, breast sonography is advised as an initial investigation prior to mammography in women younger than 30 years or in female patients that are lactating or pregnant [38]. This is recommended both to prevent unnecessary radiation exposure to a population of patients who carry a low incidence of breast cancer [39] and, as women under 30 years of age, generally have a relatively higher breast tissue density [40], mammographic sensitivity is decreased [41].

5. Magnetic Resonance Imaging (MRI)

The role of MRI in breast cancer diagnosis and management continues to evolve. MRI, with the aid of contrast (Gadolinium) enhancement, offers high soft tissue distinction, multiplanar sectioning, and three-dimensional reconstructions of the breast. It affords a sensitivity (over 90%), which is more favorable than both mammography and breast sonography for breast cancer [42]. However, the specificity of lesion characterization with MRI remains low to moderate (approximately 72%) [43], rendering the distinction between cancer and benign pathology a challenge.

The value of MRI as a screening adjunct in high-risk populations has been definitively recognized [44]. In the high-risk cohorts, such as patients with BRCA1 and BRCA2 deleterious mutations, TP53 mutations (Li–Fraumeni syndrome), or rare moderate-penetrance alleles such as CHEK2, ATM, and BRIP1, breast cancer can occur at a younger age, when breast density is higher. In these cases, tumors are often of a high grade and present at an advanced clinical stage [45]. In a comprehensive, multicenter randomized control trial of 2,809 high-risk women with dense breasts, Berg et al. [46] demonstrated that the sensitivity and specificity of combined mammography, ultrasound, and breast MRI was 100% and 65%, respectively. In contrast, the sensitivity of mammography only was 52%, while the specificity was 91%.

In recent years, the clinical application of preoperative breast MRI in patients with newly diagnosed breast cancer has seen rapid expansion as the modality becomes increasingly more available to clinicians [47]. Its use, however, remains controversial. No consensus has been reached concerning the utility of breast MRI in preoperative staging of all women with newly diagnosed breast cancer, and its benefit remains the topic of unremitting debate. The publication of the COMICE trial highlighted that the addition of contrast-enhanced MRI to conventional triple assessment was not associated with reduced reoperation in a large randomized cohort of women with primary breast cancer [48]. However, these findings were counter-balanced by evidence that preoperative MRI delineates patients with additional diseases that may be indistinguishable on conventional imaging [49–52].

In 2010, the European Society of Breast Cancer Specialists (EUSOMA) working group, consisting of a panel of twenty-three experts from a spectrum of disciplines including epidemiology, genetics, oncology, radiology, radiation oncology, and surgery took steps to evaluate the evidence and establish a consensus opinion for breast MRI indications [44]. Recommendations were detailed on appropriate use for; MRI for staging before treatment planning; high-risk screening; response evaluation following neoadjuvant treatment and patients with an occult primary on conventional methods, amongst others. This position paper highlighted the need for breast cancer specialists to adhere to the recommendations with patient outcomes as the primary endpoint. Despite this, the breadth of conflicting literature regarding the use of MRI for breast cancer management demonstrates that consensus opinions are still somewhat divergent.

6. Microwave Breast Imaging (MBI)

The shortcomings of mammography, such as relatively low sensitivity, radiation exposure, and uncomfortable breast compression, have resulted in research into alternative methods of breast imaging. Microwave breast imaging (MBI) has been highlighted as an exciting method for the detection of diseased breast tissue, offering a potential non-ionizing, non-compressive approach to breast cancer diagnosis [53] and monitoring the effect of neoadjuvant chemotherapy [54]. The potential of microwave imaging for clinical application has been researched over the last forty years [55]. Despite considerable efforts, only limited progress has been made in translating this potential into a clinically useful modality, as demonstrated by review articles from 1982 and 2016 describing microwave imaging as a "promising imaging modality" [56,57].

Microwave imaging uses electromagnetic radiation with frequencies between 0.3 and 9.0 GHz to deduce the dielectric properties (permittivity and conductivity) or contrast within a set volume, termed the imaging domain. To acquire data, the imaging volume is illuminated with electromagnetic radiation which propagates through the imaging domain and is scattered by dielectric contrasts in the imaging domain. The backscattered data is then recorded and used for image formation. A variety of systems exist, some which reconstruct a 3D volume, and others reconstruct repeated coronal slices of the breast to reduce the imaging algorithm complexity and to accelerate image reformatting [58]. Quantitative or qualitative image reconstruction algorithms are then used to estimate the dielectric contrast within the imaging domain. Qualitative algorithms, such as radar-based imaging, detect regions within the imaging domain where the dielectric properties fluctuate from the surrounding tissue, while quantitative algorithms, such as tomography, establish the actual dielectric properties for specific foci from the propagation paths through the imaging domain.

Microwave imaging is mostly analogous to sonography, where microwave energy is used instead of high-frequency sound, and scattering is based on the dielectric properties of tissues instead of the acoustic impedance. However, many differences exist between the two modalities which warrant further investigation:

- Respective beam widths of the transducer and the antennas;
- The relative dielectric properties and acoustic properties of the tissues of interest which is not well-studied;
- Importance of contact between the skin and the transducer and the antenna.

The dielectric properties, and hence the propagation, reflection, and attenuation of the electromagnetic waves in the microwave frequency range is sensitive to water, and accordingly, the water content in tissue plays a crucial factor in tissue characterization with microwave imaging [59]. Tissue water content has been shown to be higher in carcinogenesis due to a progressive increase in cell hydration induced by successive genetic and epigenetic changes [60]. Morphologically, cytoskeletal filaments are highly dynamic structures mainly involved in cell movements and proliferation. However, in the setting of an undifferentiated tumor cell, the cytoskeleton has a preponderance to be imperfect and dysfunctional due to a reduction in the quantity and organization of microtubules and microfilaments. This can result in the loss of normal cell structure and an altered cell membrane permeability. As a result, the tumor cells preserve more fluid than healthy cells, and this additional fluid alters the dielectric properties of the tissue [61].

Plasma constitutes 60% of blood content and is largely made up of water (92% by volume) [62]. In a tumor microenvironment, neoangiogenesis occurs to facilitate and nourish cell proliferation. This results in a network of new capillaries, and as the tumor increases in dimension, these networks can develop into small vessels that connect to major blood vessels, resulting in a significantly higher throughput of blood in the region. This increased volume of water in the tumor microenvironment is responsible for greater electromagnetic conductivity and permittivity. The dielectric contrast of the cancerous tissue against the surrounding healthy tissue results in increased scattering at the site of the tumor, thus enabling the detectability of the cancerous tissue with microwave imaging [63].

At least seven operational systems have been employed for numerous trials to investigate the clinical utility of MBI. These studies include healthy control volunteers or patients with benign breast disease or invasive carcinoma and are briefly summarized.

In 2000, the first of five clinical trials employing a tomography-based operational system developed at Dartmouth College (DC), USA, was described [64]. With this prototype, the breast is actively illuminated with a 16-element transceiving monopole antenna array in the 300–1000 MHz range. These trials ranged in size from 23 patients to 150 patients with and without breast disease and included a study investigating the role of the DC system in neoadjuvant chemotherapy monitoring [54,64–67]. In the cohort investigated undergoing neoadjuvant chemotherapy ($n = 8$), a positive correlation was identified between conductivity and 30-day response pathological response in all patients [54].

Outcomes from the Multistatic Array Processing for Radiowave Image Acquisition (MARIA®) systems, developed at the University of Bristol, UK, have been published since 2010, and report the largest outcomes from operational MBI systems. Six clinical studies have been reported describing the use of this radar-based system ranging in size from 86 patients [53] to 223 patients [68]. This system was designed with a 60-element antenna array system that consists of 60 wide-slot antenna elements positioned in a hemispherical arrangement. The antennas operate over a frequency range of 3 to 8 GHz in a cavity loaded slot arrangement. The most up-to-date system, the MARIA®5, was redesigned to improve the clinical utility of the system: with a reduced data acquisition time, immediate data processing to allow a DICOM compatible image reconstruction in less than 2 min. The sensitivity of this system is claimed to be as high as 86% for cancers in dense tissue [68]. This system has been made commercially available by Micrima Ltd. and has been deployed in several symptomatic breast units in the North Bristol Trust as part of the undergoing clinical evaluation of the system [66]. At least seven further operational systems had been employed for numerous trials to investigate the clinical utility of MBI, each reporting favorable outcomes [68].

In 2013 the first clinical report was published assessing a system developed by the University of Calgary, Canada, called the Tissue Sensing Adaptive Radar (TSAR) system. In this pilot study, the findings from eight patients were reported. The images showed responses consistent with the known clinical history in five patients, while various degrees of ambiguity surrounded the remaining three patients due to patient complexity and technical issues during data acquisition [69]. While the number of patients included in the initial trial was small, further clinical trials are planned with a new generation system [70,71].

In 2017, a group from the Southern University of Science and Technology, China, described the early results of a radar-based system which has been employed in Phase I clinical trials of 11 female Asian patients, aged between 22 and 47, with varying levels of hyperplasia [72]. Further phases of trials are scheduled using this system. As Asian women have denser breast parenchyma than their European counterparts, these results will be essential in assessing the clinical utility of microwave imaging in dense breasts. Also, in 2017, a group from Hiroshima University, Japan, described early results of a handheld, radar-based system [73]. This study included five patients, all of whom had either IDC or DCIS. Images were reconstructed without insight into the tumor location or clinical history of the patient. Despite this, the group demonstrated that the pathology could be located and that their findings were consistent with the clinical history of the patient.

In 2016, a wearable device system was described by Porter et al. at McGill University, Quebec, Canada [74]. In this study, 13 healthy control patients were evaluated. Imaging using this device was found to be comfortable, and measurements were reproducible, although sources of variability, such as patient positioning, were highlighted. As this study was confined to healthy control volunteers, the need for further clinical evaluation of the system is clear.

A system developed at Shizuoka University, Japan, has been described [75]. This ultra-wideband radar system had between 6 and 30 antennae to accommodate various breast sizes. This study, however, was limited to two participants, and as such, the clinical utility of this system will require further investigation.

Early reports from an ongoing clinical study at the Clinical Research Facility of Galway University Hospital (CRFG) have been described [76,77]. The Wavelia system is a low-power electromagnetic wave operational system consisting of two subsystems, both performing a non-compressive, non-invasive breast examination. The first subsystem, the optical breast contour detection (OBCD) subsystem, serves to gather information to help increase the accuracy of the subsequent microwave breast imaging subsystem. The OBCD subsystem consists of a 3D optical camera placed at 15–20 cm below an examination table and determines the volume and boundary outline of the subject breast. An azimuthal scan of the 3D camera allows the contour of the breast to be reconstructed, and the breast volume deduced. The second subsystem, microwave breast imaging, is performed on a separate examination table, where a vertical scan of the pendulous breast is performed, and consecutive coronal sections obtained. Multistatic radar detection technology is employed to detect and localize Regions-Of-Interest (ROIs) of breast tissue, with significant dielectric contrast on each coronal slice of the scanned breast. The Wavelia microwave imaging system operates using 18 wideband Vivaldi-type antennas arranged in a circle in a horizontal plane outside the cylinder containing the coupling fluid. Preliminary results from this study were favorable, with initial MBI demonstrating unambiguous detectability of cancerous lesions, with clusters of significant radar target echoes in the region of known underlying carcinoma [77]. The first phase of this clinical investigation has been completed, consisting of patients with benign and malignant breast disease. The findings of this study will determine the potential and potential clinical utility of the Wavelia system.

7. Prospects for Microwave Breast Imaging

Despite its limitations, mammography remains the gold standard against which new imaging technologies are measured. The adjunct of sonography and, more recently, tomosynthesis into clinical practice have improved breast cancer detection, while the increasing use of breast MRI is having a favorable impact when used in the appropriate setting. Although technological advances have brought about improvements in imaging quality and developments in modalities, there remains a chasm between current and optimal breast cancer detection levels, with approximately 2.4–6% of patients still being identified with de novo stage-IV breast cancer at the time of initial diagnosis [78]. While mortality rates are declining, the incidence of this multifaceted disease continues to increase with survival dependent on the stage at diagnosis [5]. Microwave imaging is rapid and inexpensive and may offer an additional adjunct to mammography, or perhaps a stand-alone modality in the future. If the exciting preliminary results of several operating systems are substantiated, the non-ionizing, non-invasive, and painless characteristics of this modality will popularize its implementation in routine diagnostic breast care. While several study populations to date have been too small to determine clinical efficacy accurately, the favorable preliminary results from the larger trials such as the DC and MARIA® have indicated that microwave imaging may have an integrated role in breast imaging in the near future [66,68]. From a clinical perspective, further clinical trials will require a significantly higher number of patients to validate the true potential of the systems. Ideally, these trials should have a variety of breast pathology to represent the heterogeneity of breast disease, including invasive ductal carcinoma, invasive lobular carcinoma, fibroadenoma, and cystic breast disease.

As we approach an age where the translation of microwave breast imaging systems into the clinical setting has become a reality, it will be imperative that the findings from microwave breast imaging studies are interrogated by breast radiologists with an aim to determine consensus opinions about multiple factors. These will include issues like reporting methods and terminology for describing findings, image presentation for the radiologist (i.e., 3D representation or standard anatomical planes such as coronal, axial and sagittal), imaging features (e.g., clusters/ foci of signal) and limits of signal that may suggest malignancy or benign disease. Furthermore, it will be crucial that the overseeing physician (radiologist), will play a role in developing standard operating procedures to limit any psychological or physical side-effects of MBI on a patient, considering the sensitivity of cancer imaging.

Author Contributions: Conceptualization, B.M.M., D.O.'L, S.A.E., and M.J.K.; writing—original draft preparation, B.M.M., D.O.'L and S.A.E., writing—review and editing, B.M.M., D.O.'L, S.A.E., and M.J.K.; supervision, M.J.K.; funding acquisition, M.J.K.; All authors have read and agreed to the published version of the manuscript.

References

1. Ferlay, J.; Soerjomataram, I.; Dikshit, R.; Eser, S.; Mathers, C.; Rebelo, M.; Parkin, D.M.; Forman, D.; Bray, F. Cancer incidence and mortality worldwide: sources, methods and major patterns in GLOBOCAN 2012. *Int. J. Cancer* **2015**, *136*, E359–E386. [CrossRef] [PubMed]
2. Feuer, EJ.; Wun, L.M.; Boring, C.C.; Flanders, W.D.; Timmel, M.J.; Tong, T. The lifetime risk of developing breast cancer. *J. Natl. Cancer Inst.* **1993**, *85*, 892–897. [CrossRef] [PubMed]

3. Levi, F.; Bosetti, C.; Lucchini, F.; Negri, E.; La Vecchia, C. Monitoring the decrease in breast cancer mortality in Europe. *Eur. J. Cancer Prev.* **2005**, *14*, 497–502. [CrossRef] [PubMed]
4. Myers, E.R.; Moorman, P.; Gierisch, J.M.; Havrilesky, L.J.; Grimm, L.J.; Ghate, S.; Davidson, B.; Mongtomery, R.C.; Crowley, M.J.; McCrory, D.C.; et al. Benefits and Harms of Breast Cancer Screening: A Systematic Review. *JAMA* **2015**, *314*, 1615–1634. [CrossRef]
5. Siegel, R.L.; Miller, K.D.; Jemal, A. Cancer statistics, 2016. *CA Cancer J. Clin.* **2016**, *66*, 7–30. [CrossRef]
6. Gold, R.H.; Bassett, L.W.; Widoff, B.E. Highlights from the history of mammography. *Radiographics* **1990**, *10*, 1111–1131. [CrossRef]
7. Warren, S.L. A Roentgenologic Study of the Breast. *Am. J. Roentgenol.* **1930**, *24*, 113–124.
8. Keemers-Gels, M.E.; Groenendijk, R.P.; van den Heuvel, J.H.; Boetes, C.; Peer, P.G.; Wobbes, T.H. Pain experienced by women attending breast cancer screening. *Breast Cancer Res. Treat.* **2000**, *60*, 235–240. [CrossRef]
9. Bartella, L.; Smith, C.S.; Dershaw, D.D.; Liberman, L. Imaging breast cancer. *Radiol. Clin. North Am.* **2007**, *45*, 45–67. [CrossRef]
10. Walter, L.C.; Schonberg, M.A. Screening mammography in older women: A review. *JAMA* **2014**, *311*, 1336–1347. [CrossRef]
11. Drukteinis, J.S.; Mooney, B.P.; Flowers, C.I.; Gatenby, R.A. Beyond mammography: New frontiers in breast cancer screening. *Am. J. Med.* **2013**, *126*, 472–479. [CrossRef] [PubMed]
12. Autier, P.; Hery, C.; Haukka, J.; Boniol, M.; Byrnes, G. Advanced breast cancer and breast cancer mortality in randomized controlled trials on mammography screening. *J. Clin. Oncol.* **2009**, *27*, 5919–5923. [CrossRef] [PubMed]
13. Weedon-Fekjaer, H.; Romundstad, P.R.; Vatten, L.J. Modern mammography screening and breast cancer mortality: Population study. *BMJ* **2014**, *348*, g3701. [CrossRef] [PubMed]
14. Shapiro, S. Periodic screening for breast cancer: The HIP Randomized Controlled Trial. Health Insurance Plan. *J. Natl. Cancer Inst. Monogr.* **1997**, *22*, 27–30. [CrossRef]
15. Tabár, L.; Vitak, B.; Chen, H.H.; Duffy, S.W.; Yen, M.F.; Chiang, C.F.; Krusemo, U.B.; Tot, T.; Smith, R.A. The Swedish Two-County Trial twenty years later. Updated mortality results and new insights from long-term follow-up. *Radiol. Clin. North Am.* **2000**, *38*, 625–651. [CrossRef]
16. Andersson, I.; Nystrom, L. Mammography screening. *J. Natl. Cancer Inst.* **1995**, *87*, 1263–1264.
17. Nystrom, L.; Andersson, I.; Bjurstam, N.; Frisell, J.; Nordenskjold, B.; Rutqvist, L.E. Long-term effects of mammography screening: Updated overview of the Swedish randomised trials. *Lancet* **2002**, *359*, 909–919. [CrossRef]
18. Bjurstam, N.; Bjorneld, L.; Warwick, J.; Sala, E.; Duffy, S.W.; Nystrom, L.; Walker, N.; Cahlin, E.; Eriksson, O.; Hafstrom, L.O.; et al. The Gothenburg Breast Screening Trial. *Cancer* **2003**, *97*, 2387–2396. [CrossRef]
19. Miller, A.B.; To, T.; Baines, C.J.; Wall, C. The Canadian National Breast Screening Study-1: Breast cancer mortality after 11 to 16 years of follow-up. A randomized screening trial of mammography in women age 40 to 49 years. *Ann. Intern. Med.* **2002**, *137*, 305–312. [CrossRef]
20. Miller, A.B.; To, T.; Baines, C.J.; Wall, C. Canadian National Breast Screening Study-2: 13-year results of a randomized trial in women aged 50–59 years. *J. Natl. Cancer Inst.* **2000**, *92*, 1490–1499. [CrossRef]
21. Moss, S.M.; Cuckle, H.; Evans, A.; Johns, L.; Waller, M.; Bobrow, L. Effect of mammographic screening from age 40 years on breast cancer mortality at 10 years' follow-up: A randomised controlled trial. *Lancet* **2006**, *368*, 2053–2060. [CrossRef]
22. Early Breast Cancer Trialists' Collaborative Group. Effects of adjuvant tamoxifen and of cytotoxic therapy on mortality in early breast cancer. An overview of 61 randomized trials among 28,896 women. *New Engl. J. Med.* **1988**, *319*, 1681–1692. [CrossRef] [PubMed]
23. Bleyer, A.; Welch, H.G. Effect of three decades of screening mammography on breast-cancer incidence. *New Engl. J. Med.* **2012**, *367*, 1998–2005. [CrossRef] [PubMed]
24. Gotzsche, P.C.; Nielsen, M. Screening for breast cancer with mammography. *Cochrane Database Syst. Rev.* **2006**, *6*, CD001877.
25. Biller-Andorno, N.; Juni, P. Abolishing mammography screening programs? A view from the Swiss Medical Board. *New Engl. J. Med.* **2014**, *370*, 1965–1967. [CrossRef]
26. Swiss Medical Board stellt systematisches Mammographie-Screening in Frage. *Bulletin des médecins suisses* **2014**, *95*, 196.

27. De Koning, H.J.; Heijnsdijk, E.A. Swiss Medical Board Mammography screening predictions for Switzerland: Importance of time-periods. *J. Med. Screen.* **2015**, *22*, 201–206. [CrossRef]
28. Independent UK Panel on Breast Cancer Screening. The benefits and harms of breast cancer screening: An independent review. *Lancet* **2012**, *380*, 1778–1786. [CrossRef]
29. Nelson, H.D.; O'Meara, E.S.; Kerlikowske, K.; Balch, S.; Miglioretti, D. Factors Associated With Rates of False-Positive and False-Negative Results From Digital Mammography Screening: An Analysis of Registry Data. *Ann. Intern. Med.* **2016**, *164*, 226–235. [CrossRef]
30. US Preventive Services Task Force. Screening for breast cancer: U.S. Preventive Services Task Force recommendation statement. *Ann. Intern. Med.* **2009**, *151*, 716. [CrossRef]
31. BreastCheck. Annual Report 2017/8. Available online: https://www.breastcheck.ie/content/annual_reports (accessed on 1 November 2019).
32. Hanley, J.A.; Hannigan, A.; O'Brien, K.M. Mortality reductions due to mammography screening: Contemporary population-based data. *PLoS ONE* **2017**, *12*, e0188947. [CrossRef] [PubMed]
33. Health Information and Quality Authority. *National Quality Assurance Standards for Symptomatic Breast Disease Services*; HIQA: Dublin, Ireland, 2006.
34. Helvie, M.A. Digital mammography imaging: Breast tomosynthesis and advanced applications. *Radiol. Clin. North Am.* **2010**, *48*, 917–929. [CrossRef] [PubMed]
35. Pattacini, P.; Nitrosi, A.; Giorgi Rossi, P.; Iotti, V.; Ginocchi, V.; Ravaioli, S.; Vacondio, R.; Braglia, L.; Cavuto, S.; Campari, C. Digital Mammography versus Digital Mammography Plus Tomosynthesis for Breast Cancer Screening: The Reggio Emilia Tomosynthesis Randomized Trial. *Radiology* **2018**, *288*, 375–385. [CrossRef] [PubMed]
36. Houssami, N.; Irwig, L.; Simpson, J.M.; McKessar, M.; Blome, S.; Noakes, J. Sydney Breast Imaging Accuracy Study: Comparative sensitivity and specificity of mammography and sonography in young women with symptoms. *AJR Am. J. Roentgenol.* **2003**, *180*, 935–940. [CrossRef]
37. Weinstein, S.P.; Conant, E.F.; Sehgal, C. Technical Advances in Breast Ultrasound Imaging. *Seminars in Ultrasound, CT and MRI* **2006**, *27*, 273–283. [CrossRef]
38. Joshi, S.; Dialani, V.; Marotti, J.; Mehta, T.S.; Slanetz, P.J. Breast disease in the pregnant and lactating patient: Radiological-pathological correlation. *Insights Imaging* **2013**, *4*, 527–538. [CrossRef]
39. Ciatto, S.; Bravetti, P.; Bonardi, R.; Rosselli del Turco, M. The role of mammography in women under 30. *Radiol. Med.* **1990**, *80*, 676–678.
40. Checka, C.M.; Chun, J.E.; Schnabel, F.R.; Lee, J.; Toth, H. The relationship of mammographic density and age: Implications for breast cancer screening. *AJR Am. J. Roentgenol.* **2012**, *198*, W292–W295. [CrossRef]
41. Pinsky, R.W.; Helvie, M.A. Mammographic breast density: Effect on imaging and breast cancer risk. *J. Natl. Compr. Cancer Netw.* **2010**, *8*, 1157–1164. [CrossRef]
42. Berg, W.A.; Gutierrez, L.; NessAiver, M.S.; Carter, W.B.; Bhargavan, M.; Lewis, R.S.; Ioffe, O.B. Diagnostic accuracy of mammography, clinical examination,, U.S.; and MR imaging in preoperative assessment of breast cancer. *Radiology* **2004**, *233*, 830–849. [CrossRef]
43. Menezes, G.L.; Knuttel, F.M.; Stehouwer, B.L.; Pijnappel, R.M.; van den Bosch, M.A. Magnetic resonance imaging in breast cancer: A literature review and future perspectives. *World J. Clin. Oncol.* **2014**, *5*, 61–70. [CrossRef] [PubMed]
44. Sardanelli, F.; Boetes, C.; Borisch, B.; Decker, T.; Federico, M.; Gilbert, F.J.; Helbich, T.; Heywang-Köbrunner, S.H.; Kaiser, W.A.; Kerin, M.J.; et al. Magnetic resonance imaging of the breast: Recommendations from the EUSOMA working group. *Eur. J. Cancer* **2010**, *46*, 1296–1316. [CrossRef] [PubMed]
45. Garcia, E.M.; Storm, E.S.; Atkinson, L.; Kenny, E.; Mitchell, L.S. Current breast imaging modalities, advances, and impact on breast care. *Obstet. Gynecol. Clin. North Am.* **2013**, *40*, 429–457. [CrossRef] [PubMed]
46. Berg, W.A.; Zhang, Z.; Lehrer, D.; Jong, R.A.; Pisano, E.D.; Barr, R.G.; Böhm-Vélez, M.; Mahoney, M.C.; Evans, W.P., 3rd; Larsen, L.H.; et al. Detection of breast cancer with addition of annual screening ultrasound or a single screening MRI to mammography in women with elevated breast cancer risk. *JAMA* **2012**, *307*, 1394–1404. [PubMed]
47. Bassett, L.W.; Dhaliwal, S.G.; Eradat, J.; Khan, O.; Farria, D.F.; Brenner, R.J.; Sayre, J.W. National trends and practices in breast MRI. *AJR Am. J. Roentgenol.* **2008**, *191*, 332–339. [CrossRef] [PubMed]

48. Turnbull, L.; Brown, S.; Harvey, I.; Olivier, C.; Drew, P.; Napp, V.; Hanby, A.; Brown, J. Comparative effectiveness of MRI in breast cancer (COMICE) trial: A randomised controlled trial. *Lancet* **2010**, *375*, 563–571. [CrossRef]
49. Houssami, N.; Turner, R.M.; Morrow, M. Meta-analysis of pre-operative magnetic resonance imaging (MRI) and surgical treatment for breast cancer. *Breast Cancer Res. Treat.* **2017**, *165*, 273–283. [CrossRef]
50. Brennan, M.E.; Houssami, N.; Lord, S.; Macaskill, P.; Irwig, L.; Dixon, J.M.; Warren, R.M.; Ciatto, S. Magnetic resonance imaging screening of the contralateral breast in women with newly diagnosed breast cancer: Systematic review and meta-analysis of incremental cancer detection and impact on surgical management. *J. Clin. Oncol.* **2009**, *27*, 5640–5649. [CrossRef]
51. Houssami, N.; Hayes, D.F. Review of preoperative magnetic resonance imaging (MRI) in breast cancer: Should MRI be performed on all women with newly diagnosed, early stage breast cancer? *CA Cancer J. Clin.* **2009**, *59*, 290–302. [CrossRef]
52. Morrow, M.; Waters, J.; Morris, E. MRI for breast cancer screening, diagnosis, and treatment. *Lancet* **2011**, *378*, 1804–1811. [CrossRef]
53. Preece, A.W.; Craddock, I.; Shere, M.; Jones, L.; Winton, H.L. MARIA M4: Clinical evaluation of a prototype ultrawideband radar scanner for breast cancer detection. *J. Med. Imaging* **2016**, *3*, 033502. [CrossRef] [PubMed]
54. Meaney, P.M.; Kaufman, P.A.; Muffly, L.S.; Click, M.; Poplack, S.P.; Wells, W.A.; Schwartz, G.N.; di Florio-Alexander, R.M.D.; Tosteson, T.; Li, Z.; et al. Microwave imaging for neoadjuvant chemotherapy monitoring: Initial clinical experience. *Breast Cancer Res.* **2013**, *15*, R35. [CrossRef] [PubMed]
55. O'Loughlin, D.; O'Halloran, M.; Moloney, B.M.; Glavin, M.; Jones, E.; Elahi, M.A. Microwave Breast Imaging: Clinical Advances and Remaining Challenges. *IEEE Trans. Biomed. Eng.* **2018**, *65*, 2580–2590.
56. Kwon, S.; Lee, S. Recent Advances in Microwave Imaging for Breast Cancer Detection. *Int. J. Biomed. Imaging* **2016**, *2016*, 5054912. [CrossRef] [PubMed]
57. Larsen, L.; Jacobi, J. Microwaves offer promise as imaging modality. *Diagn. Imaging* **1982**, *11*, 44–47.
58. Golnabi, A.H.; Meaney, P.M.; Epstein, N.R.; Paulsen, K.D. Microwave imaging for breast cancer detection: Advances in three–dimensional image reconstruction. In Proceedings of the 2011 Annual International Conference of the IEEE Engineering in Medicine and Biology Society, Boston, MA, USA, 30 August–3 September 2011; pp. 5730–5733.
59. Conceicao, R.C.; Mohr, J.J.; O'Halloran, M. *An Introduction to Microwave Imaging for Breast Cancer Detection*; Springer: Berlin/Heidelberg, Germany, 2015.
60. McIntyre, G.I. Increased cell hydration promotes both tumor growth and metastasis: A biochemical mechanism consistent with genetic signatures. *Med. Hypotheses* **2007**, *69*, 1127–1130. [CrossRef]
61. Modiri, A.; Goudreau, S.; Rahimi, A.; Kiasaleh, K. Review of breast screening: Toward clinical realization of microwave imaging. *Med. Phys.* **2017**, *44*, e446–e458. [CrossRef]
62. Dean, L. *Blood Groups and Red Cell Antigens*; NCBI: Bethesda, MD, USA, 2005.
63. Joines, W.T.; Zhang, Y.; Li, C.; Jirtle, R.L. The measured electrical properties of normal and malignant human tissues from 50 to 900 MHz. *Med. Phys.* **1994**, *21*, 547–550. [CrossRef]
64. Meaney, P.M. A clinical prototype for active microwave imaging of the breast. *IEEE Trans. Microwave Theory Tech.* **2000**, *48*, 12.
65. Meaney, P.M.; Fanning, M.W.; Raynolds, T.; Fox, C.J.; Fang, Q.; Kogel, C.A.; Poplack, S.P.; Paulsen, K.D. Initial clinical experience with microwave breast imaging in women with normal mammography. *Acad Radiol.* **2007**, *14*, 207–218. [CrossRef]
66. Poplack, S.P.; Tosteson, T.D.; Wells, W.A.; Pogue, B.W.; Meaney, P.M.; Hartov, A.; Kogel, C.A.; Soho, S.K.; Gibson, J.J.; Paulsen, K.D. Electromagnetic breast imaging: Results of a pilot study in women with abnormal mammograms. *Radiology* **2007**, *243*, 350–359. [CrossRef] [PubMed]
67. Poplack, S.P.; Paulsen, K.D.; Hartov, A.; Meaney, P.M.; Pogue, B.W.; Tosteson, T.D.; Grove, M.R.; Soho, S.K.; Wells, W.A. Electromagnetic breast imaging: Average tissue property values in women with negative clinical findings. *Radiology* **2004**, *231*, 571–580. [CrossRef] [PubMed]
68. Massey, H.; Ridley, N.; Lyburn, I. Radiowave Detection of Breast Cancer In The Symptomatic Clinic—A Multi-Centre Study. In Proceedings of the International Cambridge Conference on Breast Imaging, Cambridge, UK, 3–4 July 2017.

69. Fear, E.C.; Bourqui, J.; Curtis, C.F. Microwave Breast Imaging With a Monostatic Radar-Based System: A Study of Application to Patients. *IEEE Trans. Microwave Theory Tech.* **2013**, *61*, 9. [CrossRef]
70. Kurrant, D.; Bourqui, J.; Fear, E. Surface Estimation for Microwave Imaging. *Sensors* **2017**, *17*, 1658. [CrossRef] [PubMed]
71. Lavoie, B.R.; Okoniewski, M.; Fear, E.C. Estimating the Effective Permittivity for Reconstructing Accurate Microwave-Radar Images. *PLoS ONE* **2016**, *11*, e0160849. [CrossRef] [PubMed]
72. Yang, F.S.L.; Hu, Z. A Large-Scale Clinical Trial of Radarbased Microwave Breast Imaging for Asian Women: Phase, I. In Proceedings of the International Symposium on Antennas and Propagation (APSURSI), San Diego, CA, USA, 9–15 July 2017; IEEE: San Diego, CA, USA, 2017; pp. 781–783.
73. Song, H.; Sasada, S.; Kadoya, T.; Okada, M.; Arihiro, K.; Xiao, X.; Kikkawa, T. Detectability of Breast Tumor by a Hand-held Impulse-Radar Detector: Performance Evaluation and Pilot Clinical Study. *Sci. Rep.* **2017**, *7*, 16353. [CrossRef]
74. Porter, E.D.K.; Popovic, M. Investigation of Time-Domain Microwave Radar With Breast Clinic Patients. In Proceedings of the 10th European Conference on Antennas and Propagation (EuCAP), Davos, Switzerland, 10–15 April 2016; 2016; pp. 1–3.
75. Kuwahara, Y. Microwave Imaging for Early Breast Cancer Detection. *New Perspect. Breast Imaging*. IntechOpen. 2017, pp. 45–71. Available online: https://www.intechopen.com/books/new-perspectives-in-breast-imaging/microwave-imaging-for-early-breast-cancer-detection (accessed on 4 October 2017).
76. Fasoula, A.; Duchesne, L.; Gil Cano, J.D.; Lawrence, P.; Robin, G.; Bernard, J.G. On-Site Validation of a Microwave Breast Imaging System, before First Patient Study. *Diagnostics* **2018**, *8*, 53. [CrossRef]
77. Fasoula, A.; Moloney, B.M.; Duchesne, L.; Cano, J.D.G.; Oliveira, B.L.; Bernard, J.G.; Kerin, M. Super-Resolution Radar Imaging for Breast Cancer Detection with Microwaves: The Integrated Information Selection Criteria. In Proceedings of the 2019 41st Annual International Conference of the IEEE Engineering in Medicine and Biology Society (EMBC), Berlin, Germany, 2019; pp. 1868–1874.
78. Siegel, R.L.; Miller, K.D.; Jemal, A. Cancer statistics, 2019. *CA Cancer J. Clin.* **2019**, *69*, 7–34. [CrossRef]

3

The Application of an Iterative Structure to the Delay-and-Sum and the Delay-Multiply-and-Sum Beamformers in Breast Microwave Imaging

Tyson Reimer [1,*], Mario Solis-Nepote [2] and Stephen Pistorius [1,2]

1 Department of Physics and Astronomy, University of Manitoba, Winnipeg, MB R3T 2N2, Canada; stephen.pistorius@umanitoba.ca
2 Research Institute in Oncology and Hematology, University of Manitoba, Winnipeg, MB R3E 0V9, Canada; mario.solis.n@gmail.com
* Correspondence: reimert5@myumanitoba.ca

Abstract: Breast microwave imaging (BMI) is a potential breast cancer screening method. This manuscript presents a novel iterative delay-and-sum (DAS) based reconstruction algorithm for BMI. This iterative-DAS (itDAS) algorithm uses a forward radar model to iteratively update an image estimate. A variation of the itDAS reconstruction algorithm that uses the delay-multiply-and-sum (DMAS) beamformer was also implemented (the itDMAS algorithm). Both algorithms were used to reconstruct images from experimental scans of an array of 3D-printed MRI-based breast phantoms performed with a clinical BMI system. The signal-to-clutter ratio (SCR) and signal-to-mean ratio (SMR) were used to compare the performance of the itDAS and itDMAS methods to the DAS and DMAS beamformers. While no significant difference between the itDAS and itDMAS methods was observed in most images, the itDAS algorithm produced reconstructions that had significantly higher SMR than the non-iterative methods, increasing contrast by as much as 19 dB over DAS and 13 dB over DMAS. The itDAS algorithm also increased the SCR of reconstructions by up to 5 dB over DAS and 4 dB over DMAS, indicating that both high-intensity and background clutter are reduced in images reconstructed by the itDAS algorithm.

Keywords: microwave imaging; image reconstruction; breast imaging; microwave radar

---

1. Introduction

Breast microwave imaging (BMI) has emerged as a potential breast cancer detection technique [1]. This modality uses non-ionizing microwave radiation to interrogate the breast tissues, and measurements of the resultant field produced after scattering from the tissues can be used to reconstruct an image of the breast. While X-ray mammography is the current breast imaging standard, its sizable false-positive rate (the cumulative risk of a false-positive after ten mammograms is estimated to be between 20–60% [2]), use of ionizing X-ray radiation and need for a highly trained operator make it less than ideal as a screening technique, particularly in remote rural communities. Because BMI systems use non-ionizing microwave radiation and are relatively low-cost, the modality has been proposed as a potential breast cancer screening method [1,3].

BMI systems use an antenna to illuminate the breast with a microwave signal. The tissues within the breast scatter this signal, and the resultant field can be measured using an antenna or array of antennas. The dielectric properties of the tissues govern the interaction of the microwave signal within the breast, and the contrast in the properties of malignant and healthy tissues [4,5] allows for the detection of malignant lesions by BMI systems.

Radar-based image reconstruction techniques in BMI aim to reconstruct a reflectivity map of the breast in which regions of strong reflections are prominently displayed. The primary reconstruction method in radar-based BMI is the delay-and-sum (DAS) beamformer [6]. This technique synthetically focuses the time domain signals collected by a radar system to reconstruct an image. Several derivatives of the DAS beamformer have been developed, including delay-multiply-and-sum (DMAS) [7], improved delay-and-sum (IDAS) [8], coherence-factor based delay-and-sum (CF-DAS) [9], and channel-ranked delay-and-sum (CR-DAS) [10]. The DAS-derivative algorithms have primarily been designed to reward coherence between measured radar signals [7–9] or account for path-dependent effects [10].

The DAS beamformer and its derivatives have been widely used and the image reconstruction method used in many patient imaging studies in radar-based BMI systems has been the DAS beamformer or its derivatives [11–24]. While other image reconstruction techniques have been proposed (microwave imaging via space time in [25,26] and data-adaptive methods in [27,28]), the DAS beamformer and its derivatives have been used as standards of comparison [29,30]. Recent patient and phantom investigations have found that only one DAS-derivative, the DMAS beamformer [7], reduced both background and high-intensity clutter while accurately localizing the tumor response in reconstructions [29,30].

This manuscript presents a novel iterative DAS-based reconstruction method. The functional form of the maximum-likelihood expectation-maximization (MLEM) algorithm used in positron emission tomography [31,32] is applied to the DAS beamformer. The iterative structure of the algorithm [31] was first presented for use in breast microwave radar imaging in a preliminary investigation [32]. The initial work in [32] did not apply the iterative algorithm to the DAS beamformer, and this investigation bridges the gap between the MLEM-based method described in [32] and the DAS method [6], resulting in the itDAS algorithm.

A second novel iterative algorithm is presented herein, in which the iterative structure is applied to the DMAS beamformer (resulting in the itDMAS algorithm). The iterative structure of the algorithm rewards signal coherence using multiple iterations and, through improvements to the forward signal model, allows for the modeling of path-dependent effects.

This work presents results on an array of anthropomorphic MRI-based breast phantoms (derived from the numerical models from [33]) that are representative of the four BI-RADS breast density classification categories [34]. The performance of the reconstruction methods as a function of breast density is discussed, and the results obtained with the iterative methods are compared to those obtained using the DAS and DMAS beamformers. To facilitate reproducibility and transparency, the code used to perform the analysis and produce the figures presented herein is open-source and available at Supplementary Materials https://github.com/TysonReimer/itDAS.

2. Methods

2.1. The itDAS Reconstruction Algorithm

The iterative DAS-based algorithm presented herein is referred to as the itDAS algorithm. The itDAS beamformer adopts the iterative form of the MLEM reconstruction algorithm used in positron emission tomography (PET) [31]. The MLEM algorithm in PET is derived from the Poisson statistics of both the emission and detection events characteristic of PET [31]. This algorithm has a functional form that references only the forward and back projections of the imaging system. This functional form is displayed in Equation (1) with an additional normalization factor $\hat{\mathbf{F}}[U]$ multiplying the dataset D,

$$I^{n+1} = \frac{I^n}{\hat{\mathbf{B}}[U]}\hat{\mathbf{B}}\left[\frac{D \cdot \hat{\mathbf{F}}[U]}{\hat{\mathbf{F}}[I^n]}\right] \tag{1}$$

where $\hat{\mathbf{B}}$ denotes the back-projection operator, $\hat{\mathbf{F}}$ denotes the forward projection operator, D denotes the set of experimentally measured data, U is a unity matrix, and I^n is the image estimate at the nth

iteration. The back-projection operator transforms data from the data domain (in breast microwave radar imaging, this is the time domain) to the spatial domain of the image-space, and the forward projection operator simulates the dataset that would be obtained if the system scanned an object that would reproduce the image estimate. A flowchart of the functional form of the itDAS algorithm is displayed in Figure 1.

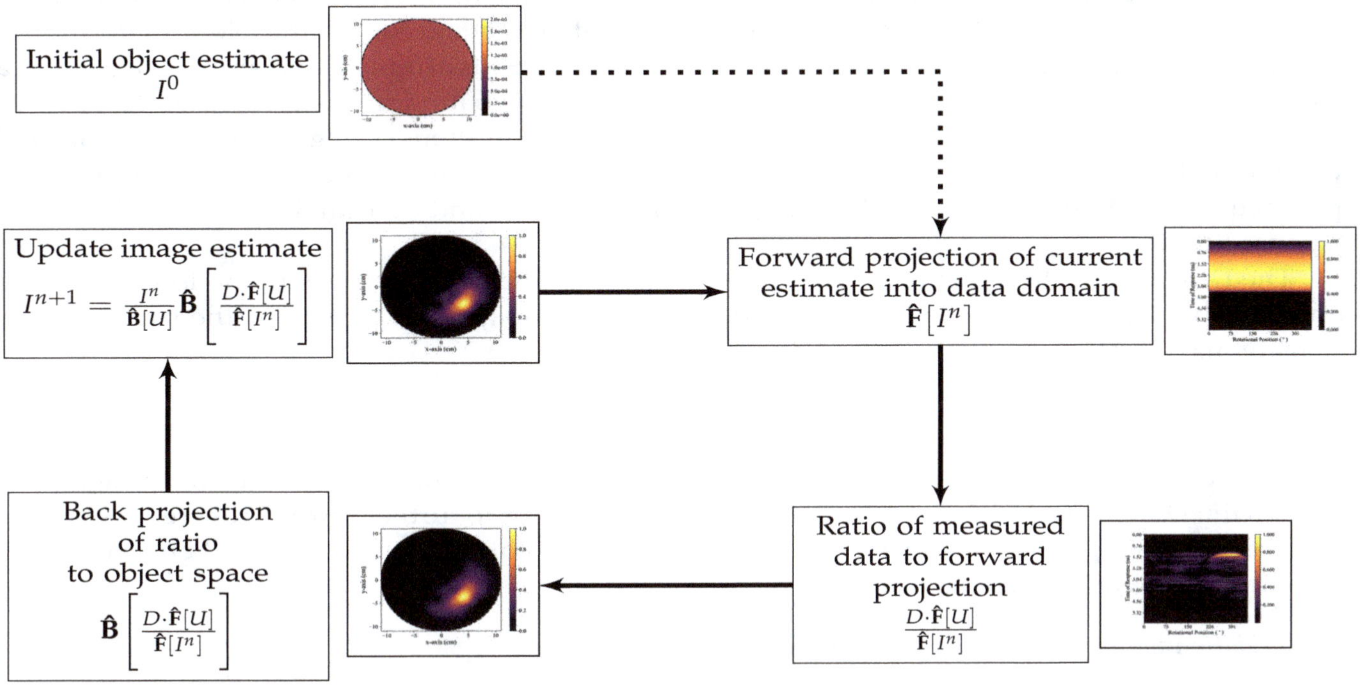

Figure 1. Flow chart of the functional form of the itDAS algorithm. The initial object estimate is forward-projected into the data domain, and the ratio between the measured data and this forward projection is determined. This ratio is then back-projected to the object space and the new image estimate is obtained by multiplying the previous image estimate by this back-projected ratio.

The iterative structure of Equation (1) was adopted for use in breast microwave radar imaging using the DAS beamformer as the back-projection operator. The initial image estimate was set to be a homogeneous map. For both the itDAS and itDMAS algorithms, the sixth iteration was the optimal balance of image contrast and noise and was selected as the stopping iteration.

A radar signal model, described in Equation (2), was used to compute the forward projection

$$\mathbf{s}_m(t) = \sum_{i=1}^{N} \sigma_i \delta(t - t_m(\mathbf{r}_i)) \tag{2}$$

where $\mathbf{s}_m$ is the radar signature measured at the mth antenna position, σ_i is the reflectivity of the ith pixel, $\mathbf{r}_i$ is the position of the ith pixel, and the sum is over all pixels in the object space. The time-of-flight t_m is defined to be

$$t_m(\mathbf{r}) = 2\frac{|\mathbf{r} - \mathbf{r}_m|}{v} \tag{3}$$

where v is the estimated average propagation speed of the signal in the object space, and $\mathbf{r}_m$ is the mth antenna position.

The DAS beamformer was used as the back-projection operator $\hat{\mathbf{B}}$ in Equation (1). This method synthetically focuses the recorded radar signatures from each antenna position during a scan,

$$I(\mathbf{r}) = \sum_{m=1}^{M} \mathbf{s}_m(t_m(\mathbf{r})) \tag{4}$$

where $I(\mathbf{r})$ is the intensity value at point $\mathbf{r}$ in the reconstructed image, and the sum is over all M antenna positions used in the scan. After determining the intensity for each $\mathbf{r}$, the reconstructed image is then presented as the squared intensity map.

2.2. The itDMAS Reconstruction Algorithm

While the itDAS algorithm uses the DAS beamformer as the back-projection operator, alternative techniques could be used. This work presents one alternative method, where the DMAS algorithm is used as the back-projection operator (resulting in the itDMAS algorithm). Two studies presented a comparison between radar-based reconstruction algorithms, evaluating six methods (the DAS, DMAS, IDAS, CF-DAS, CR-DAS, and robust capon beamformer [27] algorithms) using phantom data [30] and patient data [29]. The results in both studies indicate that among these algorithms, only the DMAS approach reduced both background and high-intensity clutter and accurately localized the tumor response [29,30].

The DMAS algorithm first performs antenna-pair multiplication before summation, rewarding coherence between measured signals. The reconstructed image is displayed as the square of the intensity map $I(\mathbf{r})$,

$$I(\mathbf{r}) = \sum_{m=1}^{M-1} \sum_{n=m+1}^{M} \mathbf{s}_m(t_m(\mathbf{r})) \cdot \mathbf{s}_n(t_n(\mathbf{r})). \tag{5}$$

The itDMAS algorithm shares the functional form described in Equation (1) with the itDAS algorithm but uses the DMAS beamformer as the back-projection operator to further reward coherence between measured antenna-pair signals. In a monostatic radar system, this rewards coherence between signals measured at different antenna positions.

2.3. Validation with a Clinical BMI System and Breast Phantoms

A rotating radar-based BMI system [35] was used to perform experimental scans of anthropomorphic breast phantoms to evaluate the itDAS and itDMAS algorithms. The system uses a vector network analyzer (VNA) (Planar 804/1, Copper Mountain Technologies, Indianapolis, IN, USA) to generate a stepped-frequency continuous-waveform microwave signal over 1–8 GHz at 1001 frequency points. This signal is supplied to a double-ridged horn antenna (LB-20200-SF, A-INFO, Chengdu, China) that was used to illuminate the scan chamber with the microwave signal. The system operates in air, without the use of a coupling medium.

When performing a scan, the VNA recorded the S_{11} scattering parameters at 72 equally spaced positions along a circular trajectory centered at the axis of rotation of the imaging chamber. The S_{11} measurements were collected in the frequency domain, and the inverse chirp z-transform was used to convert the data to the time domain using 700 points between 0 ns and 6 ns. These time-domain signals were then used directly with the reconstruction approaches to produce images of the scanned phantoms. The measured frequency-domain S_{11} parameters for each phantom used in this investigation can be accessed at Supplementary Materials https://bit.ly/itDAS-data.

An array of 3D-printed MRI-based breast phantoms were used in these experimental scans. The phantoms were derived from the publicly available phantom repository hosted by the University of Wisconsin-Madison [33] and were fabricated using the methods described in [36]. A photograph of the phantom array is displayed in Figure 2. The array consists of three adipose shells and five fibroglandular shells.

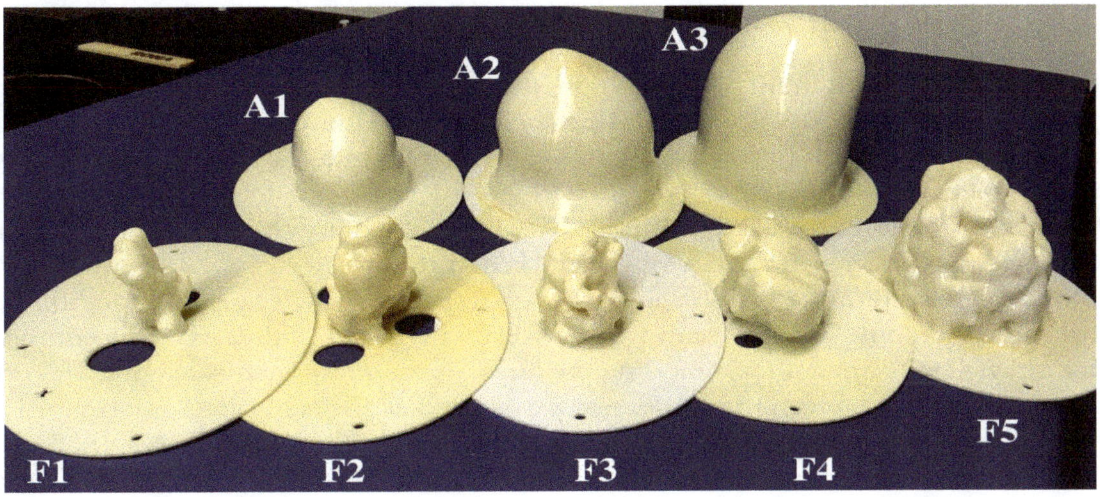

Figure 2. The array of 3D-printed MRI-derived breast phantoms. Adipose shells labeled A1 through A3, fibroglandular shells labeled F1 through F5.

3D-printed phantoms allow for reproducible and controlled experimentation and have been used throughout the literature [33,36–42]. While the low-permittivity plastic layers are undesirable, they allow for the printing of morphologically accurate phantoms. To facilitate reproducibility, the 3D-printable .stl files used to produce the phantoms in Figure 2 are available at Supplementary Materials https://bit.ly/itDAS-phantoms.

When in use, a fibroglandular shell is inserted into an adipose shell. Each is then filled with a liquid designed to mimic the dielectric properties of the corresponding tissue. Glycerin was used to mimic adipose tissue, and a 30% Triton X-100 solution was used to mimic fibroglandular tissue [36]. Spherical glass bulbs of 15 mm and 10 mm radii filled with a saline solution were used as tumor analogs during the scans. The dielectric properties of the tissue analogs are described in [36].

Nine different adipose-fibroglandular shell combinations were experimentally scanned in this study. These phantoms are representative of all four of the BI-RADS breast density classification categories [34]. Table 1 displays the fibroglandular content by percent-volume of each of the phantom combinations used in this investigation. Eighteen scans were performed; each phantom was scanned once containing a 10 mm radius lesion and once containing a 15 mm radius lesion. The tumor analogs were positioned at the same height as the antenna (within an estimated uncertainty of 10 mm).

Table 1. Breast density and BI-RADS classifications of phantom combinations used in this manuscript.

	Fibroglandular Shell	**Fibroglandular Volume**	**BI-RADS Classification**
Small Adipose Shell (A1)	F1	4.4%	Class II
	F3	19.9%	Class III
	F4	37.2%	Class IV
Medium Adipose Shell (A2)	F1	1.8%	Class I
	F3	8.1%	Class II
	F4	15.0%	Class III
	F5	38.2%	Class IV
Large Adipose Shell (A3)	F2	2.7%	Class I
	F4	9.8%	Class II

2.4. Skin Response Suppression and Propagation Speed Estimation

While the phantoms used in this investigation do not have a skin surrogate, large reflections occur at the air-plastic interface and at the plastic-adipose interface. Without the use of a coupling medium, the reflections at the air-phantom interface are sufficiently large to obscure the responses from the inner tissue structures.

Ideal skin suppression was used in this study to remove these air-tissue reflections and allow a direct comparison of the performance of the proposed iterative reconstruction methods and the literature standard non-iterative counterparts. Ideal suppression was implemented by performing two scans of each phantom. The first scan was performed with all phantom tissue components and the second scan was performed after removing the inner tissue components, leaving only the adipose surrogate. The difference between these two scans was used as the calibrated dataset.

An average propagation speed was used to compute the time-delays (in Equation (3)) for each beamformer. The permittivity in the breast was assumed to be that of the adipose tissue-mimicking material at the central scan frequency, $\epsilon = 6.4$. The propagation speed used in the reconstruction algorithms was the average permittivity in the scan region assuming a circular breast. Accurate permittivity estimation in BMI is an active area of work [22,43,44], but the relatively straight forward approach of using an average estimated permittivity also allows for the direct comparison of the four reconstruction methods, without the influence of a sophisticated propagation speed correction, and has been used in other works comparing reconstruction methods [7,8,26,29].

2.5. Image Quality Metrics

Two image quality metrics were employed to quantitatively analyze the reconstructions produced by each of the four algorithms. These metrics were selected to measure the contrast present in an image. The signal-to-mean ratio (SMR) was defined as

$$\text{SMR} = 20\log_{10}\left(\frac{S_{max}}{C_{mean}}\right) \tag{6}$$

where S_{max} was the maximum response in the region known to belong to the tumor, and C_{mean} was the mean response in the clutter region (defined to be the region of the image known to belong to the phantom, but not to the tumor). The region belonging to the tumor was assumed to be a circle of radius $r = r_t + 5$ mm centered on the known tumor position, where r_t was the radius of the spherical glass bulb used as the tumor surrogate. This was done to account for estimated positioning errors of the tumor during experimental scans. The signal-to-clutter ratio (SCR) was defined as

$$\text{SCR} = 20\log_{10}\left(\frac{S_{max}}{C_{max}}\right) \tag{7}$$

where C_{max} was the maximum response in the clutter region.

While no standard image quality metric is used throughout the literature, the definition of SMR in Equation (6) is the same as the definition of SCR in [37] and the same as in [45], and the definition of the SCR in Equation (7) is the same as in [45]. The SMR and SCR are measures of the contrast between the tumor response and the clutter in the image. The SCR provides a measure of the contrast between the tumor reflections and the strongest reflections in the image that belong to structures other than the tumor. A negative SCR indicates that the largest reflections in the image belong to a region outside of the known tumor location, while a large SCR indicates the tumor response is dominant in the reconstruction. A reconstruction with a negative SCR (indicating that the strongest response in the image was outside of the tumor location) was defined to be a reconstruction in which the tumor response was not identifiable.

While the SCR gives a measure of the contrast between the tumor response and high-intensity clutter, the SMR is a measure of the contrast between the tumor response and the average response within the breast region, indicating how easily the tumor response can be identified within the image with respect to the low-intensity clutter.

The localization error of the tumor response in reconstructions was also determined and was defined as the distance between the maximum-intensity response in the image and the center of the known tumor location.

To determine the uncertainty in the SMR and SCR, it was assumed that the uncertainty in C_{mean} was zero and the estimated uncertainty in S_{max} was defined to be the standard deviation of the intensities of the pixels with intensities within the 75th percentile of all pixels within the known tumor region. The estimated uncertainty in C_{max} was defined to be the standard deviation of the intensities of the pixels with intensities within the 95th percentile of all clutter pixels.

3. Results and Discussion

3.1. Comparison of itDAS, itDMAS, DAS, and DMAS Methods

The DAS, DMAS, itDAS, and itDMAS beamformers were used to reconstruct images of each of the phantom scans. All beamformers produced 12 reconstructions that had identifiable tumour responses. For comparison, only these reconstructions are considered for analysis.

Figure 3 displays representative reconstructions produced by each algorithm for (a–d) a Class I phantom, (e–h) a Class II phantom, (i–l) a Class III phantom, and (m–p) a Class IV phantom. The reconstructed images were 2D coronal slices, at the same plane as the tumor location, and the approximate breast and tumor boundaries are indicated in the reconstructions. Table 2 displays the SMR and SCR for each reconstruction in Figure 3.

In all reconstructions, across all density classes, the itDAS and itDMAS algorithms produced images with higher SMR and SCR than either the DAS and DMAS methods, indicating that the iterative methods produce reconstructions with both reduced high-intensity and reduced low-intensity clutter, as shown in Figure 3. The iterative beamformers maintain the tumor response while significantly reducing the clutter intensity in the reconstructed images (as indicated in the SCR and SMR in Table 2).

The clinical system used to perform the scans of the breast phantoms operates in air without the use of a coupling medium. While ideal calibration of the air-tissue interface reflections was performed, the mismatch at the air-tissue interface results in clutter responses that are significant in the DAS and (to a lesser degree) the DMAS reconstructions.

All reconstructions of Class I phantoms prominently display the tumor response, as in Figure 3a–d. The iterative methods significantly reduced both the high-intensity clutter responses near the tumor location and the low-intensity background responses, compared to the non-iterative beamformers.

In the Class II and Class III reconstructions displayed in Figure 3e,f,i,j, the tumor response is not significantly greater than the high-intensity clutter responses (as indicated in the SCR in Table 2). The high-intensity clutter is present near the air-tissue boundary of the phantoms and near the center of the phantom. While the outer reflections are likely due to imperfect air-tissue reflection calibration, the central clutter response may be due to the fibroglandular tissues which are in the center of the phantoms.

The low contrast between this central response and the tumor response of the Class III reconstruction produced by both the DAS and DMAS methods; SCRs of (1 ± 1) dB and (2 ± 2) dB for the DAS and DMAS beamformers, respectively, makes the identification of the tumor response challenging. The itDAS and itDMAS reconstructions have higher SCRs; (4 ± 2) dB and (5 ± 3) dB, respectively.

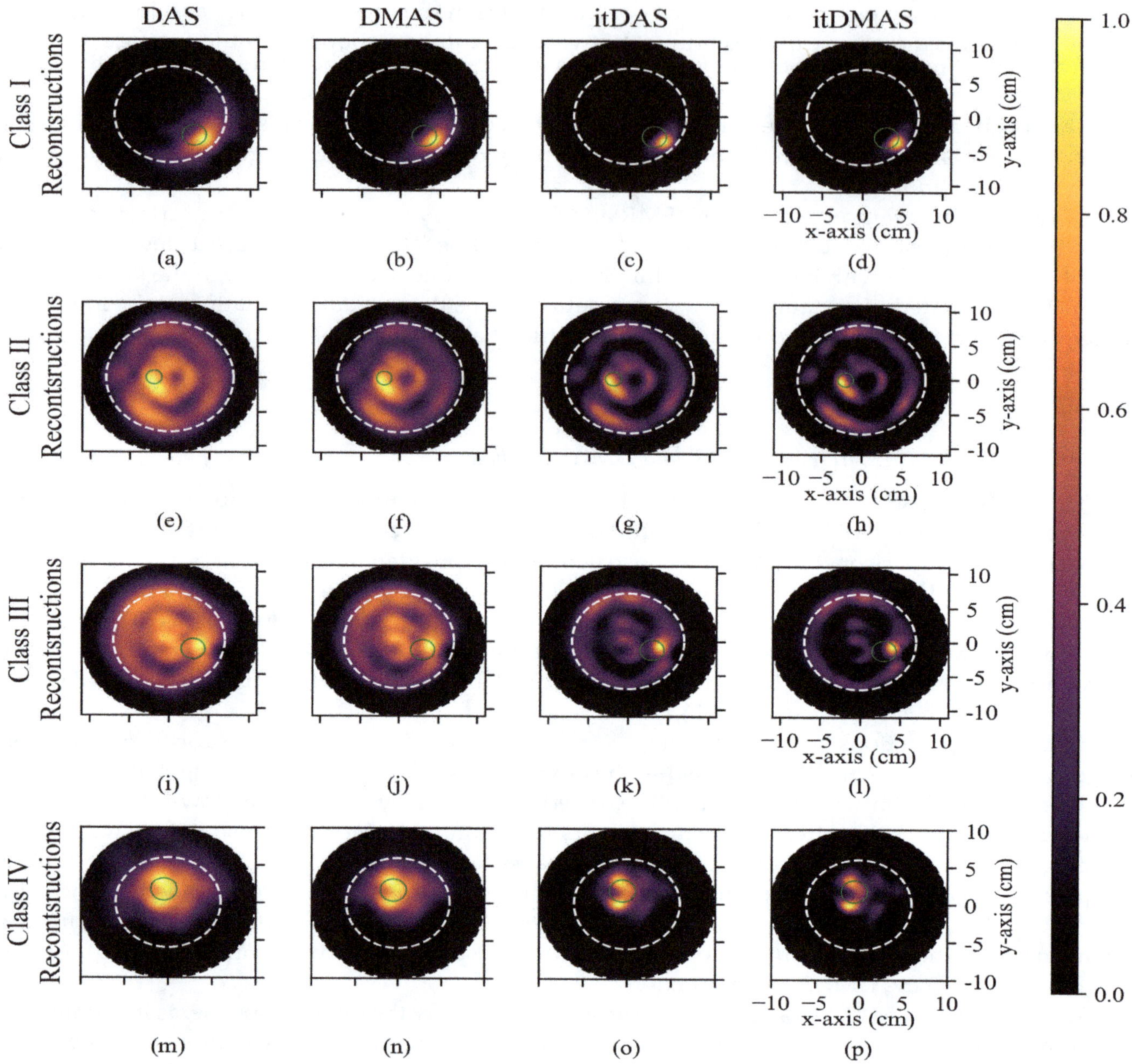

Figure 3. Reconstructions of breast phantoms by (left to right) the DAS, DMAS, itDAS, and itDMAS beamformers. (**a–d**) display the reconstructions of a 15 mm radius lesion in a Class I (A2F1) phantom, (**e–h**) display the reconstructions of a 10 mm radius lesion in a Class II (A3F4) phantom, (**i–l**) display the reconstructions of a 15 mm radius lesion in a Class III (A2F4) phantom, and (**m–p**) display the reconstruction of a 15 mm radius lesion in a Class IV (A1F4) phantom. Each image is normalized to its maximum intensity. The dotted black circle indicates the antenna trajectory during the scan, the dotted white line indicates the approximate breast phantom boundary, and the solid green circle indicates the known tumor position.

Table 2. Image Quality Metrics of Reconstructions Displayed in Figure 3.

		DAS	DMAS	itDAS	itDMAS
Class I Images	SMR (dB)	11 ± 1	19 ± 2	29 ± 2	30 ± 3
	SCR (dB)	1 ± 2	1 ± 2	2 ± 3	2 ± 3
Class II Images	SMR (dB)	4.2 ± 0.5	7.7 ± 0.9	13 ± 2	16 ± 2
	SCR (dB)	0 ± 1	0 ± 2	1 ± 2	1 ± 2
Class III Images	SMR (dB)	3.2 ± 0.6	6 ± 1	12 ± 2	16 ± 2
	SCR (dB)	1 ± 1	2 ± 2	4 ± 2	5 ± 3
Class IV Images	SMR (dB)	6.5 ± 0.4	10.7 ± 0.6	18 ± 1	22 ± 1
	SCR (dB)	0 ± 2	1 ± 2	0 ± 2	0 ± 2

While none of the reconstruction methods accurately reconstruct the lesion size, the tumor response is visible in the itDAS and itDMAS reconstructions and is localized within the expected region. No significant differences were observed in the localization error of the tumor response in the four examined reconstruction algorithms. The localization error of reconstructions produced by the DAS and DMAS methods was (11 ± 4) mm, (12 ± 5) mm for itDAS, and (11 ± 4) mm for itDMAS.

The average computation time required for image reconstruction with the itDAS algorithm was compared to that of the DAS and DMAS beamformers using a Ryzen 2700X central processing unit. When reconstructing 500×500 images (as presented in this article) from the 72×700 time-domain S_{11} array (700 time points per antenna position) used to represent each scan, the DAS algorithm required (13.1 ± 0.1) s to reconstruct an image, DMAS required (14.6 ± 0.2) s, and itDAS required (149 ± 2) s. While the ratio of computation time of itDAS compared to DAS was (11 ± 1):1, the total computation time was under 3 minutes and is not prohibitive.

itDAS requires the computation of forward and back projections at each iteration. The back projections are nearly equivalent to a complete DAS reconstruction with respect to computation time, requiring (11.9 ± 0.1) s. The forward projections required (9.1 ± 0.1) s. itDAS also requires the initialization of the forward and back projections of a unity dataset, $\hat{\mathbf{F}}[U]$ and $\hat{\mathbf{B}}[U]$ respectively. This initialization required (22.4 ± 0.1) s to complete. The majority of the computation time of itDAS is due to this initialization and the computation of the forward and back projections at each iteration.

The number of radar signals N_s used to create the image is one factor that is expected to affect the algorithmic complexity of DAS-based reconstruction methods. As described in [46], DAS requires N_s summations to reconstruct an image using N_s measured radar signals, resulting in an algorithmic complexity of $O(N_s)$ with respect to the number of measured radar signals used to produce the reconstruction. itDAS requires N_s summations at each iteration to compute the back-projection and N_s summations to compute the forward-projection, in addition to the $2N_s$ summations required for the initialization of the forward and back projections of unity arrays. With respect to the number of measured radar signals, DAS has an algorithmic complexity of $O(N_s)$ while itDAS has an algorithmic complexity of $O(2(N_{iter} + 1)N_s)$, where N_{iter} is the number of iterations used to produce the reconstruction.

This model assumes that the summations used to compute the forward projections are the same as those used to produce the back projections, but the measured computation times indicate that forward-projection can be performed faster than back-projection. This model is therefore an overestimate of the algorithmic complexity of itDAS, but demonstrates that the algorithmic complexity is approximately linearly related to that of DAS with respect to the number of radar signals used for reconstruction. This model, in combination with the absolute and relative measured computation times stated above, demonstrate that while itDAS is more computationally complex and requires greater computation time to produce a reconstruction, these effects are not prohibitive.

Figure 4 displays the average SMR and SCR for reconstructions of each of the BI-RADS density classification categories with an identifiable tumor response (a reconstructed image was defined to have an identifiable tumor response if the SCR of the image was greater than zero) for each of the reconstruction algorithms. While a relatively small number of phantoms were used to represent each density classification category, the observed trend of decreasing SMR in higher-density breasts (excluding the Class IV phantom where only one of the four Class IV phantom reconstructions had an identifiable tumor response) agrees with the expected model of denser breasts presenting a more challenging reconstruction scenario for tumor detection.

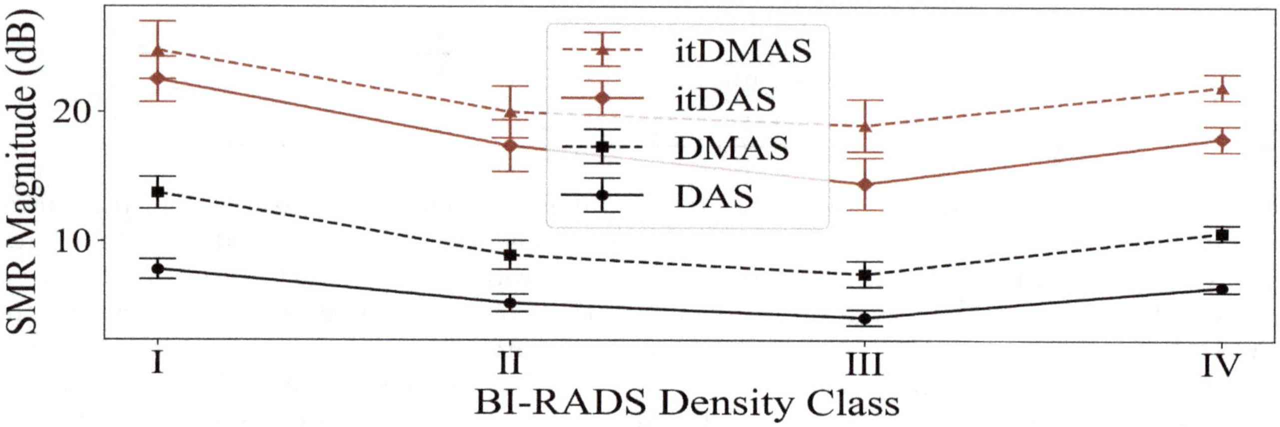

(a)

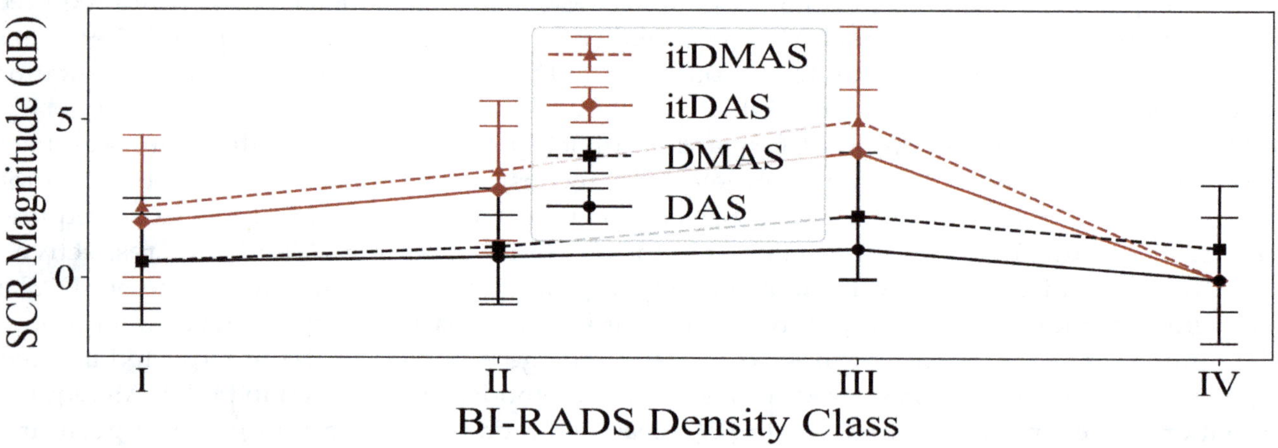

(b)

Figure 4. (**a**) Average SMR and (**b**) average SCR for the reconstruction algorithms using scans of phantoms representative of the four BI-RADS density classification categories.

This univariate analysis displays that in all density classes, the itDAS and itDMAS methods produced reconstructions with higher SMR and SCR than the DAS or DMAS beamformers. A multivariate analysis of contrast as a function of breast density, tumor size, tumor position, and breast size is outside the scope of this work, which aims to present the itDAS and itDMAS algorithms and make a comparison to the DAS and DMAS standards, but may be performed in future work using the phantom array.

As was found in phantom [30] and patient studies [29], images produced by the DMAS method consistently had higher SMR and SCR than reconstructions by the DAS algorithm. The DMAS beamformer produced reconstructions with an average increase in SMR of 75% relative to the DAS beamformer on Class I phantoms, 70% on Class II phantoms, and 81% on Class III phantoms, and 64% on Class IV phantoms.

While the DMAS reconstructions resulted in a 64–81% increase in SMR on average and a 0–111% increase in SCR on average, the iterative methods provided an even greater increase in contrast. The itDAS beamformer increased SMR by an average of 188% for Class I phantoms (relative to the DAS images), 231% for Class II, 249% for Class III, and 177% for Class IV. Improvements in SCR were as large as 321% for Class III phantoms. However, the itDMAS algorithm offered the greatest improvement over the DAS beamformer-increasing the SMR by as much as 358% in Class III phantoms and the SCR by 426% in Class III phantoms, on average.

The DMAS beamformer initially presented a significant improvement in clutter reduction in reconstructions for radar-based BMI [7] over the DAS beamformer [6]. The pair-wise signal multiplication rewards signal coherence while punishing incoherence [7]. Just as the DMAS method provided significant improvements over DAS, so too does the itDAS algorithm over DMAS. The multiplicative iterative structure further rewards signal coherence while punishing incoherence during reconstruction, resulting in images that prominently display tumor responses with significantly reduced low-intensity background clutter, and reduced high-intensity clutter. However, unlike the DMAS method, the itDAS and itDMAS algorithms have the potential to improve the forward signal model by accounting for path-dependent effects.

Both iterative algorithms resulted in significant increases in both SMR and SCR relative to the non-iterative beamformers, but the SCR and SMR of most reconstructions produced by the itDAS and itDMAS algorithms were not significantly different. This indicates that while the signal-pair multiplication in the DMAS beamformer rewards coherence between signals and results in higher contrast metrics in the DMAS images relative to the DAS images, the impact of this pairwise multiplication on the final reconstructed image is insignificant when combined with the effect of the iterative structure of Equation (1). The iterative structure is the dominant cause of the higher contrast present in the iterative reconstructions-for both the itDAS and itDMAS algorithms.

3.2. Future Work and Improving the Signal Model

Future work can investigate the impact of using other DAS-based methods as the back-projection operator in the iterative structure, including the IDAS [8], CF-DAS [9], and CR-DAS [10] methods. This investigation of the itDAS algorithm explored the use of the DMAS beamformer as the back-projection operator in the itDMAS algorithm due to its performance in [29,30], but alternative methods can also be explored.

Just as several DAS-derivative algorithms aimed to reward signal coherence [7–9], the iterative structure of the algorithm inherently rewards signal coherence (through multiplicative updates at each iteration) while punishing incoherence. While other DAS-derivatives have aimed at accounting for path-dependent effects [10] (and other radar-based reconstruction methods more broadly [26,27,32,37]), the itDAS algorithm is capable of both rewarding signal coherence and correcting for path-dependent effects through improvements to the forward model.

The measured sinogram (after ideal skin suppression) for one of the phantom scans and the forward projection of the image estimate at each of the first six iterations during the itDAS reconstruction is displayed in Figure 5. While the tumour response is more apparent in later iterations, the differences between the forward projections and the measured sinogram highlight the limitations of the current radar signal model. Signal attenuation and inhomogeneous signal propagation affect the measured data but are not incorporated into the forward projection model presented herein.

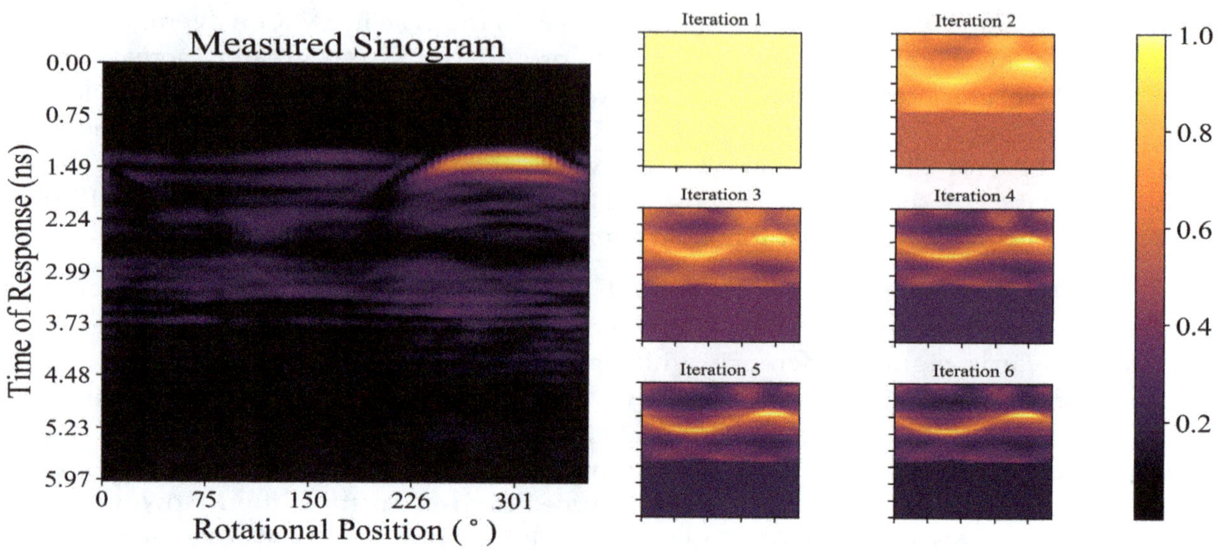

Figure 5. The measured sinogram (after ideal skin suppression) and the forward projection of the image estimate at each of the first six iterations during the itDAS reconstruction (displayed in Figure 3c) of the Class I phantom. Each sinogram and forward projection has been normalized to have a maximum value of unity.

Despite the limitations in the current forward projection model, the contrast improvements provided by the iterative structure of the itDAS method are significant, and the improvements in the reconstructions in Figure 3 are evident. The implementation of correction factors to improve the signal model used in the forward and back-projection operators will be explored in future work. Corrections for the antenna characteristics [32,37], the non-uniform propagation speed [37], and other path-dependent effects can be investigated. Previous work that had adapted the functional form of the MLEM algorithm from PET for use in BMI [32,37] found that the implementation of correction factors improved image contrast, and the impact of these corrections when this functional form is applied to the DAS beamformer will be investigated in future work.

The iterative structure of the itDAS algorithm requires the use of a stopping rule. The sixth iteration was selected as the final iteration for all reconstructions examined in this work, and future work should investigate more rigorous stopping rules based on phantom scans.

4. Conclusions

This work presents a novel iterative image reconstruction algorithm for use in breast microwave radar imaging. The presented itDAS method applies the functional form of the MLEM algorithm from PET [31] to the DAS beamformer [6], using the DAS beamformer as the back-projection operator and a radar signal model as the forward operator. A derivative of the itDAS algorithm using the DMAS method as the back-projection operator was also presented.

The DAS, DMAS, itDAS, and itDMAS algorithms were used to reconstruct images of eighteen tumor-containing experimental scans of 3D-printed MRI-based breast phantoms. In all cases, the itDAS and itDMAS algorithms produced images with higher SMR and SCR than either the DAS or DMAS methods.

The iterative structure of the itDAS algorithm inherently rewards signal coherence while punishing incoherence (through multiplicative image estimate updates) and has the potential to correct for path-dependent effects (through improvements to the forward model and modifications to the back-projection operator). Even without corrections for path-dependent effects, the itDAS algorithm produced reconstructions that had significantly higher SMR than the non-iterative methods, increasing contrast by as much as 19 dB over DAS and 13 dB over DMAS. The itDAS algorithm also increased the SCR of reconstructions by up to 5 dB over DAS and 4 dB over DMAS. No significant difference in the contrast of itDAS and itDMAS images was observed in the majority of reconstructions, indicating the rewarded coherence through the iterative structure is more significant than the effects of signal-pair multiplication present in the DMAS method. The promising results presented herein for an air-operated BMI system demonstrate the advantages of using the iterative beamforming methods.

Author Contributions: Conceptualization, S.P.; methodology, T.R. and S.P.; software, T.R.; validation, T.R., M.S.-N., and S.P.; writing—original draft preparation, T.R.; writing—review and editing, T.R., M.S.-N., and S.P.; supervision, M.S.-N., and S.P. All authors have read and agreed to the published version of the manuscript.

References

1. Nikolova, N.K. Microwave imaging for breast cancer. *IEEE Microw. Mag.* **2011**, *12*, 78–94. [CrossRef]
2. Gøtzsche, P.C.; Jørgensen, K.J. Screening for breast cancer with mammography. *Cochrane Database Syst. Rev.* **2013**, *22*, CD001877. [CrossRef] [PubMed]
3. Fear, E.; Meaney, P.; Stuchly, M. Microwaves for breast cancer detection? *IEEE Potentials* **2003**, *22*, 12–18. [CrossRef]
4. Lazebnik, M.; Popovic, D.; McCartney, L.; Watkins, C.B.; Lindstrom, M.J.; Harter, J.; Sewall, S.; Ogilvie, T.; Magliocco, A.; Breslin, T.M.; et al. A large-scale study of the ultrawideband microwave dielectric properties of normal, benign and malignant breast tissues obtained from cancer surgeries. *Phys. Med. Biol.* **2007**, *52*, 6093–6115. [CrossRef] [PubMed]
5. Sugitani, T.; Kubota, S.I.; Kuroki, S.I.; Sogo, K.; Arihiro, K.; Okada, M.; Kadoya, T.; Hide, M.; Oda, M.; Kikkawa, T. Complex permittivities of breast tumor tissues obtained from cancer surgeries. *Appl. Phys. Lett.* **2014**, *104*, 1–5. [CrossRef]
6. Hagness, S.C.; Taflove, A.; Bridges, J. Two-dimensional FDTD analysis of a pulsed microwave confocal system for breast cancer detection: fixed-focus and antenna-array sensors. *IEEE Trans. Biomed. Eng.* **1998**, *45*, 1470–1479. [CrossRef]
7. Lim, H.B.; Nhung, N.T.T.; Li, E.P.; Thang, N.D. Confocal microwave imaging for breast cancer detection: Delay-multiply-and-sum image reconstruction algorithm. *IEEE Trans. Biomed. Eng.* **2008**, *55*, 1697–1704. [CrossRef]
8. Klemm, M.; Craddock, I.J.; Leendertz, J.A.; Preece, A.; Benjamin, R. Improved delay-and-sum beamforming algorithm for breast cancer detection. *Int. J. Antennas Propag.* **2008**, *2008*. [CrossRef]
9. Klemm, M.; Leendertz, J.A.; Gibbins, D.; Craddock, I.J.; Preece, A.; Benjamin, R. Microwave radar-based breast cancer detection: Imaging in inhomogeneous breast phantoms. *IEEE Antennas Wirel. Propag. Lett.* **2009**, *8*, 1349–1352. [CrossRef]
10. O'Halloran, M.; Glavin, M.; Jones, E. Improved Confocal Microwave Imaging of the breast using path-dependent signal weighting. In Proceedings of the 2011 URSI General Assembly and Scientific Symposium, Istanbul, Turkey, 13–20 August 2011; pp. 1–4. [CrossRef]
11. Porter, E.; Coates, M.; Popovic, M. An early clinical study of time-domain microwave radar for breast health monitoring. *IEEE Trans. Biomed. Eng.* **2016**, *63*, 530–539. [CrossRef]
12. Preece, A.; Craddock, I.; Shere, M.; Jones, L.; Winton, H.L. MARIA M4: Clinical evaluation of a prototype ultrawideband radar scanner for breast cancer detection. *J. Med. Imag.* **2016**, *3*, 033502. [CrossRef] [PubMed]
13. Porter, E.; Kazemi, R.; Santorelli, A.; Popović, M. Study of daily tissue changes through breast monitoring with time-domain microwave radar. In Proceedings of the 2015 9th European Conference on Antennas and Propagation (EuCAP), Lisbon, Portugal, 13–17 April 2015; pp. 1–5.
14. Porter, E.; Santorelli, A.; Popovic, M. Time-domain microwave radar for breast screening: Initial testing with volunteers. In Proceedings of the 8th European Conference on Antennas and Propagation (EuCAP 2014), The Hague, The Netherlands, 6–11 April 2014; pp. 104–107. [CrossRef]
15. Porter, E.; Santorelli, A.; Popovic, M. Time-domain microwave radar applied to breast imaging: Measurement reliability in a clinical setting. *Prog. Electromagn. Res.* **2014**, *149*, 119–132. [CrossRef]

16. Sasada, S.; Masumoto, N.; Song, H.; Kajitani, K.; Emi, A.; Kadoya, T. Portable impulse-radar detector for breast cancer: A pilot study. *J. Med. Imag.* **2018**, *5*, 025502. [CrossRef] [PubMed]
17. Fear, E.C.; Bourqui, J.; Curtis, C.; Mew, D.; Docktor, B.; Romano, C. Microwave breast imaging with a monostatic radar-based system: A study of application to patients. *IEEE Trans. Microw. Theory Tech.* **2013**, *61*, 2119–2128. [CrossRef]
18. Song, H.; Sasada, S.; Kadoya, T.; Okada, M.; Arihiro, K.; Xiao, X.; Kikkawa, T. Detectability of breast tumor by a hand-held impulse-radar detector: Performance evaluation and pilot clinical study. *Sci. Rep.* **2017**, *7*, 16353. [CrossRef]
19. Lavoie, B.R.; Bourqui, J.; Fear, E.C. Metrics for assessing the similarity of microwave breast imaging scans of healthy volunteers. *IEEE Trans. Med. Imag.* **2018**, *37*, 1788–1798. [CrossRef]
20. Curtis, C.; Lavoie, B.R.; Fear, E. An analysis of the assumptions inherent to near-field beamforming for biomedical applications. *IEEE Trans. Comp. Imag.* **2017**, *3*, 953–965. [CrossRef]
21. Curtis, C.; Fear, E. Coherent summation of monostatic radar signals. In Proceedings of the 2013 7th European Conference on Antennas and Propagation (EuCAP), Gothenburg, Sweden, 8–12 April 2013; pp. 628–629.
22. Lavoie, B.R.; Okoniewski, M.; Fear, E.C. Estimating the effective permittivity for reconstructing accurate microwave-radar images. *PLoS ONE* **2016**, *11*, e0160849. [CrossRef]
23. Porter, E.; Santorelli, A.; Kazemi, R.; Popovic, M. Microwave time-domain radar: Healthy tissue variations over the menstrual cycle. *IEEE Antennas Wirel. Propag. Lett.* **2015**, *14*, 1310–1313. [CrossRef]
24. Porter, E.; Bahrami, H.; Santorelli, A.; Gosselin, B.; Rusch, L.A.; Popovic, M. A wearable microwave antenna array for time-domain breast tumor screening. *IEEE Trans. Med. Imag.* **2016**, *35*, 1501–1509. [CrossRef]
25. Kuwahara, Y.; Miura, S.; Nishina, Y.; Mukumoto, K.; Ogura, H.; Sakahara, H. Clinical test of microwave mammography. In Proceedings of the 2013 IEEE Antennas and Propagation Society International Symposium (APSURSI), Orlando, FL, USA, 7–13 July 2013; pp. 2028–2029. [CrossRef]
26. Bond, E.; Li, X.; Hagness, S.; Van Veen, B.D. Microwave imaging via space-time beamforming for early detection of breast cancer. *IEEE Trans. Antennas Propag.* **2003**, *51*, 1690–1705. [CrossRef]
27. Guo, B.; Wang, Y.; Li, J.; Stoica, P.; Wu, R. Microwave imaging via adaptive beamforming methods for breast cancer detection. *J. Electromagn. Waves Appl.* **2006**, *20*, 53–63. [CrossRef]
28. Byrne, D.; Craddock, I.J. Time-domain wideband adaptive beamforming for radar breast imaging. *IEEE Trans. Antennas Propag.* **2015**, *63*, 1725–1735. [CrossRef]
29. Elahi, M.A.; O'Loughlin, D.; Lavoie, B.R.; Glavin, M.; Jones, E.; Fear, E.C.; O'Halloran, M. Evaluation of image reconstruction algorithms for confocal microwave imaging: Application to patient data. *Sensors* **2018**, *18*, 1678. [CrossRef]
30. Elahi, M.A.; Lavoie, B.R.; Porter, E.; Glavin, M.; Jones, E.; Fear, E.C.; O'Halloran, M. Comparison of radar-based microwave imaging algorithms applied to experimental breast phantoms. In Proceedings of the 2017 General Assembly and Scientific Symposium of the International Union of Radio Science (URSI GASS), Montreal, QC, Canada, 19–26 August 2017; pp. 1–4. [CrossRef]
31. Shepp, L.A.; Vardi, Y. Maximum Likelihood Reconstruction for Emission Tomography. *IEEE Trans. Med. Imag.* **1982**, *1*, 113–122. [CrossRef] [PubMed]
32. Reimer, T.; Rodriguez Herrera, D.; Solis Nepote, M.; Pistorius, S. The use of a novel microwave radar reconstruction algorithm to image lesions in realistic 3D breast phantoms. In Proceedings of the 12th European Conference on Antennas and Propagation (EuCAP 2018), London, UK, 9–13 April 2018; pp. 1–5. [CrossRef]
33. Burfeindt, M.J.; Colgan, T.J.; Owen Mays, R.; Shea, J.D.; Behdad, N.; Van Veen, B.D.; Hagness, S. MRI-derived 3-D-printed breast phantom for microwave breast imaging validation. *IEEE Antennas Wirel. Propag. Lett.* **2012**, *11*, 1610–1613. [CrossRef]
34. Sickles, E.; D'Orsi, C.; Basset, L.; Appleton, C.; Berg, W.; Burnside, E.; Feig, S.; Gavenonis, S.; Newell, M.; Trinh, M. ACR BI-RADS®Mammography. In *ACR BI-RADS®Atlas, Breast Imaging Reporting and Data System*; American College of Radiology: Reston, VA, USA, 2013.
35. Solis-Nepote, M.; Reimer, T.; Pistorius, S. An Air-Operated Bistatic System for Breast Microwave Radar Imaging: Pre-Clinical Validation. In Proceedings of the 2019 41st Annual International Conference of the IEEE Engineering in Medicine and Biology Society (EMBC), Berlin, Germany, 23–27 July 2019; pp. 1859–1862. [CrossRef]

36. Herrera, D.R.; Reimer, T.; Solis Nepote, M.; Pistorius, S. Manufacture and testing of anthropomorphic 3D-printed breast phantoms using a microwave radar algorithm optimized for propagation speed. In Proceedings of the 2017 11th European Conference on Antennas and Propagation (EUCAP), Paris, France, 19–24 March 2017; pp. 3480–3484. [CrossRef]
37. Reimer, T.; Nepote, M.S.; Pistorius, S. Initial results using an MLEM-based reconstruction algorithm for breast microwave radar imaging. In Proceedings of the 2018 18th International Symposium on Antenna Technology and Applied Electromagnetics (ANTEM), Waterloo, ON, Canada, 19–22 August 2019; pp. 1–2. [CrossRef]
38. Joachimowicz, N.; Duchene, B.; Conessa, C.; Meyer, O. Reference phantoms for microwave imaging. In Proceedings of the 2017 11th European Conference on Antennas and Propagation (EUCAP), Paris, France, 19–24 March 2017; pp. 2719–2722. [CrossRef]
39. Rydholm, T.; Fhager, A.; Persson, M.; Meaney, P. A first evaluation of the realistic supelec-breast phantom. *IEEE J. Electromagn. RF Microw. Med. Biol.* **2017**, *1*, 59–65. [CrossRef]
40. LoVetri, J.; Asefi, M.; Abdollahi, N.; Brown, K.; Geddert, N.; Jeffrey, I. Phantom study of a flat-faceted air-based microwave breast imaging system. In Proceedings of the 12th European Conference on Antennas and Propagation (EuCAP 2018), London, UK, 9–13 April 2018; pp. 1–2. [CrossRef]
41. Tobon-Vasquez, J.; Vipiana, F.; Casu, M.; Vacca, M.; Sarwar, I.; Scapaticci, R.; Joachimowicz, N.; Duchene, B. Experimental assessment of qualitative microwave imaging using a 3-D realistic breast phantom. In Proceedings of the 2017 11th European Conference on Antennas and Propagation (EUCAP), Paris, France, 19–24 March 2017; pp. 2728–2731. [CrossRef]
42. Kumari, V.; Sheoran, G.; Kanumur, T. SAR analysis of directive antenna on anatomically real breast phantoms for microwave holography. *Microw. Opt. Technol. Lett.* **2020**, *62*, 466–473. [CrossRef]
43. Rodriguez-Herrera, D.; Flores-Tapia, D.; Pistorius, S. Comparison of image quality metrics for electromagnetic wave propagation speed estimation in breast microwave radar imaging scenarios. In Proceedings of the 8th European Conference on Antennas and Propagation (EuCAP 2014), The Hague, The Netherlands, 6–11 April 2014; pp. 516–519. [CrossRef]
44. Modiri, A.; Kiasaleh, K. Permittivity estimation for breast cancer detection using particle swarm optimization algorithm. In Proceedings of the 2011 Annual International Conference of the IEEE Engineering in Medicine and Biology Society, Boston, MA, USA, 30 August–3 September 2011; pp. 1359–1362. [CrossRef]
45. Hazarika, P.; Santorelli, A.; Popovic, M. Investigation of antenna array configurations for microwave radar breast screening. In Proceedings of the 2016 17th International Symposium on Antenna Technology and Applied Electromagnetics (ANTEM), Montreal, QC, Canada, 10–13 July 2016; pp. 1–2. [CrossRef]
46. KaramFard, S.; Asl, B.M. Fast delay-multiply-and-sum beamformer: Application to confocal microwave imaging. *IEEE Antennas Wirel. Propag. Lett.* **2020**, *19*, 14–18. [CrossRef]

4

Challenges and Potential Solutions of Psychophysiological State Monitoring with Bioradar Technology

Lesya Anishchenko

Remote Sensing Laboratory, Bauman Moscow State Technical University, Moscow 105005, Russia; anishchenko@rslab.ru

Abstract: Psychophysiological state monitoring provides a promising way to detect stress and accurately assess wellbeing. The purpose of the present work was to investigate the advantages of utilizing a new unobtrusive multi-transceiver system on the accuracy of remote psychophysiological state monitoring by means of a bioradar technique. The technique was tested in laboratory conditions with the participation of 35 practically healthy volunteers, who were asked to perform arithmetic and physical workload tests imitating different types of stressors. Information about any variation in vital signs, registered by a bioradar with two transceivers, was used to detect mental or physical stress. Processing of the experimental results showed that the designed two-channel bioradar can be used as a simple and relatively easy approach to implement a non-contact method for stress monitoring. However, individual specificity of physiological responses to mental and physical workloads makes the creation of a universal stress-detector classifier that is suitable for people with different levels of stress tolerance a challenging task. For non-athletes, the proposed method allows classification of calm state/mental workload and calm state/physical workload with an accuracy of 89% and 83% , respectively, without the usage of any additional a priori information on the subject.

Keywords: stress detection; bioradar; psychophysiological state monitoring; unobtrusive monitoring

---

1. Introduction

Stress is a normal organism response to changing environmental conditions, as defined by Selye [1]. In [2], Selye differentiated between "dis- and eustress", or pathological stress (negative, distress) vs. health-promoting stress (positive, eustress). While eustress helps us deal successfully with everyday challenges, distress leads to physiological and psychological health problems. In the short term, distress may result in fatigue, decrease in the ability to work, anxiety, etc. However, chronic stress, which is one of the fundamental problems of today's society, may result in irreversible physiological and psychological shifts that increase, in the long-term perspective, the risk of socially-significant health problems such as cardiovascular diseases [3,4], obesity [5], diabetes [6], sleep disorders [7,8], different types of psychosis [9,10] and depression [11]. That is why stress detection techniques may be helpful tools allowing the prevention of health problems associated with prolonged stress. These methods should provide scientifically reliable results as well as be comfortable for the user.

At present, to detect stress and estimate its level, numerous psychological questionnaires are used. The main drawback of their usage is the necessity to interpret results by an expert (professional psychologist). Moreover, there are stress detection techniques based on measuring physiological parameters, such as level of cortisol [12,13], event-related brain potential [14], electrodermal activity or galvanic skin response [15,16], blood pressure [17], heart rate variability (HRV) [18], respiration [19], etc. The main drawback of these methods is their need for direct contact such as electrodes or sensors with the human body or taking saliva samples (in the case of measuring cortisol level), which makes them inappropriate for everyday usage.

Some stress detection methods are based on analyzing information about pupil diameter [20], eye movements [19] and facial expression [21] extracted from the video data. In comparison to contact methods, these are much more comfortable for the user; however, they are known to be extremely sensitive to lighting conditions as all methods are based on analyzing data from video cameras. Therefore, the reliability of their results is questionable.

Furthermore, there are mobile applications and wearables that claim to be able to monitor mental stress [22]. For the majority of them, the main limitation is that they only consider HRV registered by a smartphone camera. Moreover, in the majority of cases, there is no data about the accuracy of HRV and stress detection algorithm verification in realistic conditions for these apps, which reduce the confidence held in the reliability of the results.

One of the methods that can be used for prolonged daily unobtrusive stress detection and monitoring is the bioradar technique [23]. This method has been known since the 1970s [24,25]. It is based on the modulation of a radar probing signal reflected from the human by the movement of a body's surface, which may be caused by respiration, heartbeat, vocalization, gut motility, limb movements, etc. The main advantage of bioradiolocation is its non-contact nature, since any direct physical contact with the user is not required. Over the last decade, the scientific community and manufacturers have experienced a growing interest in non-contact methods thanks to its high acceptance by patients and users [26].

Research activities dealing with the application of bioradars for the estimation of user's psychophysiological states and detection of mental stress have been carried out at the Remote Sensing Laboratory of Bauman Moscow State Technical University (BMSTU) since 2011 [27,28].

It should be noted that, until now, the majority of work dealing with the monitoring of a human psychophysiological state by means of bioradars has been mainly focused on bioradar signal processing, which allows the registration of heartbeat and respiration patterns [29–31]. In the present paper, we propose using the features of vital signs registered by bioradar for detecting the presence of external stress factors by analyzing them.

This paper deals with two main challenges that arise while applying the proposed technique in realistic conditions and suggests methods for their solution by using the experience of previous works along with new experimental data. The first one is caused by a high impact of the subject orientation toward radar on the level of the desired signal and the accuracy of the estimation of vital signs. The second challenge is determined by the variability of subjects' reaction to a stressor, which depends on the level of individual stress tolerance.

The purpose of the present study was to investigate the advantages of utilizing a multi-transceiver system on the accuracy of psychophysiological state monitoring by means of a bioradar technique. This is explicitly due to the capability of such bioradar architecture to overcome one of the challenges that arise while applying the proposed technique in realistic conditions, which is a high impact of the subject orientation toward radar antennae on the level of the desired signal and the accuracy of the estimation of vital signs from previous works [32]. The novelty of the present work lies in the proposed architecture of the bioradar using two transceivers, which allows the observation of the subject from different angles, and thus increases classification accuracy compared to using a standard bioradar with a single transceiver. Moreover, the present paper discusses the method to overcome another challenge of using a bioradar for stress detection, which is determined by the variability of subjects' reaction to a stressor due to individual stress tolerance.

2. Materials and Methods

2.1. Experimental Setup

The architecture of the bioradar used in the present work is shown in Figure 1.

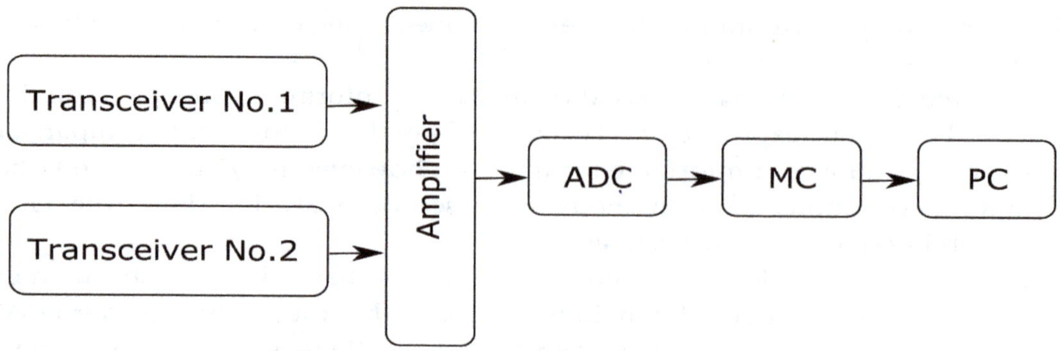

Figure 1. Two-channel bioradar scheme.

The bioradar was designed using two single-chip, high-sensitivity, dual-channel transceivers K-LC5 (RFbeam) [33], a photo of which is shown in Figure 2. The transceivers operate at a frequency of 24 GHz and provide output signals of two quadratures (I and Q). To prevent interference between the probing signals of two transceivers, we use VCO input of the second transceiver to make the probing frequency 24.2 GHz. As the K-LC5 sensors do not have an integrated amplifier, we designed a variable gain amplifier adapted to monitor human vital signs by limiting bandwidth to around 0.1–15 Hz. The gain can be adjusted in the range of 0–30 dB, depending on the range to the examinee and his orientation towards the transceiver antenna.

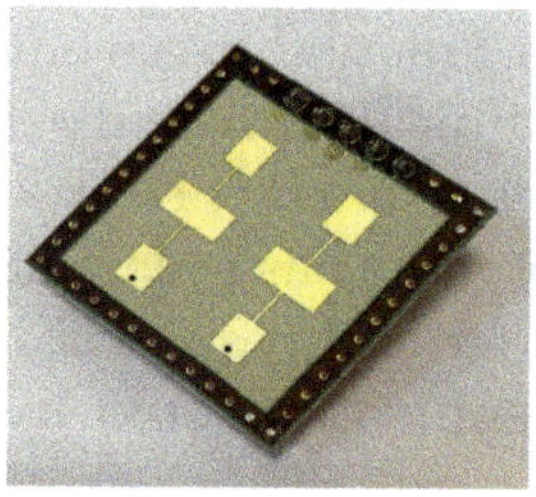

Figure 2. K-LC5 transceiver [33].

As an analog-to-digital converter (ADC), we used a higher-precision ADC ADS1115, which provides 16-bit precision at 860 samples/second over I2C and can be configured as four single-ended input channels. As a micro-controller (MC) board, an Arduino UNO board was used, which sent the data registered by the bioradar via Serial Port to the personal computer (PC) for further off-line analysis.

The maximum power density radiated by the radar is less than 3 μW/cm^2, which satisfies the Russian standard for microwave emission, which is 25 μW/cm^2 in the frequency range 3–300 GHz (for 24 h exposure).

2.2. Description of the Experimental Procedure

Experiments were conducted to determine whether the usage of a bioradar with two spaced transceivers increases the accuracy of detecting mental and physical stress in humans as compared to a single transceiver bioradar and to evaluate the corresponding accuracy gain. Using spaced transceivers should allow the observation of a biological object from different angles, which results in different amplitude levels of a received signal. Moreover, such architecture allows separating the vital signs patterns of two different, simultaneously observed humans if needed, which is described in [34].

During the experiment, a subject sat in front of the bioradar at a distance of 0.5–1.0 m from the antennas. The distance to the subject varied depending on the individual anthropomorphic features of the subject and the way he/she sat in the chair during the experiment. Each transceiver was oriented to the surface of the examinee's chest, and the distance between centers of the transceiver antennas was 0.3 m. The scheme of the experiment is given in Figure 3.

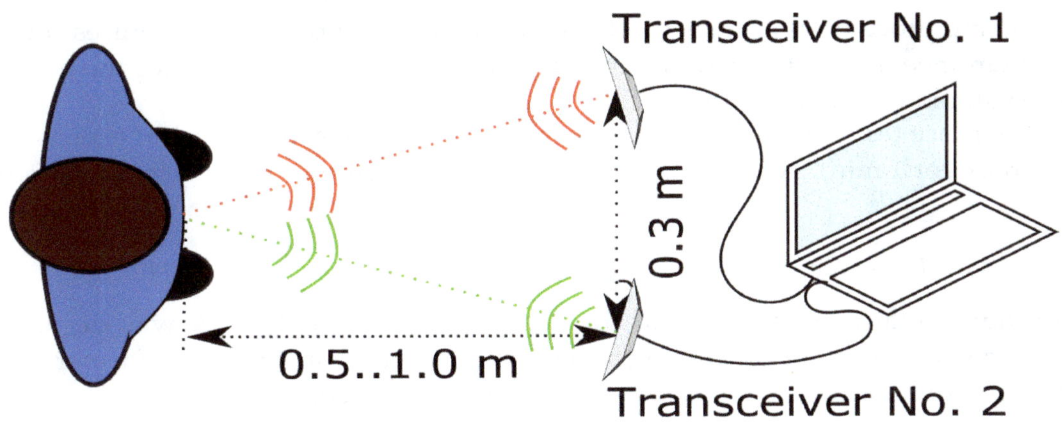

Figure 3. Scheme of the experiment.

Experiments were carried out at BMSTU from March to April 2018. For the experiments involving human participants, an ethical approval was obtained on 1 March 2018 from the ethics committee of BMSTU. The test population of 35 young healthy adults consisted of 14 males and 21 females in the age group of 19–22 years. All subjects gave their oral as well as written informed consent prior to the start of the experiments. In addition, each volunteer provided information about his/her individual fitness state, which may affect an organism individual reaction to stress. Four examinees turned out to be athletes.

In the previous work [35], we found that estimates of vital signs made by bioradars are less accurate for overweight people than for people with a normal weight. This is reasonable because the movements of the subjects' thorax caused by respiration and heartbeat are damped by a subcutaneous fat layer. That is why, in the present work, height and weight measurements were taken for each subject prior to the experiment to calculate their Body Mass Index (BMI). Information about the studied subjects is given in Table 1.

Table 1. Information about the studied subjects.

Dataset Characteristics	Values
Male : Female	14 : 21
Age (Years)	20.1 $\pm$ 0.6 (19–22)
Body Mass Index (kg/m^2)	22.0 $\pm$ 3.6 (17.4–30.4)
Respiration rate (breath per minute)	16.9 $\pm$ 5.0 (7–36)

For each volunteer, experiments of three of the following types were carried out.

- Calm breathing test: During this test, an examinee was asked to sit relaxed and breathe normally. If the subject was in a state of psycho-emotional agitation, then vital signs estimation should be performed only after the respiratory and heart rates dropped stationary levels, which corresponded to the calm state of the examinee. It took, in general, between 1 and 2 min for vital signs to stabilize after the beginning of the experiment as shown in [27]. That is why, to prevent the influence of the psycho-emotional agitation of some examinees at the start of the experiment, 2 min were added to the experiment duration. In total, calm breathing test lasted for 5 min; however, only the last 3 min of data were used in further analysis.
- Mental workload test: The volunteer was asked to perform a mental arithmetic task, which was more complex that the one from our previous papers dealing with mental stress monitoring [27,28]. The usage of a more complex arithmetic task was needed to present a challenge that resulted in a physiological response (increasing of cerebral oxygen consumption) in the examinees. The duration of this experimental stage was 3 min for each subject. We did not use standard

stress-inducing procedures such as the Trier social stress test because it requires communication with the examinee during the experiments, which may significantly reduce the quality of useful signals registered by the bioradar.

- Exercise tolerance test: Each volunteer was asked to perform some physical exercises (30 bobs or plank exercise for 1 min). After that, the examinee's vital signs were registered by a bioradar for 3 min.

2.3. *Signal Processing Technique*

The bioradar signal processing algorithm used in the present work was designed utilizing Matlab2018a. It consisted of pre-processing and classification algorithms. The former is required for accurate extraction of the features that are used by the latter for detection of stress.

2.3.1. Pre-Processing Algorithm

The scheme summarizing the steps of the signal pre-processing algorithm is depicted in Figure 4.

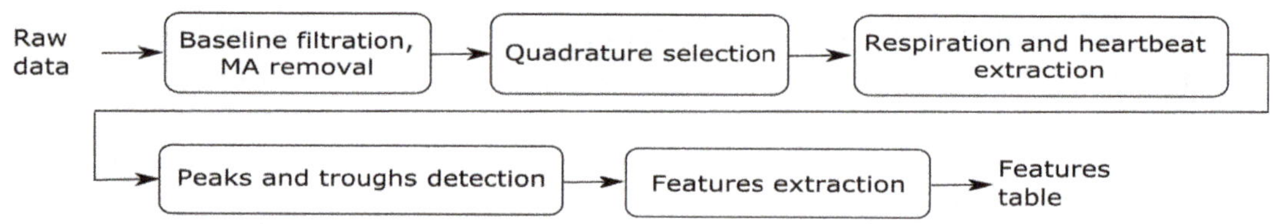

Figure 4. Scheme of the pre-processing algorithm.

The first stage consists of the baseline trend and movement algorithm suppression. These tasks are performed utilizing a highpass Butterworth filter with a cut-off frequency of 0.05 Hz for baseline trend filtering, and the algorithm proposed in [36] for movement artifact (MA) removal. In Figure 5, raw quadratures delivered by a single transceiver with the detected movement artifact are shown. After that, the examinee vital signs were registered by a bioradar for 3 min. The artifact periods were excluded from further analysis of the signal.

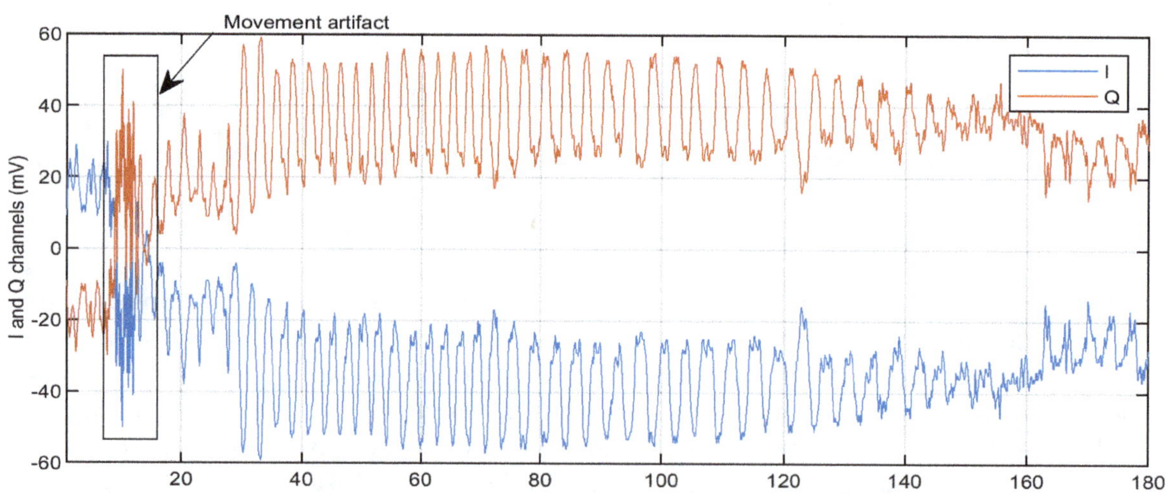

Figure 5. Raw bioradar quadratures.

The second stage deals with the selection quadrature for further analysis over the I and Q channels for two transceivers. As is known, in realistic conditions, phase demodulation of two quadratures received by the radar does not always provide good results due to the clutter caused by reflections from surrounding objects and the walls of the room where the examination takes place. Thus, in the present work, we did not use phase demodulation. Instead, we picked one quadrature with a higher peak-to-peak variation for each transceiver. Selected quadratures were used for further analysis.

After that, respiration and heartbeat patterns were extracted from chosen quadratures by sixth-order bandpass Butterworth filters with bandwidth [0.05; 0.7] Hz and [0.7; 2.0] Hz, respectively.

After filtration, peaks and troughs were detected in extracted respiration and heartbeat patterns by a search of local maximums and minimums using the function findpeak from Signal Processing Toolbox in Matlab. Peaks were detected as turning points in the signal with the minimum distance of 0.5 s and 1.5 s for heartbeat and respiratory patterns, respectively. In Figure 6, the respiration signal filtered from the chosen quadrature is shown. Moreover, the ends of inhaling and exhaling phases, corresponding to the local minimums and maximums of the filtered signal, are depicted.

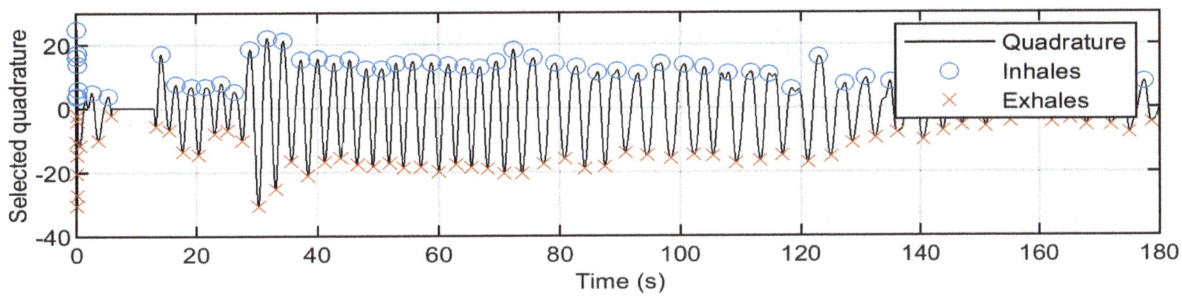

Figure 6. Respiration pattern with detected peaks and troughs.

Time and frequency domain features of respiration and heartbeat patterns filtered from the bioradar signal were extracted for further classification.

Time Features: The number of positive peaks was computed in a time window of 30 s and 10 s to estimate respiration and heartbeat rates, respectively. For these variables, the average, median, Inter Quartile Range (IQR), median-IQR rate, variance and skewness were computed. In addition, we estimated the same parameters for respiration circles (intervals between peaks), exhaling (time between peaks and troughs) and inhaling (time between troughs and peaks) periods. For more details, see Figure 7.

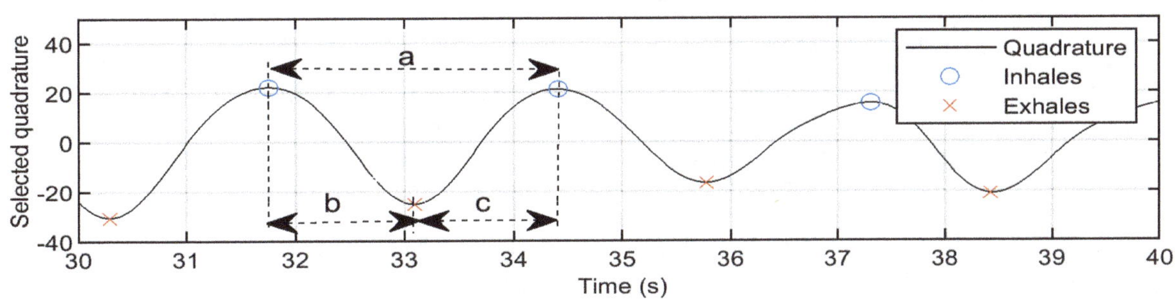

Figure 7. Time features for respiration pattern: respiration circle (a), exhaling (b) and inhaling (c) intervals.

Frequency Features: The average respiration and heartbeat frequencies were detected by frequency spectrum analysis. A standard Matlab function providing Discrete Fourier Transform was used for this purpose. Estimation of respiratory and heartbeat frequencies was done in a time window of 30 s and 10 s, respectively, by detecting a global maximum in a frequency spectrum in corresponding filtered signals. Such widths of time windows allow considering the analyzed fragments as being quasi-stationary.

2.3.2. Classification Algorithm

To discriminate between the calm breathing test and workload of different types (mental and physical), we used a support vector machine (SVM) classifier with a linear kernel realized in MATLAB. We chose this classifier because it showed the best performance using the cross-validation k-folds technique with $k = 5$, which was applied to prevent overfitting.

3. Results

The classifier was trained to distinguish between the calm state of the examinee and his/her state under mental or physical stress. Firstly, training was carried out using features extracted from data recorded by transceivers No. 1 and 2 (F_{tr1} , F_{tr2}, respectively) independently. After that, the same was done using a superposition of features for both transceivers ($F_{tr1\&2}$). To estimate the performance of the proposed classifier, the confusion matrix and accuracy were calculated. The results listed below show how usage of additional transceivers may help to improve the accuracy of examinees psychophysiological state classification.

3.1. Classification Calm State/Mental Workload

Table 2 presents the results of classification of steady state/mental stress for using data for a transceiver No. 1. In Table 3, the accuracies of classifiers trained on F_{tr1}, F_{tr2}, and $F_{tr1\&2}$ are listed. It can be seen that the accuracy of the classifier using features for both transceivers $F_{tr1\&2}$ is slightly higher than for classifiers using features for a single transceiver.

Table 2. Classification results for transceiver No. 1.

		Predicted Class	
		Steady State	**Mental Stress**
True Class	**Steady state**	26	9
	Mental stress	9	26
	Accuracy, %		
	Sensitivity, %	74.3	
	Specificity, %		

Table 3. Steady state/mental stress classification results.

	F_{tr1}	F_{tr2}	$F_{tr1\&2}$
Accuracy, %	74.3	64.7	77.5

The classifiers' relatively low accuracies (less than 80%) were caused by nine "outliers"; persons whose reactions to the mental stress was completely different from the other 26 subjects. Their cardiorespiratory system reacted by increasing frequencies of respiration and heartbeat.

Four outliers were experienced swimmers, which is why their cardiorespiratory system responded to the mental workload by increasing amplitudes of respiratory and heart muscles contractions, while the frequencies of these processes remained mostly unchanged, which is typical for trained persons.

Five other outliers had tachypnea. Their respiration rate during the calm breathing test was higher than 0.5 Hz, which is known to be too high for normal calm breathing. These examinees' respiration and heartbeat systems react to the mental workload by decreasing the analyzed vital signs frequencies. Moreover, eight out of nine outliers had BMI > 25, which may cause less accurate detection of respiration and heartbeat patterns, and thus influence the classifier accuracy.

The re-trained classifier for experimental dataset without nine outliers showed much better performance (Table 4) than the previous one (88.5% for dataset without nine outliers vs. 77.5% for the whole dataset). Moreover, it should be noted that using classification data for both transceivers resulted in higher accuracy than the same estimation using singe transceiver data (88.5% vs. 84.6%).

Table 4. Steady state/mental stress classification results (dataset without nine outliers).

	$\mathbf{F}_{tr1}$	$\mathbf{F}_{tr2}$	$\mathbf{F}_{tr1\&2}$
Accuracy, %	84.6	78.8	88.5

3.2. Classification Calm State/Physical Workload

Table 5 presents the results of classification of steady state/physical stress using F_{tr1}, F_{tr2}, and $F_{tr1\&2}$. It can be seen that the accuracy of classifiers using features for both transceivers $F_{tr1\&2}$ is higher than for classifiers using features for a single transceiver (F_{tr1} and F_{tr2}).

Table 5. Steady state/physical stress classification results.

	$\mathbf{F}_{tr1}$	$\mathbf{F}_{tr2}$	$\mathbf{F}_{tr1\&2}$
Accuracy (dataset for all 35 examinees), %	69.1	73.5	77.9
Accuracy (dataset without 9 outliers), %	75.0	80.8	82.7

4. Discussion

Psychophysiological state monitoring provides a promising way for detecting stress and accurate assessment of wellbeing. The major advantage of the proposed technique, compared to other stress detection methods, is its unobtrusive nature that does not require any direct contact between the device and the person. The technique was tested in laboratory conditions with the participation of 35 young, healthy volunteers who were asked to perform arithmetic and physical workload tests that imitated different types of stressors. The information about variations of vital signs registered by a bioradar with two transceivers was used to detect mental or physical workload. The usage of two transceivers provides the benefit of observing a subject from different angles, which results in increasing classification accuracy as compared to using a bioradar with a single transceiver. A drawback of the proposed approach might be given by the increasing complexity of the device architecture.

The analysis of the experimental results showed that the physiological responses to mental and physical workload differ for trained and untrained persons as well as for persons with tachypnea. This individual specificity of physiological responses to mental and physical workload makes the creation of a universal stress detector suitable for people with different level of stress tolerance a challenging task. One of the possible solutions of this issue may be training different classifiers for athletes and non-athletes without tachypnea. In the present paper, using such an approach allows increasing accuracy for classification of the calm state/mental workload from 78% to 89% as well as increasing AUC values (Figure 8).

The achieved results should be accepted with caution because the experimental data used for the classifier training are only for young, practically healthy examinees. The relatively low number of volunteers who were declared to be athletes or having tachypnea does not allow the training of the classifier for these groups; however, in the future, we are planning to enrich the experimental dataset and add heuristics to make the classifier consider individual information of the person (BMI, chronic tachypnea, etc.), which should increase the accuracy of psychophysiological monitoring.

The work might contribute to the development of a noncontact system for evaluating individual reactions of a user to mental stress factors in everyday life.

In future work, it is planned to extend the research to the evaluation of different stress levels using standard stress-inducing procedures. This activity will be carried out in cooperation with psychologists and medical researchers from Lomonosov Moscow State University (Moscow, Russia).

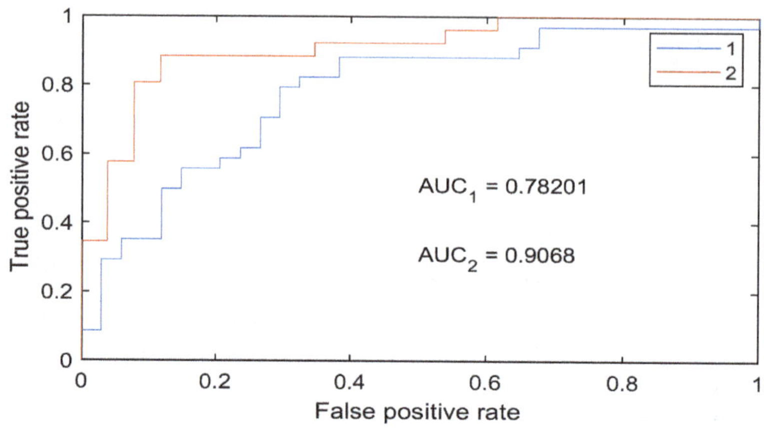

Figure 8. ROC curve of the calm state/mental workload classifier for the whole dataset (1), and for non-athletes dataset (2).

Acknowledgments: The author would like to thank A. Turetskaya and K. Kaleyeva for their help with conducting the experiments.

Abbreviations

The following abbreviations are used in this manuscript:

ADC	Analog-to-Digital Converter
AUC	Area Under the Curve
BMI	Body Mass Index
BMSTU	Bauman Moscow State Technical University
HRV	Heart Rate Variability
I2C	Inter-Integrated Circuit
MA	Movement Artifact
MC	Micro-Controller
PC	Personal Computer
ROC	Receiver Operating Characteristic
SVM	Support Vector Machine
VCO	Voltage-Controlled Oscillator

References

1. Selye, H. The Evolution of the stress concept. The originator of the concept traces its development from the discovery in 1936 of the alarm reaction to modern therapeutic applications of syntoxic and catatoxic hormones. *Am. Sci.* **1973**, *61*, 692–699. [PubMed]
2. Selye, H. Stress and Distress. *Compr. Ther.* **1975**, *1*, 9–13. [PubMed]
3. Steptoe, A.; Kivimäki, M. Stress and cardiovascular disease. *Nat. Rev. Cardiol.* **2012**, *9*, 360–370. [CrossRef] [PubMed]
4. Colquhoun, D.M.; Bunker, S.J.; Clarke, D.M.; Hare, D.L.; Hickie, I.B.; Tatoulis, J.; Thompson, D.R.; Wilson, A.; Branagan, M.G. Psychosocial risk factors for coronary heart disease. *Med. J. Aust.* **2013**, *199*, 179–180.
5. Scott, K.A, Melhorn, S.J.; Sakai, R.R. Effects of Chronic Social Stress on Obesity. *Curr. Obes. Rep.* **2012**, *1*, 16–25. [CrossRef] [PubMed]

6. Kelly, S.J.; Ismail, M. Stress and type 2 diabetes: A review of how stress contributes to the development of type 2 diabetes. *Annu. Rev. Public Health* **2015**, *18*, 441–462. [CrossRef] [PubMed]
7. Han, K.S.; Kim, L.; Shim, I. Stress and Sleep Disorder. *Exp. Neurobiol.* **2012**, *21*, 141–150 [CrossRef] [PubMed]
8. Sanford, L.D.; Suchecki, D.; Meerlo, P. Stress, arousal, and sleep. *Curr. Top Behav. Neurosci.* **2015**, *25*, 379–410. [PubMed]
9. Van Winkel, R.; Stefanis, N.C.; Myin-Germeys, I. Psychosocial Stress and Psychosis. A Review of the Neurobiological Mechanisms and the Evidence for Gene-Stress Interaction. *Schizophr. Bull.* **2008**, *34*, 1095–1105. [CrossRef] [PubMed]
10. McKlveen, J.M.; Morano, R.L.; Fitzgerald, M.; Zoubovsky, S.; Cassella, S.N.; Scheimann, J.R.; Ghosal, S.; Mahbod, P.; Packard, B.A.; Myers, B.; et al. Chronic Stress Increases Prefrontal Inhibition: A Mechanism for Stress-Induced Prefrontal Dysfunction. *Biol. Psychiatry* **2016**, *80*, 754–764. [CrossRef] [PubMed]
11. Slavich, G.M.; Irwin, M.R. From stress to inflammation and major depressive disorder: A social signal transduction theory of depression. *Psychol. Bull.* **2014**, *140*, 774–815. [CrossRef] [PubMed]
12. Dickerson, S.S.; Kemeny, M.E. Acute Stressors and Cortisol Responses: A Theoretical Integration and Synthesis of Laboratory Research. *Psychol. Bull.* **2004**, *130*, 355–391. [CrossRef] [PubMed]
13. Van Eck, M.; Berkhof, H.; Nicolson, N.; Sulon, J. The Effects of Perceived Stress, Traits, Mood States, and Stressful Daily Events on Salivary Cortisol. *Psychosom. Med.* **1996**, *58*, 447–458. [CrossRef] [PubMed]
14. Kramer, A.F. Physiological Metrics of Mental Workload: A Review of Recent Progress. In *Multiple-Task performance*; Damos, D.L., Ed.; Taylor and Francis: London, UK, 1991; pp. 279–328, ISBN 0-85066-757-7.
15. Setz, C.; Arnrich, B.; Schumm, J.; La Marca, R.; Tröster, G.; Ehlert, U. Discriminating Stress from Cognitive Load using a Wearable EDA Device. *IEEE Trans. Inf. Technol. Biomed.* **2010**, *14*, 410–417. [CrossRef] [PubMed]
16. Hernandez, J.; Morris, R.R.; Picard, R.W. Call Center Stress Recognition with Person-Specific Models. In Proceedings of the 2011 International Conference on Affective Computing and Intelligent Interaction, Memphis, TN, USA, 9–12 October 2011; pp. 125–134.
17. Vrijkotte, T.G.; Van Doornen, L.J.; De Geus, E.J. Effects of Work Stress on Ambulatory Blood Pressure, Heart Rate, and Heart Rate Variability. *Hypertension* **2000**, *35*, 880–886. [CrossRef] [PubMed]
18. Dishman, R.K.; Nakamura, Y.; Garcia, M.E.; Thompson, R.W.; Dunn, A.L.; Blair, S.N. Heart Rate Variability, Trait Anxiety, and Perceived Stress among Physically Fit Men and Women. *Int. J. Psychophysiol.* **2000**, *137*, 121–133. [CrossRef]
19. Fairclough, S.H. Fundamentals of physiological computing. *Interact. Comput.* **2009**, *21*, 133–145. [CrossRef]
20. Mokhayeri, F.; Akbarzadeh-T, M.R.; Toosizadeh, S. Mental Stress Detection using Physiological Signals based on Soft Computing Techniques. In Proceedings of the 18th IEEE Iranian Conference of Biomedical Engineering (ICBME), Tehran, Iran, 18–20 December 2013; pp. 232–237.
21. Deschênes, A.; Forget, H.; Daudelin-Peltier, C.; Fiset, D.; Blais, C. Facial Expression Recognition Impairment following Acute Social Stress. *J. Vis.* **2015**, *15*, 1383. [CrossRef]
22. Peake, J.M.; Kerr, G.; Sullivan, J.P. A Critical Review of Consumer Wearables, Mobile Applications, and Equipment for Providing Biofeedback, Monitoring Stress, and Sleep in Physically Active Populations. *Front. Physiol.* **2018**, *9*, in press. [CrossRef] [PubMed]
23. Anishchenko, L.; Alekhin, M.; Tataraidze, A.; Ivashov, S.; Bugaev, A.S.; Soldovieri, F. Application of step-frequency radars in medicine. In Proceedings of the SPIE 9077 Radar Sensor Technology XVIII, Baltimore, MD, USA, 29 May 2014.
24. Lin, J.C. Non-invasive microwave measurement of respiration. *Proc. IEEE* **1975**, *63*, 557–565. [CrossRef]
25. Lin, J.C. Microwave apexcardiography. *IEEE Trans. Microw. Theory Tech.* **1979**, *27*, 618–620. [CrossRef]
26. Kranjec, J.; Beguš, S.; Geršak, G.; Drnovšek, J. Non-contact Heart Rate and Heart Rate Variability Measurements: A Review. *Biomed. Signal Process. Control* **2014**, *13*, 102–112. [CrossRef]
27. Anishchenko, L.; Bugaev, A.; Ivashov, S.; Zhuravlev, A. Bioradar for Monitoring of Human Adaptive Capabilities. In Proceedings of the General Assembly and Scientific Symposium of International Union of Radio Science (XXXth URSI), Istanbul, Turkey, 13–20 August 2011; pp. 1–4.
28. Fernandez, J.R.M.; Anishchenko, L. Mental stress detection using bioradar respiratory signals. *Biomed. Signal Process. Control* **2018**, *43*, 244–249. [CrossRef]
29. Droitcour, A.D.; Boric-Lubecke, O.; Lubecke, V.M.; Lin, J.; Kovacs, G.T. Range correlation and I/Q performance benefits in single-chip silicon Doppler radars for noncontact cardiopulmonary monitoring. *IEEE Trans. Microw. Theory Tech.* **2004**, *52*, 838–848. [CrossRef]

30. Lazaro, A.; Girbau, D.; Villarino, R. Analysis of vital signs monitoring using an IR-UWBradar. *Prog. Electromagn. Res.* **2010**, *100*, 265–284. [CrossRef]
31. Pittella, E.; Bottiglieri, A.; Pisa, S.; Cavagnaro, M. Cardio-respiratory frequency monitoring using the principal component analysis technique on UWB radar signal. *Int. J. Antennas Propag.* **2017**, *2017*, 4803752. [CrossRef]
32. Anishchenko, L.N.; Demendeev, A.A.; Ivashov, S.I. Use of Radiolocation for Non-contact Estimation of Patterns of Respiration and Motion Activity in Sleeping Humans. *Biom. Eng.* **2013**, *47*, 7–11. [CrossRef]
33. K-LC5 High Sensitivity Dual Channel Transceiver. Available online: https://www.rfbeam.ch/product?id=9 (accessed on 6 September 2018).
34. Anishchenko, L.; Razevig, V.; Chizh, M. Blind separation of several biological objects respiration patterns by means of a step-frequency continuous-wave bioradar. In Proceedings of the 2017 IEEE International Conference on Microwaves, Antennas, Communications and Electronic Systems (COMCAS), Tel-Aviv, Israel, 13–15 November 2017; pp. 1–4.
35. Anishchenko, L.N.; Razevig, V.V. Two-channel Bioradar for Stress Monitoring. In Proceedings of the 2018 Progress In Electromagnetics Research Symposium (PIERS), Toyama, Japan, 1–4 August 2018; pp. 1–4, in press.
36. Anishchenko, L.; Gennarelli, G.; Tataraidze, A.; Gaisina, E.; Soldovieri, F.; Ivashov, S. Evaluation of rodents' respiratory activity using a bioradar. *IET Radar Sonar Navig.* **2015**, *9*, 1296–1302. [CrossRef]

5

Diagnosing Breast Cancer with Microwave Technology: Remaining Challenges and Potential Solutions with Machine Learning

Bárbara L. Oliveira [1,*], Daniela Godinho [2], Martin O'Halloran [3], Martin Glavin [1], Edward Jones [1] and Raquel C. Conceição [2]

1 Electrical and Electronic Engineering, National University of Ireland Galway, H91 TK33 Galway, Ireland; martin.glavin@nuigalway.ie (M.G.); edward.jones@nuigalway.ie (E.J.)

2 Instituto de Biofísica e Engenharia Biomédica, Faculdade de Ciências da Universidade de Lisboa, Campo Grande, 1749-016 Lisboa, Portugal; dgodinho94@gmail.com (D.G.); raquelcruzconceicao@gmail.com (R.C.C.)

3 Translational Medical Device Lab, National University of Ireland Galway, H91 TK33 Galway, Ireland; martin.ohalloran@nuigalway.ie

* Correspondence: b.oliveira1@nuigalway.ie

Abstract: Currently, breast cancer often requires invasive biopsies for diagnosis, motivating researchers to design and develop non-invasive and automated diagnosis systems. Recent microwave breast imaging studies have shown how backscattered signals carry relevant information about the shape of a tumour, and tumour shape is often used with current imaging modalities to assess malignancy. This paper presents a comprehensive analysis of microwave breast diagnosis systems which use machine learning to learn characteristics of benign and malignant tumours. The state-of-the-art, the main challenges still to overcome and potential solutions are outlined. Specifically, this work investigates the benefit of signal pre-processing on diagnostic performance, and proposes a new set of extracted features that capture the tumour shape information embedded in a signal. This work also investigates if a relationship exists between the antenna topology in a microwave system and diagnostic performance. Finally, a careful machine learning validation methodology is implemented to guarantee the robustness of the results and the accuracy of performance evaluation.

Keywords: machine learning; automated breast diagnosis; microwave imaging

---

1. Introduction

1.1. Motivation

Microwave Breast Imaging (MBI) for breast cancer detection has seen significant academic and commercial development in recent years. At least 4 studies have reported findings from clinical trials [1–7], indicating that MBI has the potential to match state-of-the-art breast imaging methods, such as mammography. To date, the main goal of microwave imaging and signal processing algorithms has been the detection of tumours, i.e., to identify the presence of tumours within the breast, as shown by the literature in the area [8–12].

The development of automated breast diagnosis systems is relevant to the clinical environment, particularly considering recent reports showing minimal benefit of continuous mammographic screening in terms of long-term survival rates [13,14]. Many automated breast diagnosis systems have been proposed, and usually integrate signal or image pre-processing and segmentation, and diagnosis through machine learning [15,16]. Such systems have proved useful in aiding clinicians diagnose breast cancer, as they can identify features in a signal or image that may otherwise be missed through visual inspection. Automated diagnosis systems for microwave breast systems could play a key role in further establishing MBI as an early-stage breast cancer screening and monitoring method.

In the context of microwave breast diagnosis, a number of possibilities theoretically allow diagnosing breast tumours as benign or malignant. For example, the presence of microcalcifications in areas of the breast representing malignancy [17–20] and the difference in the dielectric properties between benign and malignant breast tumours [2,21]; however, further investigations characterising microcalcifications, and benign and malignant tissues in the microwave range are needed before microwave diagnosis systems based solely on these properties are viable. Finally, the shape and spiculation of tumours are widely recognised markers for their malignancy [22–25].

Benign tumours are roughly elliptical and usually have well circumscribed margins, and malignant tumours have irregular shapes and are surrounded by a radiating pattern of spikes, commonly referred to as spicules [22–26]. Previous studies have already shown how microwave backscattered signals may change if tumours of different sizes or shapes are present within the breast [27–38]. These studies have also demonstrated that classification and machine learning algorithms are able to learn from the shape differences in backscattered signals, albeit in relatively simple datasets. It is yet to be determined whether the performance of classification algorithms is adequate in clinically-complex scenarios.

This paper presents a comprehensive analysis into the fundamentals of microwave breast cancer diagnosis—as opposed to detection—systems. The main challenges are addressed, such as those arising from complex backscattered signals and appropriate machine learning methodology, and potential solutions are identified to overcome them. This work investigates, for the first time, whether a relationship exists between the predictive power of backscattered signals and the distribution of antennas in a microwave scan.

In the remainder of Section 1, the findings from previous studies using machine learning with microwave technology are reviewed in Section 1.2, and the main challenges still to be addressed in diagnosing breast tumours with microwaves are discussed in Section 1.3. The methodology is discussed in Section 2, which proposes a three-stage diagnosis system for addressing some of the primary challenges. The results are listed in Section 3 and Section 4 discusses and concludes the study.

1.2. Machine Learning and Microwave Technology: State-of-the-Art

With microwave breast prototype systems, a patient may sit or lie down while the breast is illuminated with low energy microwaves, and the resultant backscattered signals are recorded. In principle, it is possible to diagnose the type of tumour (benign or malignant) by examining the backscattered signals and recovering the tumour signature therein contained; in fact, previous studies indicate that backscattered signals may change if tumours of different sizes or shapes are present within the breast. In this section, a review is presented of the most significant studies to date to propose the use of machine learning to diagnose breast tumours based on their signatures.

In [29–32], several feature extraction methods (principal component analysis, discrete wavelet transforms, and independent component analysis) were used in combination with different classifiers (linear discriminant analysis, quadratic discriminant analysis, and supoprt vector machines) to diagnose breast tumours with backscattered signals. The analysis was based on numerical breast models composed mostly of adipose tissue; tumours were modelled with several sizes and shapes, and were located in the centre of the breast. These studies showed promise in using backscattered signals to diagnose tumours, and suggested that classifying tumour size ahead of tumour shape may improve diagnostic performance.

The suitability of neural networks to classify backscattered signals was also assessed. A combination of genetic algorithms and neural networks with discrete wavelet transforms was proposed in [33,34], and tested on a similar numerical dataset to the study above. As before, diagnostic performance was improved by separating tumours based on their size ahead of classification, and by investigating which transmit-receive antenna pairs provide the most useful information.

The same numerical dataset was also used in [35] to investigate the potential of self organising maps to track the development of a tumour from a benign state to different levels of malignancy. This study showed promise in distinguishing between different shapes of tumours.

In 2015, the authors of the present paper investigated the effect of signal pre-processing on diagnostic performance, by windowing the backscattered signal to contain only the tumour signature [38]. Clinically-realistic breast models were derived from the University of Wisconsin Computational Electromagnetics (UWCEM) repository [39], and tumour models of several sizes and shapes were located in various positions within the breast. The classification framework relied on principal component analysis in combination with support vector machines. The authors noted that the windowing methodology helped improve diagnostic performance when examining more complex and heterogeneous breast models.

Experimental datasets have also been used to assess the performance of diagnosis systems, namely by using principal component analysis in combination with support vector machines, linear discriminant analysis and quadratic discriminant analysis. In [36,37], tumour phantoms with various sizes and shapes were immersed in a breast phantom with dielectric properties matching those of adipose tissue. Importantly, the experimental results presented in these studies are in general agreement with previous numerical data.

The breast tumour diagnosis studies summarised in this section indicate that the shape of a breast tumour influences its signature within a backscattered signal, potentially allowing machine learning models to learn how to distinguish between benign and malignant tumours. These studies have also looked at the effect of intelligently using the most informative transmit-receive antenna pairs. In addition, these studies have concluded that it is beneficial to separate tumours according to size before final diagnosis, and also, that further signal pre-processing methodologies should be explored when dealing with more complex breast models, for example, breast models with increased content of glandular tissue.

Additionally, other authors have implemented comparable machine-learning approaches for detection, i.e., to determine whether a tumour is present in the breast [40–49]. While an in-depth review of the detection studies based on machine learning performed to date is beyond the scope of this work, their main findings are summarised here for completeness. Detection studies indicate that there is sufficient information in the backscattered signals to inform about the presence of a tumour. These studies show that detection performance can be improved by using differential signals which highlight the tumour signature and by extracting time-frequency features of the signals ahead of classification. Similarly to the diagnosis studies discussed above, selecting the transmit-receive antenna pairs with the most meaningful classification information also seems to positively impact detection performance.

1.3. Challenges with Microwave Breast Diagnosis Systems

In the previous section, a review was presented of the main microwave studies that use machine learning to diagnose breast tumours as benign or malignant. In this section, the remaining challenges in the development of microwave breast diagnosis systems are discussed, as well as potential solutions, from two perspectives: addressing the complexity of backscattered signals gathered in clinically-realistic conditions; and developing a validation methodology for the classification models.

1.3.1. Complexity of Clinically-Realistic Data

Benign and malignant tumours may present a wide range of sizes, shapes and spiculations at their margin, which can change the backscattered energy received at a given antenna. In addition, the shape of the human breast changes from person to person, and so does the distribution of adipose and glandular tissues inside the breast, which effectively alters the attenuation along each propagation path. This diversity leads to equally diverse backscattered signals, making the design of a single platform for diagnosis a complex task. Some of the challenges related to breast and tumour composition can be summarised as follows:

(i) Difficulty in capturing the tumour signature from the backscattered signal due to: (1) presence of skin, the response of which can be orders of magnitude larger than the tumour signature; (2) presence of glandular tissue clusters, which can be confused with tumour tissue, due to similarities in composition (water content and generally higher dielectric properties); (3) tumours can occur in different locations within the breast, embedded in various breast structures.

(ii) Differences in the tumour signature for a given transmit-receive antenna pair due to: (1) tumours of different shapes, meaning antennas in different locations have a different view of the tumour; (2) various angles between transmit and receive antennas, which can affect the phase of the tumour signature; (3) varying distances between the antennas and the edge of the tumour.

Particularly regarding Section 1.3.1, a number of strategies have already been proposed in previous studies. Artefact removal algorithms have been proposed, which deal with large skin reflections and decrease the glandular tissue influence on the backscattered signals, for example [50,51]. As mentioned in Section 1.2, previous studies have also suggested that: pre-processing signals by means of windowing could highlight and time-align the tumour signature [38]; extracting features based on time-frequency representations of the data could further capture the essence of the tumour signature while disregarding the background noise [48,49]; and classifying a dataset according to tumour size before attempting at classification based on the level of malignancy [29–31,33].

Concerning Section 1.3.1, while some studies have observed an improvement in diagnostic performance by restricting the classification to the backscattered signals captured with the most informative transmit-receive antenna pairs [33,41,43,45–47], no thorough investigation of optimal antenna topology and optimal use of the information from each channel was found in the literature.

A further set of challenges exists in translating microwave breast diagnosis systems to experimental and clinical evaluation: patient positioning and movement; intra-patient variation due to menstrual cycle and hormonal changes; inter-patient variation in breast size, shape and composition.

1.3.2. Challenges in Building Robust Machine Learning Classification Models

Ideally, a machine learning algorithm trained with a particular dataset should be generalisable to new, unseen datasets. Common practice is that a model should first be trained on a subset of the data, and then tested on another unseen subset of the data. The training set should be as large as possible, to minimise the variance in training the model, but the unseen subset of the data should also be representative of the original dataset, so the performance evaluation is meaningful.

However, performance evaluation commonly observed in the literature is prone to variations in approach, and often some degree of error, leading to overly-optimistic performance reports. Poor model validation is often due to: (1) overfitting of the learning model during the training phase; (2) overfitting during model selection; and (3) contamination of the information across the dataset.

Cross-validation has long been regarded as a good method to prevent overfitting of the model during training, and it is widely used as the basis for model selection. However, it has also been shown that using the performance obtained from cross-validation during model selection as the overall performance of the model might be overly-optimistic, and not generalisable. This effect is often referred to as selection bias [52,53].

Careful construction of a machine learning-based system should also consider the type of pre-processing and feature-based algorithms applied to the original dataset. As noted in the previous section, the extraction of features from the original dataset could be key to diagnostic performance; however, pre-processing or feature-based methods could also play a part in the contamination of information between the training and test sets. Typically, to prevent contamination, any method involving computation of the relationship across multiple observations, should first be applied to the train set, and the training transformations should then be applied onto the test set.

Many of the issues listed above have not been explicitly addressed in previous studies proposing detection or diagnosis algorithms through machine learning for microwave breast systems. Implementing careful and consistent methodologies for model validation and performance evaluation should, however, become best practice. Ultimately, creating learning models without proper validation methodologies could compromise the usability of microwave breast diagnosis systems.

2. Materials and Methods

In this study, the authors have implemented an integrated methodology of detecting and diagnosing breast tumours using backscattered signals. The proposed methodology is 3-fold, comprising data acquisition, data processing and diagnosis. The overall diagnostic architecture is depicted in Figure 1.

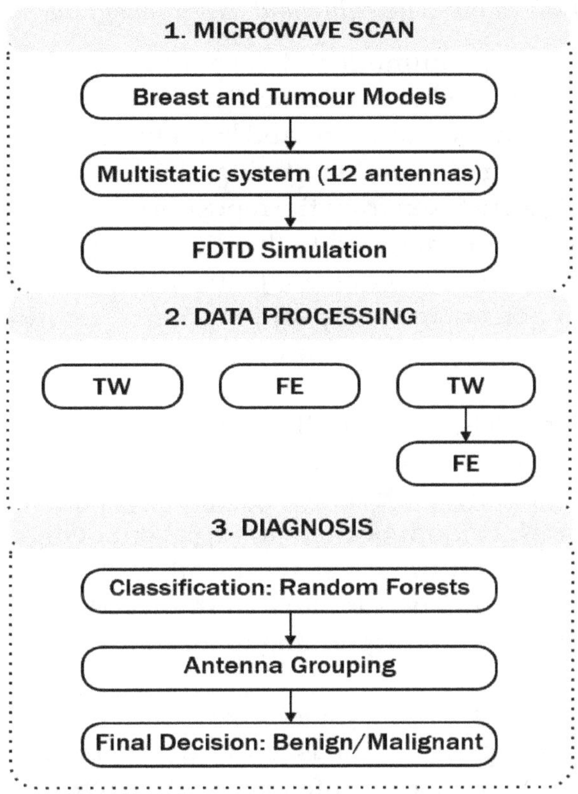

Figure 1. 3-stage diagnosis platform implemented in this study. Stage 1 consists of data collection in a microwave breast prototype. Stage 2 consists of data processing by means of tumour windowing (TW) and feature extraction (FE); the relative importance of each algorithm is compared by applying TW in combination with FE, or TW only, or FE only. Stage 3 is the diagnosis stage, which uses random forests as the classifier, includes an antenna grouping algorithm, and ends with a final diagnosis of benign or malignant.

Stage 1 consists of the microwave breast scan. To address some of the issues in dealing with clinically-realistic datasets (as highlighted in Section 1.3.1), a data processing stage was implemented next (Stage 2), comprising a tumour windowing approach to select signal segments of interest, combined with feature extraction. The relative benefits of both algorithms are analysed by comparing the diagnostic performance of applying one of the following: only tumour windowing; only feature extraction; tumour windowing in combination with feature extraction, i.e., feature extraction performed after the tumour signature is windowed from the original backscattered signal.

Stage 3 consists of the diagnosis and encompasses classification of the dataset through a range of techniques, including random forests, antenna grouping, and final decision as benign or malignant. The authors explore the concept introduced in previous studies that some channels (i.e., transmit-receive antenna pairs) might be more useful to improve diagnostic performance, by implementing three classification models, where each classification model makes different use of the information from each channel. The three classification model types will be described in greater detail in Section 2.3.2. With the algorithms implemented in Stage 3, this study aims to understand: (1) if the angular distance between the transmit and receive antennas in a channel determines its predictive power; (2) if the distance between the tumour and the channel has an impact on diagnostic performance; (3) finally, how to better use the information from each channel while adhering to best machine learning practices. In addition, a careful model validation methodology was implemented in Stage 3, to prevent issues like the ones detailed in Section 1.3.2. The three stages of the proposed microwave breast diagnosis platform will be described in greater detail in the following sub-sections.

2.1. Microwave Scan—Breast and Tumour Modelling and Electromagnetic Simulation

For the purposes of this study, a numerical dataset of breast and tumour models was created through electromagnetic simulation with the Finite-Difference Time-Domain (FDTD) formulation. This method is well-established in the literature and widely used in the field of microwave breast cancer imaging to model the propagation and scattering of microwave signals within the breast [54].

MRI-derived breast models were taken from the repository created by the UWCEM laboratory [39]. All breast models in the repository are mapped to the dielectric properties of normal and malignant breast tissues as established by Lazebnik et al. [55]. In total, 3 heterogeneous breast models were used in this study. In terms of percentage composition, the breast models used in this study range between 1% to 27% of glandular tissue by volume of breast, with the remainder percentage of tissue corresponding to adipose tissue.

For the creation of tumour models, the clinically-informed tumour modelling algorithm previously developed by the authors [56] was used to generate 72 unique tumour models, with average sizes ranging from 6 mm to 20 mm in diameter. Several degrees of spiculation were used to create tumours grouped into two distinct classes: smooth borders to represent benign tumours (with $0 \leq s \leq 0.25$), and spiculated borders for malignant tumours (with $0.50 \leq s \leq 0.90$), where s is the spiculation parameter from [56] with $0 \leq s \leq 1$. The tumours were placed in 5 different positions within the breast as described in medical reports, corresponding to locations in the four breast quadrants and the central portion.

The electromagnetic measurement system was modelled with a concentric ring of equally-distanced 12 Hertzian dipole antennas around the breast in a fully multistatic setup (which means the angle between two adjacent antennas is 30°. Each antenna element is modelled as an electric current source. The antennas were immersed in a medium with dielectric properties equivalent to those of adipose tissue. The FDTD simulations were performed using a differentiated Gaussian pulse with centre frequency of 6 GHz and a −3 dB) bandwidth (of 6 GHz). The spatial resolution of the system is 1 mm, and the sampling frequency is 600 GHz. Additionally, a reference simulation was also performed. This reference signal is later used to remove antenna effects in the backscattered signals from simulations of the full breast with tumours.

Figure 2 displays a schematic representation of the acquisition setup designed for FDTD simulation in this study, where the antennas are represented by the black diamonds surrounding the breast. A coronal slice of one of the breast models used in the study is shown, including fibroglandular tissue in the interior, and a malignant tumour in one of the lower quadrants (the spiculated shape in black). To aid the visualisation of the setup, the path from one transmitting antenna (Tx) to the tumour and from the tumour to the receiving antenna (Rx) is shown in dash and dot-dash lines, respectively.

With the proposed setup, one microwave breast scan is composed of backscattered signals collected from 78 independent channels. In total, 1080 microwave scans were performed (3 breast models each combined with 72 tumour models in 5 different positions within the breast). A dataset containing a total of 84,240 backscattered signals is used in this study.

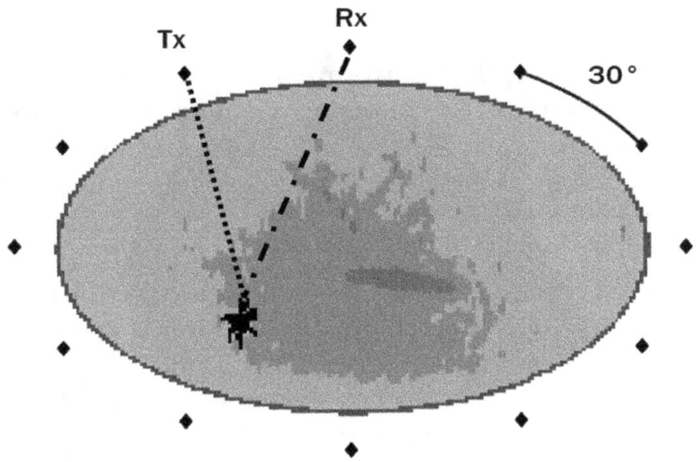

Figure 2. Representation of the acquisition setup designed for this study, where the antennas are represented by the black diamonds surrounding the breast. A coronal slice of one of the breast models is shown; the breast has fibroglandular tissue in the interior, and a malignant tumour in one of the lower breast quadrants (represented by the black spiculated shape). The path from one transmitting antenna (Tx) to the tumour and from the tumour to a receiving antenna (Rx) is shown in the dash and dot-dash lines, respectively; the 30° angle between two adjacent antennas is also shown.

2.2. Data Processing

This section describes the processing methods used to prepare the data ahead of classification. Two methods are used to process the backscattered signals, either by means of tumour windowing or feature extraction.

2.2.1. Tumour Windowing

In this paper, the authors expand on the tumour windowing concept initially proposed in [38]. Once the tumour location is identified, the round-trip propagation delay between the tumour and each channel is calculated, based on the average propagation speed through three media: immersion medium, skin and interior of the breast; the estimated tumour response is then windowed from the backscattered signal. In this paper, the ideal tumour location is used. The approximate window length was decided empirically. Visual assessment of a subgroup of backscattered signals gathered with different tumour models embedded in breast models with varying background contents found that a window length of 2.5 times the pulse width is appropriate to extract the full tumour response from the signals.

The propagation delay is highly dependent on the average dielectric properties of each medium; consequently, reflections yielding from different tumours propagating through different paths will be hard to align. To compensate for this effect, the windowing algorithm looks for the peak energy in each backscattered signal, and time-aligns the tumour responses on this basis. Each windowed tumour response is finally downsampled to a sampling frequency of 30 GHz. After downsampling, the window length of the tumour signatures consisted of 60 time samples.

By implementing the proposed tumour windowing algorithm: the reflection from the skin is eliminated; a high level of clutter resulting from the glandular clusters is potentially removed; signals collected from different channels are time-aligned. As a result, the tumour response is isolated, potentially simplifying the task given to the classification algorithm. To compensate for antenna effects in the signals, an artefact removal step can be performed prior to windowing.

When only tumour windowing is applied during Stage 2 of the 3-stage diagnosis platform (Figure 1, TW), the windowed time-domain signatures are treated as independent observations, which are then passed as input to the classification model.

2.2.2. Feature Extraction

Feature extraction is frequently applied to capture meaningful information embedded in a signal, and is helpful in reducing the dimensionality of the problem when compared to the original data.

Visual analysis of backscattered signals reveals that benign tumours result in signals that tend to preserve the original morphology of the gaussian peak, while malignant tumours result in more irregular signals, due to increased reflections from tumour spicules. Therefore, this paper examines the use of a set of features that capture signal morphology and frequency content for diagnosis. The proposed feature extraction method relies on peak analysis of different time and frequency representations of the original data, where each group of features is calculated for the signal collected by each channel of each scan. As the extraction of features is done independently on each observation, no calculations are made across the dataset and between tumour signatures, which prevents accidental data contamination issues, as those described in Section 1.3.2.

By way of example, Figure 3 displays some of the differences identified by visual analysis of benign (Figure 3a) and malignant signatures (Figure 3b). The signals were collected under ideal conditions to highlight the potential differences between types of tumours, with an adipose-only breast model; for both tumour types, two tumour models were simulated of different sizes and shapes. The resultant signals have been time-aligned and windowed. As observed in Figure 3a, the backscattered signals from the benign tumour models exhibit little distortion and the original Gaussian shape is preserved well; conversely, in Figure 3b, the malignant tumour models result in backscattered signals with a higher level of waveform distortion.

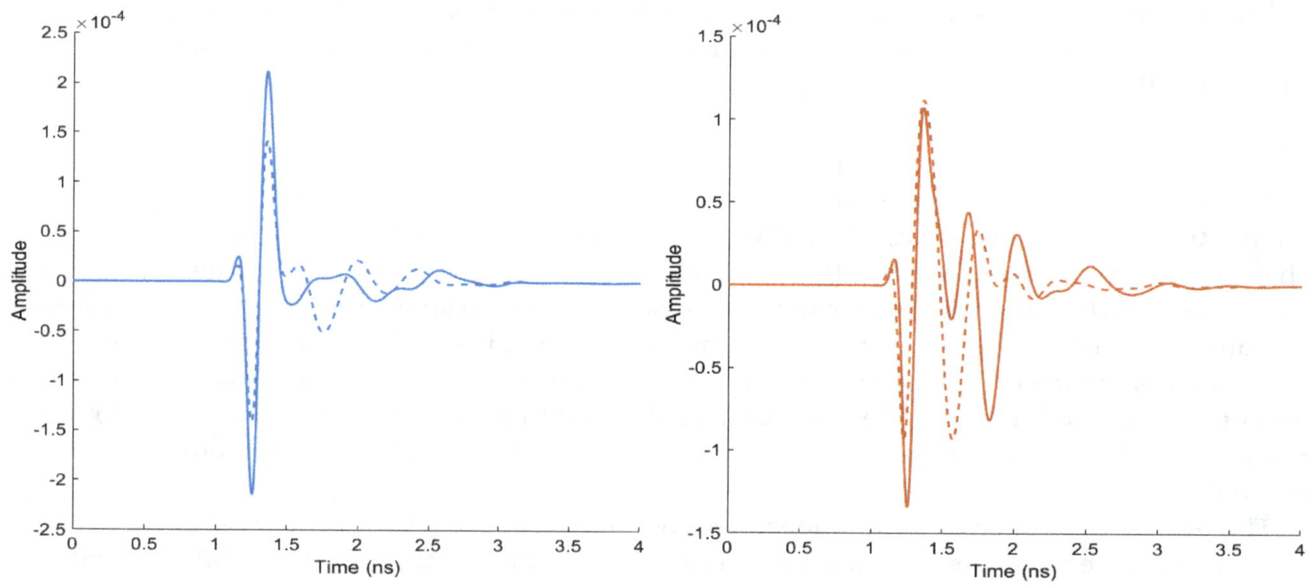

(a) (b)

Figure 3. Example of tumour signatures from benign tumour models (**a**) and malignant tumour models (**b**), captured in ideal conditions, with a fully adipose breast model. In (**a**), the benign tumour signatures are smooth, and the shape of the gaussian curve is preserved to a reasonable extent; In (**b**), the malignant tumour signatures are subject to a greater degree of irregularity, exhibiting an increased number of peaks.

In total, 30 features were extracted from each signal, divided into four sub-groups, as shown in Table 1. If feature extraction is performed on the original backscattered signals, the method is referred to as FE; if feature extraction is performed after the backscattered signals have been processed with the tumour windowing algorithm, the method is referred to as TW + FE.

Table 1. Description of all 30 features used in this study, divided into four sub-groups: Time-domain features, Autocorrelaton features, Power spectral density (PSD) features based on Welch's method, and PSD features using the periodogram method.

Time-Domain Features, Calculated From the Windowed Signals
#1–#4 Amplitudes and locations of the maximum positive and negative peaks #5 Variance #6 Root-mean-squared error #7–#8 Number of positive and negative peaks #9–#10 Mean amplitude of the positive and negative peaks #11–#12 Mean full-width half-maximum (FWHM) of the positive and negative peaks #13–#14 Mean separation between positive and negative peaks #15 Number of zero crossings #16 Integral of the signal #17 Integral of the absolute value of the signal #18 Positive percentage area of the signal #19 Negative percentage area of the signal
Autocorrelation features, which involves calculating the autocorrelation sequence of each signal [57,58]. The following features are then extracted from the autocorrelation sequence
#20 Mean value of the autocorrelation sequence #21 Number of peaks in the autocorrelation sequence #22 Mean amplitude of the peaks #23 Mean FWHM of the peaks #24 Mean separation between the peaks
PSD features—estimate of the psd of the signal, using Welch's method [59]
#25 Mean value of the Welch estimate
PSD features—estimate of the psd of the signal, using the periodogram method [60,61]
#26 Mean value of the periodogram estimate #27 Number of peaks in the periodogram #28 Mean amplitude of the peaks #29 Mean FWHM of the peaks #30 Mean separation between the peaks

2.3. Computer Aided Diagnosis

This section describes, in detail, Stage 3 (Diagnosis) of the 3-stage microwave diagnosis platform described in Figure 1. An overview of random forests, the classification algorithm, is first provided in Section 2.3.1. Section 2.3.2 describes the three types of classification models implemented in this study. The antenna grouping algorithm is detailed in Section 2.3.3. The validation methodology is described in Section 2.3.4, and the metrics to assess diagnostic performance are discussed in Section 2.3.5.

2.3.1. Classification Algorithm: Random Forests

In this study, random forests [62] were implemented to classify backscattered signals as benign or malignant.

The method of random forests is an ensemble method that essentially works by generating many single classification trees [63] and outputting the class that is the mode of the classes of all individual trees. Each tree is grown (i.e., trained) using a randomly sampled subset of observations and features from the entire dataset. Due to the inherent randomness in the process, the generated trees are uncorrelated, which ultimately contributes to the algorithm's low bias and low variance. Random forests provide generalisable models that tend not to overfit, are quick to run and are easy to interpret [62].

For the operation of a random forest, one-third of the observations in the original dataset are left out when training each tree. These observations are referred to as out-of-bag (oob) and are used as a separate set to assess the performance error of each tree. The out-of-bag error provides a measurement of the generalisation ability of the process, which is useful, for example, when optimising the internal parameters of the random forest. Random forests also allow measuring the importance of each feature in the training of each tree. In the context of diagnosing backscattered signals as benign or malignant, a measure of feature importance could provide the means to further refine classification models.

In this study, the following hyperparameters of the random forest were optimised to ensure good trained models: number of trees, number of features, leaf size. A Bayesian optimisation algorithm was implemented to perform the search for the best hyperparameters. The best hyperparameters were deemed to be those yielding the smallest out-of-bag misclassification error (that is, the hyperparameters yielding the highest accuracy).

2.3.2. Antenna Topology: Types of Classification Models

Although all channels in a given scan may contain information about a tumour, the tumour signature varies between channels depending on: the location of the tumour relative to the antennas in a channel; and the relative distance between the transmit and receive antennas in a channel. The angular distance between transmit and receive antennas in a channel is referred to as channel angle in the remainder of this work.

This variance in the tumour signatures between channels may impact the performance of the classification model, as the variance between channels may be as large as the variance between the signatures of benign and malignant tumours. To explore the significance of intra-channel variance, three types of classification models were designed, which differ in the way signals from different channel angles are utilised by the classification algorithm. The three types of classification models are shown in Figure 4. Differences in the performance of the three types of classification models may help identify if an optimal antenna pair topology exists in terms of the channel angle, which can ultimately contribute to improving diagnostic performance.

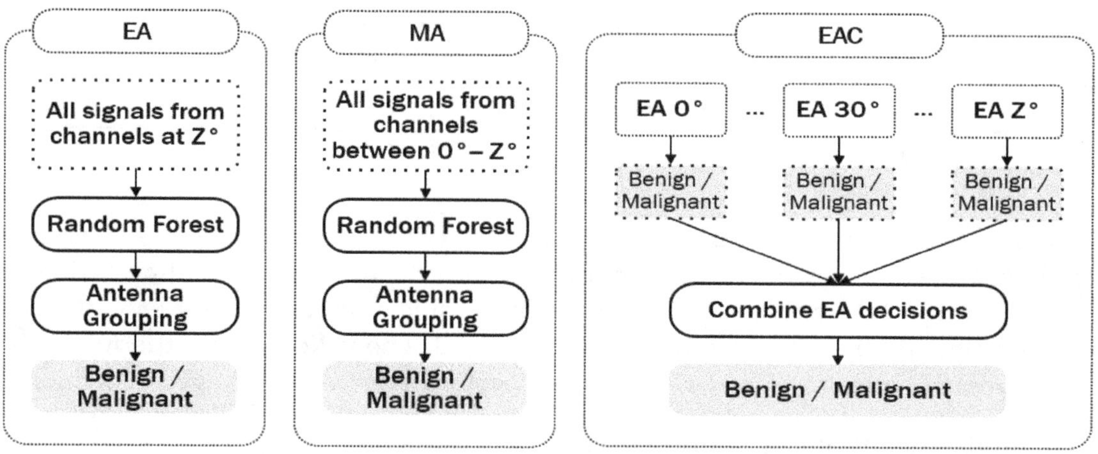

Figure 4. Description of the three types of classification models implemented: EA (equal angles), MA (multiple angles) and EAC (equal angles combined). The classification models vary in the way signals from different channel angles are utilised by the classification algorithm, where Z represents the channel angle (Z varies between 0° and 180°, and increases in steps of 30°). EA models only classify signals from a single channel angle. MA models classify signals collected at channels where the transmit and receive antennas are separated by different angles. Through majority voting, EAC models combine the predictions from multiple EA models at different channel angles to produce a final diagnosis.

The assumed system architecture is as described in Section 2.1, with one ring of 12 antennas equally distributed around the breast. Let Z be the angle between the transmit and receive antennas in a channel; here, $Z \in [0, 180]^\circ$, and Z increases by steps of 30°.

Equal Angle (EA) classification models only receive information from channels with an equal angle between transmit and receive antennas. Seven EA models were built to assess if channels with equal angles contribute to a higher diagnostic performance.

Multiple Angle (MA) models use information from channels where transmit and receive antennas are separated by different angles. If such a model underperforms, it will serve as an indication that the information captured by channels with different angles varies significantly, and that the classification model cannot adequately learn the similarities within benign and malignant tumours across signals collected at different angles. In total, six MA models were built using all antenna pairs in the interval $[0, i.Z]^\circ$, where $Z = 30^\circ$ and $i = 1, 2, ..., 6$, until all antenna pairs were used.

Equal Angle Combined (EAC) models use all possible EA models (one for each channel angle), and the predictions from each one are combined (through majority voting) at the end to produce a final diagnosis. By combining the predictions from each individual model, models which yield an incorrect result are likely to be disregarded, ultimately contributing to an increase in diagnostic performance. As before, a total of six EAC models were built using all antenna pairs in the interval $[0, i.Z]^\circ$, with $Z = 30^\circ$, until all antenna pairs were used. Table 2 summarises the models of each type, in particular the range of angles considered in this study.

Table 2. Summary of the total of number of classification models built for this study, and the channel angles used in each model. In EA models, only signals from channels at the specified angle are used in the process. In MA models, all signals from channels in the specified range are used. In EAC models, individual EA models in the specified range are combined through majority voting to produce a final diagnosis.

Classification Model Number	EA	MA	EAC
(1)	0°	–	–
(2)	30°	0–30°	0–30°
(3)	60°	0–60°	0–60°
(4)	90°	0–90°	0–90°
(5)	120°	0–120°	0–120°
(6)	150°	0–150°	0–150°
(7)	180°	0–180°	0–180°

2.3.3. Antenna Grouping

At this stage, it is important to define how backscattered signals (or the features extracted from each backscattered signal) are used in the decision-making process.

Each patient scan is comprised of signatures collected from 78 different channels (as per the system architecture described in Section 2.1), which are classified independently. However, in a realistic, clinical diagnostic system, a diagnosis is given based on a full scan, and not on the basis of a single signature. This means that the independent channel predictions need to be combined to form a final diagnosis. In the existing literature, either the procedure in determining the final diagnosis is not thoroughly discussed, or the diagnostic performance is reported based on the results from the independent channels.

To address this, an antenna grouping algorithm is implemented in this study, by which the predictions of the independent channels are grouped, and a majority vote is completed to determine if a scan is benign or malignant. The advantages of implementing such an algorithm are two-fold.

Firstly, with microwave diagnosis systems, the possibility should be considered that a signal comprises lower quality information about the tumour shape, which could result in incorrect predictions about its malignancy (e.g., signals from channels that may have poor signal-to-noise ratios). By implementing the antenna grouping algorithm, a mechanism is created that effectively allows disregarding incorrect predictions from lower quality channels.

Secondly, channels closer to a tumour should intuitively produce more useful information for its diagnosis. By implementing a ranked version of the antenna grouping algorithm, it is possible to investigate if the proximity between tumour and channel translates into higher diagnostic performances. The ranked version of the antenna grouping algorithm operates as follows. Let W be the number of channels used to perform antenna grouping, ordered by proximity to the tumour. Antenna grouping is performed by increasing W in steps of 1, until all available channels are used. For example, if $W = 3$, the majority vote is taken from the signals collected by the 3 channels closest to the tumour, before concluding on the final diagnosis.

2.3.4. Assessing Diagnostic Performance

In this study, the authors have implemented a validation methodology based on the idea of nested cross-validation [53] to assess diagnostic performance, and mitigate sources of contamination when optimising the classification model. It has been shown that nested cross-validation helps prevent overly optimistic reports of model performance [52,53]. An overview of the process is shown in Figure 5, and can be summarised as follows:

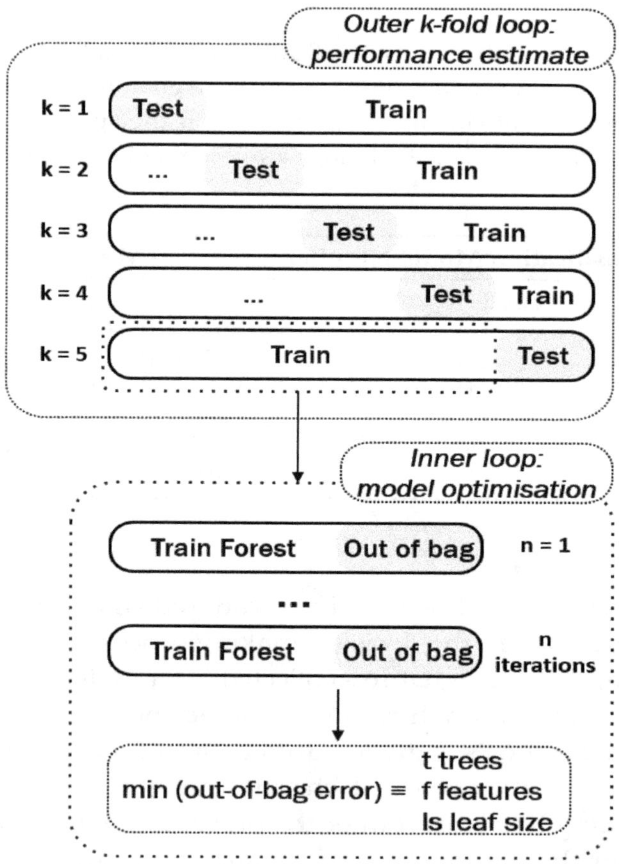

Figure 5. Nested cross-validation methodology implemented in this study to perform model optimisation and estimate model performance. In each fold, the random forest model is optimised on the train set, and new predictions are made on the test set. The predictive power of the model corresponds to the average performance obtained in the test sets across all outer folds.

- The entire dataset is divided into k stratified folds, containing equal representations of each class. In this study, the authors chose $k = 5$ outer folds as it offers a good compromise between a statistical performance analysis and speed of implementation. All signals from one breast scan are kept together when splitting each fold into training and test.

- For each outer fold, the model is trained and the classifier hyperparameters optimised. As previously detailed, random forests directly provide the out-of-bag error, which serves as an unbiased estimate of the model performance when optimising its hyperparameters. When using other classifiers another inner cross-validation loop can be implemented at this stage.
- The predictive power of the model is then reported as the average performance obtained in the test sets across all outer folds.

2.3.5. Performance Metrics

In this study, the performance of a classification model is assessed by plotting the Receiver Operating Characteristic (ROC) curves. ROC curves are created by plotting the false positive rate achieved by the classification model in the horizontal axis, against the true positive rate in the vertical axis [64]. ROC curves provide with a simple graphical representation of the diagnostic ability of the classification model, by varying the decision threshold that is used in producing the final binary decision, i.e., whether breast tumours are benign or malignant.

The Area Under the ROC Curve (AUC) is also used as a measure of classification performance. Generally, the higher the AUC, the more generalisable the model is, and the better it performs.

3. Results

This section is divided into three sub-sections. Section 3.1 discusses the issue of antenna topology and antenna grouping. Here, a relationship between the channel angle (angle between transmit and receive antennas) and predictive power is investigated, resulting in the proposal of a useful method to use the information from several multistatic scan channels. In Section 3.2, the effect of increasing tissue heterogeneity on overall diagnostic performance is discussed. Section 3.3 identifies possible avenues to expand on the knowledge gained with the extraction of features.

3.1. Antenna Topology

This section details the analysis of optimal antenna topology to be used in a breast model containing 5% of glandular tissue by volume.

Three types of classification models were defined in Section 2.3.2: EA, MA, EAC. Figure 6a–c detail the diagnostic performance achieved by all models produced, for each of the processing methods under analysis, TW, TW + FE and FE, respectively. The effect of antenna grouping (as defined in Section 2.3.3) is also investigated in Figure 6, by comparing diagnostic performance before antenna grouping (full lines) and after the antenna grouping algorithm is applied (dashed lines), using all available channels in the majority vote.

Firstly, the positive impact of antenna grouping is clearly noticeable. The diagnostic performance when antenna grouping is applied is always superior (as shown by the dashed lines in Figure 6). By taking the majority vote of all individual decisions from one single breast scan, a minority of incorrect predictions are cancelled by a majority of correct classifications. A more in-depth analysis of the effect of the ranked version of the antenna grouping algorithm (not shown in Figure 6 for conciseness) reveals that at least 3 channels are necessary to achieve a reliable diagnostic performance; above 3 channels, the performance tends to stabilise and only minor improvements are observed at the cost of more complex models. This result is seen across all classification model types (EA, MA and EAC), and by applying either of the pre-processing methods (TW, TW + FE and FE).

In Figure 6, it is also noticeable that EA and EAC models generally seem to outperform MA models. This result confirms the hypothesis that classification models perform better when dealing with signals collected under the same conditions:

- With the TW pre-processing method (Figure 6a), tumour windowing and time alignment of the signals have been performed; however, it is likely that the TW processing is not sufficient to completely neutralise the inherent differences from channels at different angles, especially considering that the intra-channel variability is likely to increase when noisy experimental or clinical data is used. One additional factor to consider with the TW processing is that knowledge of tumour location is fundamental, and localisation errors might also impact accurate time-alignment of tumour signals from different channel angles;

- In the TW + FE and FE pre-processed datasets (Figure 6b,c, respectively), comparable conclusions are observed. Models classifying signals from the same channel angles perform better. In addition, the dataset pre-processed only with FE, which does not require previous knowledge of the tumour location, slightly outperforms the TW + FE pre-processed dataset.

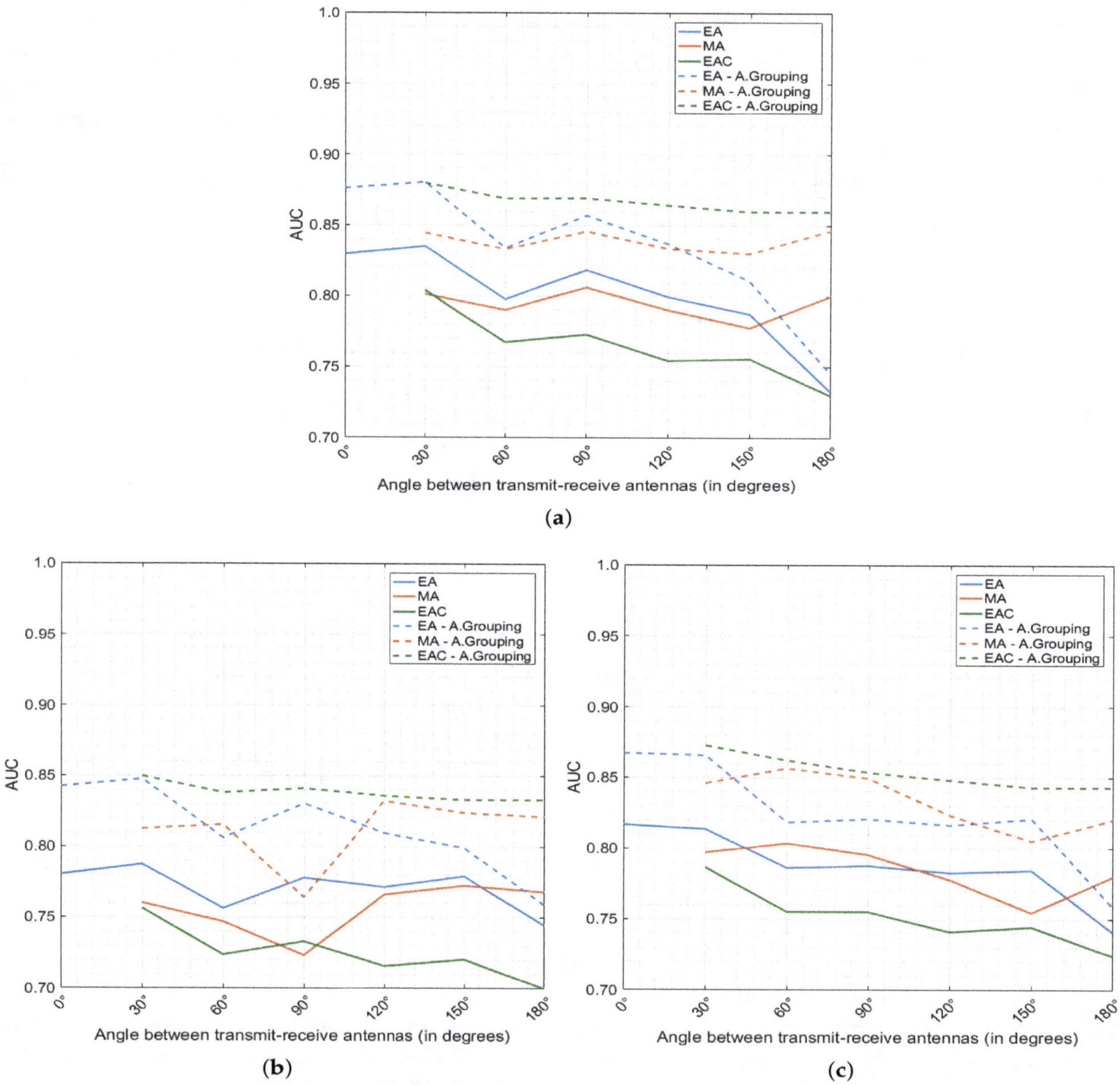

Figure 6. Diagnostic performance for the EA (blue), MA (orange) and EAC (green) models produced when features are extracted from the original dataset: (**a**) TW; (**b**) TW + FE; (**c**) FE. A.Grouping refers to the antenna grouping algorithm (using all available channels towards the majority vote). The full lines correspond to the diagnostic performance when antenna grouping was not applied, and the dashed lines when antenna grouping was applied. The horizontal axis shows the channel angles used to build each model; for the MA and EAC models, the models contain all channel angles between 0° and the angle shown in the horizontal axis.

It is also interesting to note that channel angles below 90° in the EA models lead to higher diagnostic performance when compared to channels at higher angles, which might indicate that reflected backscattered signals keep more information about tumour shape than transmitted signals. EAC models seem to benefit from this; when combining information from individual EA models, the predictions made by the EA models at lower channel angles dominate, ultimately contributing to disregarding incorrect predictions made at higher channel angles. Regardless of the pre-processing method, the best result seems to be achieved with EAC 0–30°.

In summary, optimal diagnostic performance is achieved when EAC models were used, particularly when combining channels with reflected backscattered signals. Antenna grouping is needed to achieve one final diagnosis per scan, and it helps increase diagnostic performance of the system, as it provides the means to disregard random incorrect predictions. Using all channels in the antenna grouping algorithm provides with best performance, although, the authors observed that most of the relevant information is contained in the channels closest to the tumours.

3.2. *Effect of Tissue Heterogeneity*

Increasing tissue heterogeneity is a concern when designing platforms for the diagnosis of breast cancer based on microwave backscattered signals. As glandular and tumour tissues are both characterised by higher dielectric properties, the response due to glandular clusters in the breast might sometimes be confused with the response of a tumour, causing an increased rate of false positives. In this study, the authors examine if the proposed windowing and time-alignment methodology is sufficient to handle breast heterogeneity, and if the extraction of the above-mentioned features provides meaningful and sufficient information.

From Section 3.1, one of the best performing antenna topologies was that in the EAC model at 0–30°, using all available channels when performing antenna grouping; here, the TW and FE processing methods performed the best among all considered tests. The effect of increasing tissue heterogeneity is shown in Figure 7, by plotting ROC curves obtained for the TW dataset (Figure 7a), and FE dataset (Figure 7b) using the optimal antenna topology. Separate classification models were built to diagnose scans from breast models with 1% (blue line), 5% (orange line) and 27% (green line) of glandular tissue by volume.

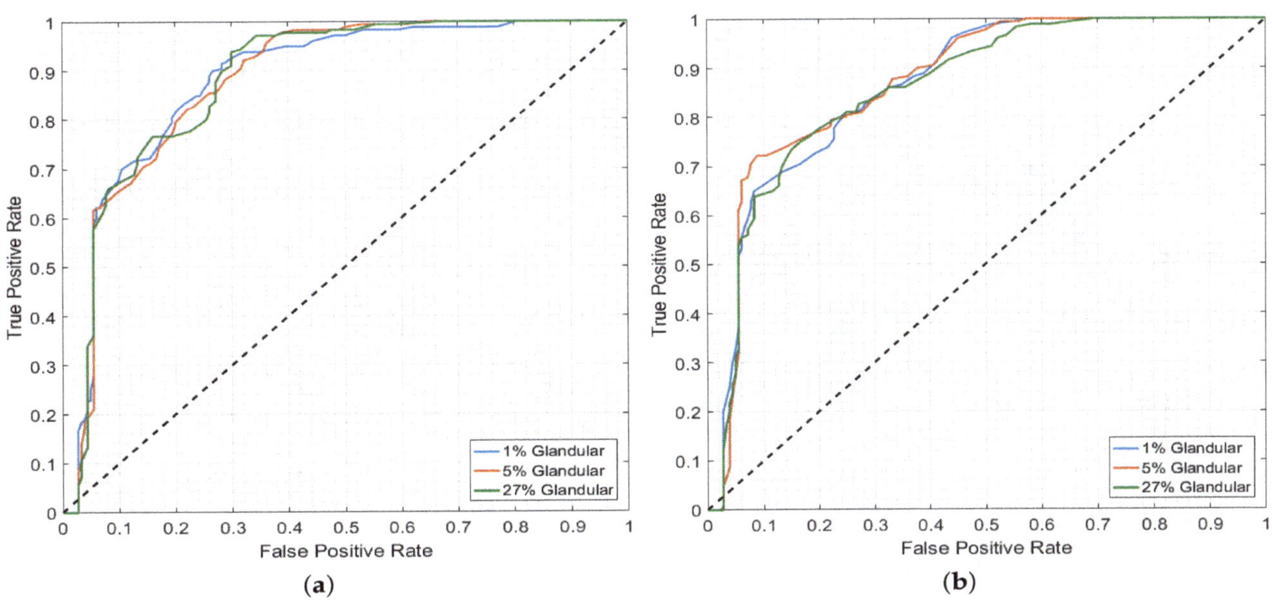

Figure 7. ROC curves showing diagnostic performance with the EAC 0–30° classification model using all channels in antenna grouping, for (**a**) TW dataset; (**b**) FE dataset. The blue line corresponds to the performance of a breast model with 1% glandular tissue by volume, orange line 5%, and green line 27%. The black dotted line represents the null hypothesis in the ROC curve.

The random forest classifier appears to be robust to tissue heterogeneity. The average performance across breast models with increasing glandular tissue content is comparable, when using either the TW or the FE methods during the pre-processing stage of the system. However, in an experimental or clinical setup, the performance of the TW pre-processed dataset is likely to decrease as tissue heterogeneity increases; noisier experimental backgrounds lead to an increased number of reflections, and the localisation of the tumour signature in the backscattered signal might be affected. Conversely, the extracted features are able to capture the differences between benign and malignant tumours, even with signals recorded in more heterogeneous breast models.

Finally, the ROC curves indicate that diagnostic performance may also be optimised by varying the decision threshold. Commonly used as a fixed threshold of 0.5, the range of optimal decision thresholds identified in this study range between 0.36 and 0.52 (not shown in Figure 7 for conciseness), which could carry further importance when translating the microwave diagnosis system to clinic.

3.3. Relative Feature Contribution

Previous sections examined the effect of antenna grouping, and the impact of tissue heterogeneity on the best performing system from initial baseline tests. In this section, an analysis of feature selection is presented, by means of the relative feature contribution map provided as one of the outputs of the random forest classifier. Investigating which features mostly contribute to the training of each tree inside a random forest could help refine the classification models, ensuring their robust and stable performance in complex scenarios, such as in experimental systems prone to high noise levels.

In Figure 8a,b, the relative feature contribution map is shown, for the breast model with 27% glandular tissue, for the TW and FE pre-processed datasets respectively. Classification was performed with the EAC 0–30° model, which uses all channels in the antenna grouping algorithm. This model is shown as an example, although the authors observed similar feature contributions across all breast and classification models.

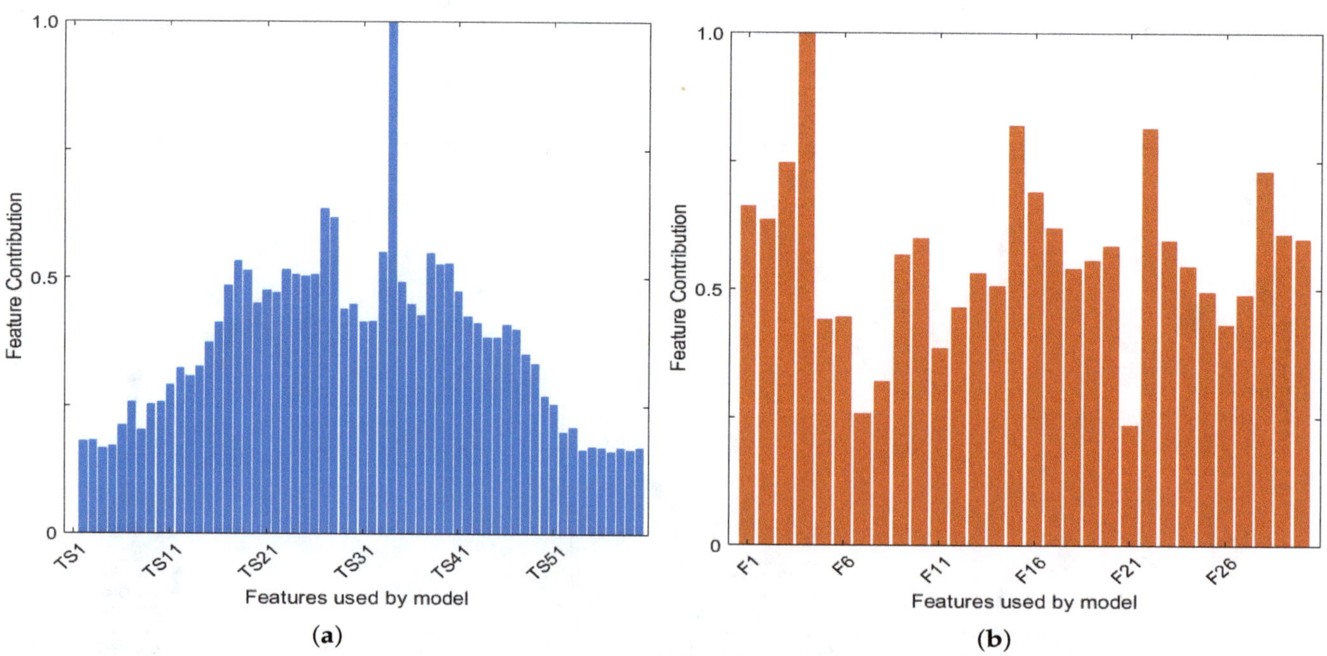

Figure 8. Map of relative feature contribution calculated during the training of the random forest model for the breast model with 27% glandular content by volume. The EAC 0–30°, with all channels in antenna grouping, is used. (**a**) refers to the dataset pre-processed with TW method; the horizontal axis shows the time samples (TS) which make up the time-domain tumour responses; (**b**) refers to the dataset pre-processed with the FE method, where F1 to F30 shown in the horizontal axis correspond to Features 1 through 30.

Firstly, Figure 8a (TW) shows that the classification model using tumour windowing is heavily reliant on one single feature. This feature is time sample 34 in the example shown. All classification models used in this study display the same reliance on one feature, which varies between time sample 33 and 36. This result suggests that any errors in the tumour windowing and alignment algorithm could indeed have a large impact in the performance of the classification.

Regarding classification with the FE method (Figure 8b), a larger number of features appear to contribute to the performance of the random forest model. Feature #4 (location of the negative peaks in the tumour signature) ranks highest, which is visible across all classification and breast models used in this study. Nine other extracted features are also identified as being particularly important in the training of the classification models. In decreasing order of contribution: amplitude of the negative peaks in the tumour signature (feature 3 shown in Figure 8b), amplitude and mean full-width half-maximum (FWHM) of positive peaks (#1, #11), mean amplitude of the peaks in the auto-correlation curve (#22), integral of the tumour signature (#16), integral of the absolute value of the signature (#17), mean power spectral density using the Welch estimate (#25), mean amplitude and FWHM of the peaks in the periodogram (#28, #29).

The features listed above were some of the features to mostly contribute to the classification of shape and spiculation of benign and malignant tumours. Particularly, the authors note the contribution of the features derived from the autocorrelation and power spectral density analysis, which reflect information otherwise not available in the time-domain tumour signatures.

4. Discussion and Conclusions

Microwave breast diagnosis systems could play a key role in further establishing microwave breast imaging and diagnosis as a tool for continuous and safe breast cancer monitoring. While diagnosis of breast tumours as benign or malignant could theoretically be performed through a number of avenues, shape and spiculation at the margin of a tumour are widely accepted as markers for malignancy, and previous studies have already demonstrated how backscattered signals are influenced by the shape of a tumour.

In this study, the authors extend previous analysis to further confirm that diagnosis of microwave backscattered signals by means of machine learning is feasible, however, there are many factors that affect performance and system optimisation must be performed with care.

Firstly, antenna grouping was identified as a key step for an increased diagnostic performance. Individual signals which compose one breast scan are independent observations, and are classified accordingly receiving a label of benign or malignant. By performing antenna grouping, those individual predictions are grouped into one final diagnosis (majority vote) for each scan. The results of this study show the benefit behind this approach, as, by doing so, a mechanism is created to disregard minor incorrect predictions. In addition, the authors observed that a relatively small number of antennas closest to the tumour guarantee the correct prediction; above this number of channels, performance tends to stabilise, but importantly, does not decrease. In this study, the 3 channels closest to the tumour were found to yield correct diagnosis; however, this may change in microwave prototypes or equipment with different setups.

Secondly, the results showed how signals collected at channels with different angles between the transmit and receive antennas have to be appropriately used by the classification model. By building individual classification models that only classify signals from channels with the same angle, diagnostic performance is increased. The predictions of individual classification models can later be combined into a fused-type model, which once again contributes to increasing the diagnostic performance. In addition, the results also showed how channels containing reflected backscattered signals performed better over channels with transmitted signals. In this study, the optimal channel angle was 0–30°.

Thirdly, data pre-processing was also shown to have an impact on diagnostic performance. When dealing with time-domain signals, knowledge of tumour location is required. With this information, a tumour windowing and time-alignment algorithm can be implemented to isolate the tumour response, while decreasing the influence of the background. A new set of 30 features was also proposed, which are extracted per backscattered signal; these features mostly rely on peak analysis of the time-domain signal, and of the frequency content of the signal. Both methods performed comparably, however, in practice, additional factors come into play which will impact performance:

- With currently available algorithms, localisation of the tumour signature in the response could be prone to error, which would impact the performance of the tumour windowing and could ultimately decrease diagnostic performance. This factor should not be neglected when building systems to classify time-domain signals.
- The extraction of features performed well, even when the time-domain signal was not pre-processed by windowing. This method appears as an alternative when exact tumour location is not available to the user. In addition, a reduced set of features of maximised contribution was identified, which could lead the way into finding an optimal set of features towards more robust classification models for microwave systems.

Finally, good machine learning practice is extremely important when designing microwave breast diagnosis systems. Without adequate feature processing methods and model validation strategies, reports of performance could be overly optimistic and not reproducible, ultimately impeding clinical acceptance of microwave diagnosis tools.

Further investigations are needed to assess the robustness of microwave breast diagnosis systems given the complexities of experimental and clinical data, such as, patient positioning and movement, intrapatient variation due to menstrual cycle and hormonal changes, and interpatient variation in breast size, shape and composition.

Author Contributions: B.L.O., D.G. and R.C.C. conceived and designed the processing tools and experiments; M.O. contributed with analysis tools; B.L.O. performed the experiments, analysed the data and wrote the paper; M.O., M.G., E.J. and R.C.C. supervised the work, including design, analysis and writing.

Acknowledgments: This work was supported by Science Foundation Ireland (Grant No. 12/IP/1523 and 11/SIRG/I2120), the MiMED COST Action (TD1301) and the European Research Council (BIOELECPRO). This paper is supported by Fundação para a Ciência e a Tecnologia—FCT/MEC (PIDDAC)—under the Strategic Programme UID/BIO/00645/2013.

Abbreviations

AUC	Area Under receiver operating characteristic Curve
EA	Equal Angle
EAC	Equal Angle Combined
FDTD	Finite-Difference Time-Domain
FE	Feature Extraction
FWHM	Full-Width Half-Maximum
MA	Multiple Angle
MBI	Microwave Breast Imaging
PSD	Power Spectral Density
ROC	Receiver Operating Characteristic
TW	Tumour Windowing
UWCEM	University of Wisconsin Computational Electromagnetics

References

1. Meaney, P.; Fanning, M.; Li, D.; Poplack, S.P.; Paulsen, K. A Clinical Prototype for Active Microwave Imaging of the Breast. *IEEE Trans. Microw. Theory Tech.* **2000**, *48*, 1841–1853, doi:10.1109/22.883861. [CrossRef]
2. Poplack, S.P.; Tosteson, T.D.; Wells, W.A.; Pogue, B.W.; Meaney, P.M.; Hartov, A.; Kogel, C.A.; Soho, S.K.; Gibson, J.J.; Paulsen, K.D. Electromagnetic Breast Imaging: Results of a Pilot Study in Women with Abnormal Mammograms. *Radiology* **2007**, *243*, 350–359, doi:10.1148/radiol.2432060286. [CrossRef] [PubMed]

3. Fear, E.C.; Bourqui, J.; Curtis, C.; Mew, D.; Docktor, B.; Romano, C. Microwave Breast Imaging with a Monostatic Radar-Based System: A Study of Application to Patients. *IEEE Trans. Microw. Theory Tech.* **2013**, *61*, 2119–2128, doi:10.1109/TMTT.2013.2255884. [CrossRef]
4. Porter, E.; Coates, M.; Popović, M. An Early Clinical Study of Time-Domain Microwave Radar for Breast Health Monitoring. *IEEE Trans. Biomed. Eng.* **2016**, *63*, 530–539, doi:10.1109/TBME.2015.2465867. [CrossRef] [PubMed]
5. Preece, A.W.; Craddock, I.J.; Shere, M.; Jones, L.; Winton, H.L. MARIA M4: Clinical Evaluation of a Prototype Ultrawideband Radar Scanner for Breast Cancer Detection. *J. Med. Imaging* **2016**, *3*, 033502, doi:10.1117/1.JMI.3.3.033502. [CrossRef] [PubMed]
6. Bannister, P. A Novel Microwave Radar Breast Imaging System in a Symptomatic Breast Clinic. In Proceedings of the BSBR Breast Imaging Research Network Workshop, Manchester, UK, 6 November 2016.
7. Fasoula, A.; Anwar, S.; Toutain, Y.; Duchesne, L. Microwave Vision: From RF Safety to Medical Imaging. In Proceedings of the 11th European Conference on Antennas and Propagation (EuCAP), Paris, France, 19–24 March 2017; pp. 2746–2750, doi:10.23919/EuCAP.2017.7928164. [CrossRef]
8. Fear, E.C.; Hagness, S.C.; Meaney, P.M.; Okoniewski, M.; Stuchly, M.A. Enhancing Breast Tumor Detection with Near-Field Imaging. *IEEE Microw. Mag.* **2002**, *3*, 48–56, doi:10.1109/6668.990683. [CrossRef]
9. Nikolova, N.K.; Webster, J.G. Microwave Biomedical Imaging. In *Wiley Encyclopedia of Electrical and Electronics Engineering*; John Wiley & Sons, Inc.: Hoboken, NJ, USA, 2014; doi:10.1002/047134608X.W8214. [CrossRef]
10. Conceição, R.C.; Mohr, J.J.; O'Halloran, M. (Eds.) *An Introduction to Microwave Imaging for Breast Cancer Detection*; Springer International Publishing: Basel, Switzerland, 2016.
11. Bolomey, J.C. Crossed Viewpoints on Microwave-Based Imaging for Medical Diagnosis: From Genesis to Earliest Clinical Outcomes. In *The World of Applied Electromagnetics*; Lakhtakia, A., Furse, C.M., Eds.; Springer International Publishing: Cham, Switzerland, 2018; pp. 369–414, doi:10.1007/978-3-319-58403-4_16.
12. O'Loughlin, D.; O'Halloran, M.J.; Moloney, B.M.; Glavin, M.; Jones, E.; Elahi, M.A. Microwave Breast Imaging: Clinical Advances and Remaining Challenges. *IEEE Trans. Biomed. Eng.* **2018**, doi:10.1109/TBME.2018.2809541. [CrossRef]
13. Gøtzsche, P.C.; Nielsen, M. Screening for Breast Cancer with Mammography. *Cochrane Database Syst. Rev.* **2011**, CD001877, doi:10.1002/14651858.CD001877.pub4. [CrossRef]
14. Biller-Andorno, N.; Jüni, P. Abolishing Mammography Screening Programs? A View from the Swiss Medical Board. *N. Engl. J. Med.* **2014**, *370*, 1965–1967, doi:10.1056/NEJMp1401875. [CrossRef] [PubMed]
15. Suri, J.S.; Rangayyan, R.M. *Recent Advances in Breast Imaging, Mammography, and Computer-Aided Diagnosis of Breast Cancer*; SPIE: Washington, WA, USA, 2006; Volume 15.
16. Jinshan, T.; Rangayyan, R.M.; Jun, X.; El Naqa, I.; Yongyi, Y. Computer-Aided Detection and Diagnosis of Breast Cancer with Mammography: Recent Advances. *IEEE Trans. Inf. Technol. Biomed.* **2009**, *13*, 236–251, doi:10.1109/TITB.2008.2009441. [CrossRef] [PubMed]
17. Olson, S.L.; Fam, B.W.; Winter, P.F.; Scholz, F.J.; Lee, A.K.; Gordon, S.E. Breast Calcifications: Analysis of Imaging Properties. *Radiology* **1988**, *169*, 329–332, doi:10.1148/radiology.169.2.3174980. [CrossRef] [PubMed]
18. Fondrinier, E.; Lorimier, G.; Guerin-Boblet, V.; Bertrand, A.F.; Mayras, C.; Dauver, N. Breast Microcalcifications: Multivariate Analysis of Radiologic and Clinical Factors for Carcinoma. *World J. Surg.* **2002**, *26*, 290–296, doi:10.1007/s00268-001-0220-3. [CrossRef] [PubMed]
19. Buchbinder, S.S.; Leichter, I.S.; Lederman, R.B.; Novak, B.; Bamberger, P.N.; Coopersmith, H.; Fields, S.I. Can the Size of Microcalcifications Predict Malignancy of Clusters at Mammography? *Acad. Radiol.* **2002**, *9*, 18–25, doi:10.1016/S1076-6332(03)80293-3. [CrossRef]
20. Cox, R.F.; Morgan, M.P. Microcalcifications in Breast Cancer: Lessons from Physiological Mineralization. *Bone* **2013**, *53*, 437–450, doi:10.1016/j.bone.2013.01.013. [CrossRef] [PubMed]
21. Ridley, N.; Iriarte, A.; Tsui, L.; Bore, C.; Shere, M.; Lyburn, I.; Bannister, P. Automatic Labelling of Lesions Using Radiofrequency Feature Discrimination. In Proceedings of the European Congress of Radiology, Vienna, Austria, 1–5 March 2017; doi:10.1594/ecr2017/C-1855.
22. Stavros, A.T.; Thickman, D.; Rapp, C.L.; Dennis, M.A.; Parker, S.H.; Sisney, G.A. Solid Breast Nodules: Use of Sonography to Distinguish between Benign and Malignant Lesions. *Radiology* **1995**, *196*, 123–134, doi:10.1148/radiology.196.1.7784555. [CrossRef] [PubMed]

23. Rangayyan, R.M.; El-Faramawy, N.M.; Desautels, J.E.L.; Alim, O.A. Measures of Acutance and Shape for Classification of Breast Tumors. *IEEE Trans. Med. Imaging* **1997**, *16*, 799–810, doi:10.1109/42.650876. [CrossRef] [PubMed]
24. Rahbar, G.; Sie, A.C.; Hansen, G.C.; Prince, J.S.; Melany, M.L.; Reynolds, H.E.; Jackson, V.P.; Sayre, J.W.; Bassett, L.W. Benign versus Malignant Solid Breast Masses: US Differentiation. *Radiology* **1999**, *213*, 889–894, doi:10.1148/radiology.213.3.r99dc20889. [CrossRef] [PubMed]
25. D'Orsi, C.; Sickles, E.; Mendelson, E.; Morris, E. *ACR BI-RADS® Atlas, Breast Imaging Reporting and Data System*; American College of Radiology: Reston, VA, USA, 2013.
26. Dorland, W.A.N. *Dorland's Illustrated Medical Dictionary*, 32nd ed.; Saunders/Elsevier: Philadelphia, PA, USA, 2012.
27. Chen, Y.; Gunawan, E.; Low, K.S.; Wang, S.C.; Soh, C.B.; Putti, T.C. Effect of Lesion Morphology on Microwave Signature in 2-D Ultra-Wideband Breast Imaging. *IEEE Trans. Biomed. Eng.* **2008**, *55*, 2011–2021, doi:10.1109/TBME.2008.921136. [CrossRef] [PubMed]
28. Davis, S.; Van Veen, B.D.; Hagness, S.C.; Kelcz, F. Breast Tumor Characterization Based on Ultrawideband Microwave Backscatter. *IEEE Trans. Biomed. Eng.* **2008**, *55*, 237–246, doi:10.1109/TBME.2007.900564. [CrossRef] [PubMed]
29. Conceição, R.; O'Halloran, M.; Byrne, D.; Jones, E.; Glavin, M. Tumor Classification Using Radar Target Signatures. In Proceedings of the Progress in Research and Electromagnetics Symposium, Cambridge, MA, USA, 5–8 July 2010; Volume 1, pp. 346–349.
30. Conceição, R.C.; O'Halloran, M.; Jones, E.; Glavin, M. Investigation of Classifiers for Early-Stage Breast Cancer Based on Radar Target Signatures. *Prog. Electromagn. Res.* **2010**, *105*, 295–311, doi:10.2528/PIER10051904. [CrossRef]
31. Conceição, R.C.; O'Halloran, M.; Glavin, M.; Jones, E. Support Vector Machines for the Classification of Early-Stage Breast Cancer Based on Radar Target Signatures. *Prog. Electromagn. Res. B* **2010**, *23*, 311–327, doi:10.2528/PIERB10062407. [CrossRef]
32. Conceição, R.C.; O'Halloran, M.; Glavin, M.; Jones, E. Evaluation of Features and Classifiers for Classification of Early-Stage Breast Cancer. *J. Electromagn. Waves Appl.* **2011**, *25*, 1–14, doi:10.1163/156939311793898350. [CrossRef]
33. O'Halloran, M.; McGinley, B.; Conceição, R.C.; Morgan, F.; Jones, E.; Glavin, M. Spiking Neural Networks for Breast Cancer Classification in a Dielectrically Heterogeneous Breast. *Prog. Electromagn. Res.* **2011**, *113*, 413–428, doi:10.2528/PIER10122203. [CrossRef]
34. O'Halloran, M.; Cawley, S.; McGinley, B.; Conceição, R.C.; Morgan, F.; Jones, E.; Glavin, M. Evolving Spiking Neural Network Topologies for Breast Cancer Classification in a Dielectrically Heterogeneous Breast. *Prog. Electromagn. Res. Lett.* **2011**, *25*, 153–162, doi:10.2528/PIERL11050605. [CrossRef]
35. Jones, M.; Byrne, D.; McGinley, B.; Morgan, F.; Glavin, M.; Jones, E.; Conceição, R.C.; O'Halloran, M. Classification and Monitoring of Early Stage Breast Cancer Using Ultra Wideband Radar. In Proceedings of the 8th International Conference on Systems (ICONS), Seville, Spain, 27 January–1 February 2013; pp. 46–51.
36. Conceição, R.C.; Medeiros, H.; O'Halloran, M.; Rodriguez-Herrera, D.; Flores-Tapia, D.; Pistorius, S. Initial Classification of Breast Tumour Phantoms Using a UWB Radar Prototype. In Proceedings of the International Conference on Electromagnetics in Advanced Applications (ICEAA), Torino, Italy, 9–13 September 2013; pp. 720–723, doi:10.1109/ICEAA.2013.6632339. [CrossRef]
37. Conceição, R.C.; Medeiros, H.; O'Halloran, M.; Rodriguez-Herrera, D.; Flores-Tapia, D.; Pistorius, S. SVM-Based Classification of Breast Tumour Phantoms Using a UWB Radar Prototype System. In Proceedings of the 31st URSI General Assembly and Scientific Symposium (URSI-GASS), Beijing, China, 16–23 August 2014; pp. 1–4, doi:10.1109/URSIGASS.2014.6930131. [CrossRef]
38. Oliveira, B.L.; Shahzad, A.; O'Halloran, M.; Conceição, R.C.; Glavin, M.; Jones, E. Combined Breast Microwave Imaging and Diagnosis System. In Proceedings of the Progress in Electromagnetics Research Symposium, Prague, Czech Republic, 6–9 July 2015; Volume 1, pp. 274–278.
39. Zastrow, E.; Davis, S.K.; Lazebnik, M.; Kelcz, F.; Van Veen, B.D.; Hagness, S.C. Development of Anatomically Realistic Numerical Breast Phantoms with Accurate Dielectric Properties for Modeling Microwave Interactions with the Human Breast. *IEEE Trans. Biomed. Eng.* **2008**, *55*, 2792–2800, doi:10.1109/tbme.2008.2002130. [CrossRef] [PubMed]

40. Kerhet, A.; Raffetto, M.; Boni, A.; Massa, A. A SVM-Based Approach to Microwave Breast Cancer Detection. *Eng. Appl. Artif. Intell.* **2006**, *19*, 807–818, doi:10.1016/j.engappai.2006.05.010. [CrossRef]
41. Byrne, D.; O'Halloran, M.; Jones, E.; Glavin, M. Support Vector Machine-Based Ultrawideband Breast Cancer Detection System. *J. Electromagn. Waves Appl.* **2011**, *25*, 1807–1816, doi:10.1163/156939311797454015. [CrossRef]
42. Byrne, D.; O'Halloran, M.; Glavin, M.; Jones, E. Breast Cancer Detection Based on Differential Ultrawideband Microwave Radar. *Prog. Electromagn. Res.* **2011**, *20*, 231–242, doi:10.2528/PIERM11080810. [CrossRef]
43. Santorelli, A.; Porter, E.; Kirshin, E.; Liu, Y.J.; Popovic, M. Investigation of Classifiers for Tumor Detection with an Experimental Time-Domain Breast Screening System. *Prog. Electromagn. Res.* **2014**, *144*, 45–57, doi:10.2528/PIER13110709. [CrossRef]
44. Conceição, R.C.; Byrne, D.; Noble, J.A.; Craddock, I.J. Initial Study for the Investigation of Breast Tumour Response with Classification Algorithms Using a Microwave Radar Prototype. In Proceedings of the 10th European Conference on Antennas and Propagation (EuCAP), Davos, Switzerland, 10–15 April 2016; pp. 1–2, doi:10.1109/EuCAP.2016.7481464. [CrossRef]
45. Li, Y.; Santorelli, A.; Laforest, O.; Coates, M. Cost-Sensitive Ensemble Classifiers for Microwave Breast Cancer Detection. In Proceedings of the IEEE International Conference on Acoustics, Speech and Signal Processing (ICASSP), Brisbane, QLD, Australia, 19–24 April 2015; pp. 952–956, doi:10.1109/ICASSP.2015.7178110. [CrossRef]
46. Li, Y.; Santorelli, A.; Coates, M. Comparison of Microwave Breast Cancer Detection Results with Breast Phantom Data and Clinical Trial Data: Varying the Number of Antennas. In Proceedings of the 10th European Conference on Antennas and Propagation (EuCAP), Davos, Switzerland, 10–15 April 2016; pp. 1–5, doi:10.1109/EuCAP.2016.7481969. [CrossRef]
47. Li, Y.; Porter, E.; Santorelli, A.; Popović, M.; Coates, M. Microwave Breast Cancer Detection via Cost-Sensitive Ensemble Classifiers: Phantom and Patient Investigation. *Biomed. Signal Process. Control* **2017**, *31*, 366–376, doi:10.1016/j.bspc.2016.09.003. [CrossRef]
48. Song, H.; Li, Y.; Coates, M.; Men, A. Microwave Breast Cancer Detection Using Empirical Mode Decomposition Features. *arXiv* **2017**, arXiv:1702.07608 [stat.ML].
49. Song, H.; Li, Y.; Men, A. Microwave Breast Cancer Detection Using Time-Frequency Representations. *Med. Biol. Eng. Comput.* **2018**, *56*, 571–582, doi:10.1007/s11517-017-1712-0. [CrossRef] [PubMed]
50. Elahi, M.A.; Shahzad, A.; Glavin, M.; Jones, E.; O'Halloran, M. Hybrid Artifact Removal for Confocal Microwave Breast Imaging. *IEEE Antennas Wirel. Propag. Lett.* **2014**, *13*, 149–152, doi:10.1109/LAWP.2014.2298975. [CrossRef]
51. Elahi, M.A.; Glavin, M.; Jones, E.; O'Halloran, M. Adaptive Artifact Removal for Selective Multistatic Microwave Breast Imaging Signals. *Biomed. Signal Process. Control* **2017**, *34*, 93–100, doi:10.1016/j.bspc.2017.01.006. [CrossRef]
52. Ambroise, C.; McLachlan, G.J. Selection Bias in Gene Extraction on the Basis of Microarray Gene-Expression Data. *Proc. Natl. Acad. Sci. USA* **2002**, *99*, 6562–6566, doi:10.1073/pnas.102102699. [CrossRef] [PubMed]
53. Cawley, G.C.; Talbot, N.L.C. On Over-Fitting in Model Selection and Subsequent Selection Bias in Performance Evaluation. *J. Mach. Learn. Res.* **2010**, *11*, 2079–2107.
54. O'Halloran, M.; Conceição, R.C.; Byrne, D.; Glavin, M.; Jones, E. FDTD Modeling of the Breast: A Review. *Prog. Electromagn. Res. B* **2009**, *18*, 1–24, doi:10.2528/PIERB09080505. [CrossRef]
55. Lazebnik, M.; Okoniewski, M.; Booske, J.; Hagness, S. Highly Accurate Debye Models for Normal and Malignant Breast Tissue Dielectric Properties at Microwave Frequencies. *IEEE Microw. Compon. Lett.* **2007**, *17*, 822–824, doi:10.1109/LMWC.2007.910465. [CrossRef]
56. Oliveira, B.L.; O'Halloran, M.; Conceição, R.C.; Glavin, M.; Jones, E. Development of Clinically Informed 3-D Tumor Models for Microwave Imaging Applications. *IEEE Antennas Wirel. Propag. Lett.* **2016**, *15*, 520–523, doi:10.1109/LAWP.2015.2456051. [CrossRef]
57. Buck, J.R.; Daniel, M.M.; Singer, A. *Computer Explorations in Signals and Systems Using MATLAB*; Prentice Hall: Upper Saddle River, NJ, USA, 2002.
58. Stoica, P.; Moses, R.L. *Spectral Analysis of Signals*; Pearson Prentice Hall: Upper Saddle River, NJ, USA, 2005.
59. Welch, P. The Use of Fast Fourier Transform for the Estimation of Power Spectra: A Method Based on Time Averaging over Short, Modified Periodograms. *IEEE Trans. Audio Electroacoust.* **1967**, *15*, 70–73, doi:10.1109/TAU.1967.1161901. [CrossRef]

60. Auger, F.; Flandrin, P. Improving the Readability of Time-Frequency and Time-Scale Representations by the Reassignment Method. *IEEE Trans. Signal Process.* **1995**, *43*, 1068–1089, doi:10.1109/78.382394. [CrossRef]
61. Fulop, S.A.; Fitz, K. Algorithms for Computing the Time-Corrected Instantaneous Frequency (Reassigned) Spectrogram, with Applications. *J. Acoust. Soc. Am.* **2006**, *119*, 360–371. [CrossRef] [PubMed]
62. Breiman, L. Random Forests. *Mach. Learn.* **2001**, *45*, 5–32, doi:10.1023/A:1010933404324. [CrossRef]
63. Breiman, L.; Friedman, J.H.; Olshen, R.A.; Stone, C.J. *Classification and Regression Trees*; Chapman & Hall: Boca Raton, FL, USA, 1984.
64. Spackman, K.A. Signal Detection Theory: Valuable Tools for Evaluating Inductive Learning. In *Proceedings of the Sixth International Workshop on Machine Learning*; Morgan Kaufmann Publishers Inc.: San Francisco, CA, USA, 1989; pp. 160–163, doi:10.1016/B978-1-55860-036-2.50047-3. [CrossRef]

6

Open-Ended Coaxial Probe Technique for Dielectric Measurement of Biological Tissues: Challenges and Common Practices

Alessandra La Gioia [1,*], Emily Porter [1], Ilja Merunka [2], Atif Shahzad [1], Saqib Salahuddin [1], Marggie Jones [1] and Martin O'Halloran [1]

1 Department of Electrical and Electronic Engineering, National University of Ireland Galway, Galway, Ireland; emily.porter@nuigalway.ie (E.P.); atifshahzad.m@gmail.com (A.S.); s.salah-ud-din1@nuigalway.ie (S.S.); marggie.jones@gmail.com (M.J.); martin.ohalloran@nuigalway.ie (M.O.)

2 Department of Electromagnetic Field, Czech Technical University in Prague, 166 27 Prague, Czech Republic; IljaMerunka@seznam.cz

* Correspondence: a.lagioia1@nuigalway.ie

Abstract: Electromagnetic (EM) medical technologies are rapidly expanding worldwide for both diagnostics and therapeutics. As these technologies are low-cost and minimally invasive, they have been the focus of significant research efforts in recent years. Such technologies are often based on the assumption that there is a contrast in the dielectric properties of different tissue types or that the properties of particular tissues fall within a defined range. Thus, accurate knowledge of the dielectric properties of biological tissues is fundamental to EM medical technologies. Over the past decades, numerous studies were conducted to expand the dielectric repository of biological tissues. However, dielectric data is not yet available for every tissue type and at every temperature and frequency. For this reason, dielectric measurements may be performed by researchers who are not specialists in the acquisition of tissue dielectric properties. To this end, this paper reviews the tissue dielectric measurement process performed with an open-ended coaxial probe. Given the high number of factors, including equipment- and tissue-related confounders, that can increase the measurement uncertainty or introduce errors into the tissue dielectric data, this work discusses each step of the coaxial probe measurement procedure, highlighting common practices, challenges, and techniques for controlling and compensating for confounders.

Keywords: dielectric measurements; biological tissues; open-ended coaxial probe; equipment-related confounders; tissue-related confounders

---

1. Introduction

The interaction of electromagnetic (EM) fields with the human body is dependent on the inherent dielectric properties of each tissue. Based on these properties, electromagnetic waves are transmitted, absorbed, and reflected by biological tissues in different ratios. Accurate knowledge of these properties is crucial for dosimetry (safety) calculations and for medical diagnostic, monitoring, and therapeutic technologies.

The dielectric properties of tissues can be incorporated into highly accurate computational and physical models, and the generated preliminary data can be used to assess the technical risk, efficacy, and safety of the medical device or treatment. For instance, numerical models based on tissue dielectric parameters are used to calculate the specific absorption rate (SAR) in biological tissues. SAR levels are regularly calculated to validate the safety of many medical technologies, including magnetic resonance imaging (MRI) and implantable devices. Since SAR is a complex function of the dielectric properties of tissue, accurate knowledge of these properties are the foundation upon which SAR safety analysis is built [1,2]. Furthermore, accurate knowledge of the dielectric properties of biological tissue have prompted the development of a wide range of novel diagnostic and therapeutic technologies.

EM imaging ranges from the low-frequency Electrical Impedance Tomography (EIT) to higher-frequency Microwave Imaging (MWI). Both of these techniques rely on dielectric contrasts between organs or on contrasts between healthy and diseased, or inflamed, tissue. These imaging methods have gained significant academic and commercial interest, since both EIT and MWI are non-invasive and low-cost techniques [3–7]. While EIT is now established commercially for lung-function monitoring applications [8,9], MWI, similarly, has made considerable progress toward clinical usage in the past two decades as tissue dielectric properties enable the differentiation of benign and malignant tissues in breast cancer imaging [10–14], the monitoring of bladder volume in the treatment of enuresis and urinary incontinence [15,16], and the detection of stroke in intracranial imaging [17–20].

From a therapeutic perspective, knowledge of the relevant dielectric properties is used in the design and optimisation of hyperthermia (HT) [21–23], radiofrequency ablation (RFA) [24–26], and microwave ablation (MWA) systems [27–31]. Hyperthermia consists of elevating the temperature of a diseased tissue to just above a normal physiological level in order to sensitise tumour cells, making the cancerous tissue more susceptible to chemotherapy and radiotherapy [32]. Targeted HT has been demonstrated to be particularly effective in the treatment of cervical cancer, breast cancer, cancers of the head and neck, and sarcoma in adults [21] and germ cell tumours in young children [23]. In EM-based hyperthermia systems, heating is achieved by coherently adding signals at the tumour location. In order to achieve coherent summing of the waves at the appropriate location, knowledge of the wave propagation speed is required, which depends on the dielectric properties of the tissues in the region. Similarly, radiofrequency ablation (RFA) and microwave ablation (MWA) are two treatments for liver, kidney, and lung cancer [33,34]. Both methods cause the direct necrosis of disease, and the relative high frequencies allow for good selectivity in terms of targeting the cancerous tissue, while protecting the surrounding healthy tissue [35]. Knowledge of the dielectric properties of tissues in the ablation region are factored into the design of ablation probes, where they are used to optimise the probe antenna efficiency and directivity, along with the size and shape of the ablation zone [36].

Thus, an accurate knowledge of the tissue dielectric properties not only has the potential to improve SAR estimates and reduce undesired tissue heating, particularly in newly developed RF-induction powered implantable sensors, but is also of key importance for the design of novel EM-based imaging and therapeutic technologies.

Due to the fast-paced development of novel, low-cost medical technologies and wearable devices, knowledge of new dielectric tissue data may be required. Thus, dielectric data may be acquired by researchers who are not specialists in the measurement of dielectric properties. For this reason, this paper reviews the most common measurement techniques for the acquisition of dielectric properties of biological tissues and references the most relevant dielectric studies in the literature.

There are several methods to measure the dielectric properties of biological tissues, including: The transmission line, cavity, tetrapolar (or multi electrode) probe, and open-ended coaxial probe techniques. Amongst these methods, the coaxial probe technique is the most commonly used [11,29,30,37–44]. Although the dielectric measurement process with an open-ended coaxial probe appears straightforward, different confounders can result in two types of errors in the measured data: Equipment-related (or system) and tissue-related errors. System errors relate to measurement equipment choice, measurement uncertainties, and measurement calibration and validation. Tissue-related errors are due to factors including: Temperature, probe-sample contact, probe-sample pressure, sample handling procedure, in vivo versus ex vivo experiments, tissue sample properties, and heterogeneity. Historically, equipment-related errors have been reduced with the development of a standard error correction calibration and good benchmarks have been defined to reduce or compensate for tissue-related errors. However, many tissue-related errors have yet to be investigated in detail. Both equipment- and tissue-related errors are addressed in this work. In particular, this paper focuses on the most common methods and best practices used to reduce or compensate for confounders affecting each step of the open-ended coaxial probe measurement process. Confounders are defined, here, as factors that affect the outcome (i.e., the measured dielectric properties) other than the intended cause (the actual tissue properties).

The remainder of the paper is organised as follows: Section 2 introduces the physical principles of the dielectric properties of biological tissues and summarises the most relevant works in the literature, highlighting the different aspects to consider in the process of tissue dielectric measurement. Section 3 describes the techniques used for dielectric measurement of biological tissues, and highlights why the open-ended coaxial probe method has, historically, been the most widely used for tissue measurements. In the following sections, the steps involved in an open-ended coaxial measurement are detailed. In Section 4, the standard calibration method is described and, in Section 5, the typical system validation procedure and the measurement uncertainty estimation are discussed. Tissue-related confounders are analysed in Sections 6 and 7. Lastly, the paper concludes in Section 8, with a discussion proposing methods to refine the dielectric characterisation of human tissues and improve the interpretation of both historical and new dielectric datasets. It is hoped that this paper will be a useful reference text for those who are not experts in the field of dielectric data acquisition, but who are interested in using the resulting dielectric data or EM-based medical technologies that rely on this data.

2. Tissue Dielectric Properties: Background and Relevant Works

This section provides the necessary theoretical background for understanding dielectric properties and their measurement. Firstly, dielectric properties are defined and their characteristics described. Then, a concise historical review of dielectric property measurements of tissues is detailed, highlighting the progress in the dielectric measurement of biological tissues to date.

2.1. Basics of Dielectric Properties

The dielectric properties of biological tissues (and polar materials) are defined by the complex permittivity, $\epsilon(\omega)^*$, which describes the interaction of the tissue with an external electric field. When an electric field is applied, a charge displacement in the tissue causes dielectric polarisation. The real and the imaginary terms of the complex permittivity are related by:

$$\epsilon(\omega)^* = \epsilon'(\omega) - j\,\epsilon''(\omega) = \epsilon'(\omega) - j\frac{\sigma(\omega)}{\omega\epsilon_0}, \quad (1)$$

where ω is the angular frequency. The real part of the complex permittivity, ϵ', also called the "dielectric constant" or "relative permittivity", expresses the ability of the tissue to store energy from an external electric field. The imaginary part of permittivity, ϵ'', reflects the dissipative nature of the tissue, which absorbs the energy and partially converts it to heat. The conductivity, $\sigma(\omega)$, is linked to the imaginary part of the complex permittivity by the relationship defined in Equation (1).

Equation (1) expresses the dependence of complex permittivity on the frequency of the applied external electric field. In particular, at specific frequencies, polarisation occurs and contributes to the tissue dielectric behaviour [45,46]. The dielectric spectrum of a tissue is characterized by three main dispersion regions, α, β, and γ, along with other minor dispersions, including the δ dispersion. These dispersion regions reflect the mechanisms occurring in various components of the biological material. Details regarding these biophysical mechanisms are thoroughly reported in [45,46].

Mathematical functions have been developed to model the dielectric behaviour of biological tissues and polar materials. These models are generally used to fit dielectric data, thus, reducing measurement data points to closed form equations and convenient graphical representations [11]. Dielectric models allow the calculation of the relative permittivity and conductivity values at any desired frequency within the range for which the relaxation equation is valid [47,48]. Importantly, these models allow for the dielectric properties of biological tissues to be easily incorporated into sophisticated computational models.

The most common models used to describe the electrical behaviour of either aqueous electrolytic solutions or tissues are the: Debye, Cole-Cole, and Cole-Davidson models [49]. In general, the Debye, Cole-Cole, and Cole-Davidson models can be represented collectively by the Havriliak–Negami relaxation, which is an empirical modification of the Debye relaxation model, accounting for the asymmetry and broadness of the dielectric dispersion curve:

$$\epsilon(\omega)^* = \epsilon_\infty + \frac{\epsilon_s - \epsilon_\infty}{\left[1 + (j\omega\tau)^{1-\alpha}\right]^{\beta}} + \frac{\sigma_s}{j\omega\epsilon_0} \quad (2)$$

where ω is the angular frequency, ϵ_∞ is the permittivity at infinite frequencies due to electronic polarizability, ϵ_s is the static (low frequency) permittivity, σ_s is the static conductivity linked to charge movements, ϵ_0 is the permittivity of the vacuum, α and β are empirical variables that account for the distribution of the relaxation time and the asymmetry of the relaxation time distribution, respectively, and τ is the characteristic relaxation time of the medium, which is the time necessary for the material molecules or dipoles to return to the relaxation state that was perturbed by the application of the electric field. When $\alpha = 0$ and $\beta = 1$, Equation (2) corresponds to the Debye model. For $0 < \alpha < 1$ and $\beta = 1$, Equation (2) results in the Cole-Cole equation, which accounts for the distribution of the relaxation time. Lastly, for $\alpha = 0$ and $0 < \beta < 1$, Equation (2) corresponds to the Cole-Davidson equation, which is characterised by an asymmetrically broadened distribution of relaxation times [49]. While all of these models are used for fitting polar aqueous solutions, biological tissue data is generally fitted with the Debye and Cole-Cole models.

Equation (2) describes a single relaxation; however, if the dielectric behaviour of a material is analysed across a wide frequency range, all dielectric relaxations occurring over that frequency range must be taken into account and more poles (corresponding to the different relaxation times of the material) should be introduced to adequately describe the material. Biological tissues are generally described in terms of multiple Cole-Cole poles, which is a physics-based compact representation of wideband frequency-dependent dielectric properties [47].

2.2. Dielectric Property Studies in the Literature

Since the late 1940s, researchers have examined the dielectric properties of human and animal tissues across different frequency ranges, often using varied measurement procedures [50–53]. In the 1980s, the dielectric relaxation processes of biological tissues were further examined and modelled [45,46], and, increasingly, the open-ended coaxial line became the most common sensor for the acquisition of the dielectric properties of animal and human tissues [38–41,54–58]. The open-ended coaxial measurement technique was preferred to the transmission line, cavity perturbation, and tetrapolar probe methods, since the open-ended coaxial technique is non-destructive and allows for ex vivo and in vivo broadband measurements [39,59–61].

In the same decade, considerable progress was made on the measurement system and procedure, and several dielectric studies were conducted. Along with the dielectric characterisation of animal and human tissues [39,54,62,63], the tissue dielectric properties were analysed as a function of their physiological properties [45,55,64]. For instance, the dependence of the dielectric properties on tissue water content at microwave frequencies was analysed [56,65], the in vivo and ex vivo dielectric properties were compared [40], the difference between healthy and malignant tissues were examined [64,65], and the change in tissue dielectric properties post-mortem were reported [55].

A decade later, in 1996, Gabriel et al. published a comprehensive literature review reporting animal and human dielectric data across ten frequency decades, from 10 Hz to 20 GHz [66]. Dielectric data from a wide literature search was gathered and compared. Some inconsistencies were noted due to the use of different equipment and samples, and, therefore, Gabriel et al. sought to supplement these datasets with newly acquired data. Gabriel et al. completed in vivo and ex vivo animal and human tissue studies over a frequency range from 10 Hz to 20 GHz [42,47,67]. With this work, Gabriel et al. bridged gaps in the literature and consolidated the available dielectric data into one large dielectric repository. The experimental measurements were performed using three different techniques, depending on the acquisition frequency. To ensure quality, wherever possible, in vivo measurements on human patients were selected in preference to ex vivo or animal measurements. Where ex vivo/in vitro tissue was used, measurements were acquired as soon as possible after death. The data collected and measured by Gabriel et al. quickly became the generally accepted standard for dielectric properties of human tissues. This work was made publicly available on, firstly, the Federal Communications Commission (FCC) website [68] and on the Italian National Research Council (CNR) website, subsequently [69]. This broad availability allowed widespread use of the data among the scientific community and contributed to its diffusion.

In the subsequent years, dielectric measurement instrumentation and procedures were further improved. Specifically, the volume of the sample interrogated by the probe was investigated to accurately assign the acquired dielectric data to the actual tissue contributing to the dielectric measurement [70–72]. Based on the analysis of the probe sensing volume, precision probes were manufactured for localised dielectric spectroscopy of both low and high permittivity tissues [73].

In 2005, following an extensive measurement programme to measure the dielectric properties of several animal tissues, Peyman et al. described many measurement challenges related to the dielectric properties of biological tissues and corresponding methods to deal with them [43]. In 2006, Gabriel and Peyman reviewed tissue dielectric properties, with the aim of examining measurement uncertainties and their effect on existing dielectric measurements. The uncertainties were divided into random ("Type A") and systematic ("Type B"), according to the guidelines defined by the National Institute of Standard and Technology (NIST) in 1994 [74,75].

In 2007, Lazebnik et al. examined the dielectric properties of breast tissue, with the aim of assessing the viability of using microwave imaging to detect early-stage breast cancer [11,76]. Through careful histological categorisation of each breast tissue sample, Lazebnik et al. found the breast to be dielectrically heterogeneous, and the dielectric contrast between fibroglandular tissue and cancerous tissue to be as little as 1.1:1 in the range between 0.5 GHz and 20 GHz. These findings were in conflict with almost all existing datasets, which had predicted considerably higher dielectric contrast (some as large as 10:1) [77,78]. The findings of Lazebnik et al. had a very significant impact in the community of researchers developing microwave breast imaging systems, since the data suggested that the dielectric contrast between healthy and cancerous tissue may be too low to clinically detect cancer using this technology. More recent works characterising healthy and cancerous breast tissue found a high variability in the properties across each tissue type and across patients, which complicates the dielectric differentiation between healthy and malignant tissue [12,58,79]. However, in Martellosio et al., a contrast in relative permittivity ranging from 1.1 to 5 was found between healthy and cancerous breast tissue across the range of 0.5–20 GHz [79], which is in broad agreement with the results of Lazebnik et al. [11,76].

In 2014, Sugitani et al. suggested that the inconsistency in the reported dielectric properties of breast tissue may be at least partially attributed to variations in the number of cells of each tissue type (e.g., fat or tumour) within a dielectric sample [12]. The findings in Sugitani et al. underscored the need to take into consideration tissue heterogeneity and histopathology within the sensing volume when completing dielectric studies.

In order to define the sensing volume to account for histological analysis of heterogeneous biological tissues, Meaney et al. and Porter et al. examined the sensing volume of the common commercial dielectric probes and evaluated the dependence of the measured dielectric properties on the sample tissue composition [80–83].

Recently, numerous studies investigating the contrast in dielectric properties between healthy and malignant tissues have been conducted in order to improve the design of existing medical devices or to expand the clinical application of both imaging and therapeutic devices [10,37,84–86]. In particular, a number of works investigated the dependence of the dielectric properties of biological tissues on temperature for the optimisation of therapeutic technologies, such as RF/MW ablation [26–31,35].

To summarise, over the last three decades, notable progress has been made in the improvement of dielectric measurement equipment and in the refinement of the measurement protocol, aimed at further improving existing dielectric repositories. However, today, there is still a need for additional dielectric data to cover all tissue types, temperatures, and frequency ranges. This data provides the foundation for safety studies involving electromagnetic fields and for the design or optimisation of novel medical technologies. Therefore, in the next sections, the dielectric measurement procedure is discussed in detail and, along with each step of the procedure, the corresponding confounders that can introduce error into the results are discussed. Compensation techniques for mitigating the impact of confounders are also provided.

3. Measurement Approaches

Different techniques have been used to measure the dielectric properties of tissue, including the transmission line and waveguide; open-ended coaxial probe; tetrapolar (or multi electrode) impedance; and perturbation cavity methods. In this section, an overview of each technique is provided, along with the known advantages and drawbacks of each. Then, the focus is on the most common method, the open-ended coaxial probe technique. This section underscores why the coaxial probe technique is the most used approach for dielectric tissue measurements. The state-of-the-art in modern open-ended coaxial probe measurement equipment is also presented.

3.1. Overview of Measurement Techniques

Among the measurement techniques used in previous dielectric studies, the most common methods are presented and briefly discussed in this subsection.

3.1.1. Transmission Line

In transmission line measurement methods, a sample is placed in a coaxial line or, in the case of anisotropic tissue, in a rectangular waveguide so that the field polarisation may be varied. The transmission line is connected to two ports of a Vector Network Analyser (VNA) in order to acquire the scattering parameters (S11 and S21) [62,87], which are then converted into the complex permittivity (dielectric properties) of the tissue. The two most commonly used conversion methods are the Nicolson-Ross-Weir (NRW) method [88,89] and the NIST iterative conversion method [90,91]. The NRW method provides a direct calculation of permittivity from the complex reflection coefficient and the complex transmission coefficient obtained from the S-parameters [88,89,91,92]. Other common conversion methods are iterative and receive the initial guess from the NRW method or users' input. The algorithm developed to implement the NIST iterative conversion method is reported in detail in Baker-Jarvis et al. [90].

The transmission line method allows measurement over a large frequency range, but only at low temperatures [87,93,94]. Waveguides are suitable for measuring larger samples (i.e., samples the size of the waveguide) at frequencies of up to 2.45 GHz, which is the frequency point normally used in microwave ablation. Smaller samples can be measured in the coaxial line, although this method also requires careful sample preparation in order to shape the sample to fit the line, and the method generally assumes that there are no air gaps in or around the sample and that the sample has smooth flat faces [95]. Thus, the transmission line method can be suitable for the measurements of biological fluids, but is unsuitable for in vivo measurements and not recommended for ex vivo measurements of semisolid or solid biological samples.

3.1.2. Cavity Perturbation

The cavity perturbation method consists of a resonant cavity that resonates at specific frequencies. The tissue samples are inserted into the cavity and analysed by measuring the resonant frequency (f) and quality factor (Q), which are altered by inserting the tissue sample [94–98]. The tissue dielectric properties are then computed using the frequency, the Q-factor, and the sample volume. Details regarding the mathematical formulation to obtain the permittivity of the sample are reported by Campbell et al. [99]. However, the resonant frequency and quality factor are generally computed with a VNA. Since the maximum change in resonant frequency is achieved when a small perturbation occurs at the maximum intensity of the cavity mode, the cavity perturbation method requires a small sample [94,97]. Dielectric measurements performed using the cavity perturbation method can be accurate, but only provide dielectric data at a single frequency (in the upper microwave frequency range of 1–50 GHz). While the equipment needed for cavity perturbation measurements is readily available and cost-effective, the sample preparation is relatively complicated, requiring an excised tissue sample to be cut and moulded to a precise size and shape to fit into the cavity [95,97]. This process may introduce air pockets within the sample or between the sample and the cavity, loss of fluid in the tissue (which would affect its properties), and an increase in density from pushing the tissue into the cavity (which could also affect its properties) [97]. Due to the required sample size and, thus, sample preparation, biological tissue measurements with the cavity perturbation method are highly challenging.

3.1.3. Tetrapolar Impedance

Unlike the previous two techniques, the tetrapolar (or multi electrode) impedance method is non-destructive and allows for in vivo tissue measurements. The tetrapolar probe is composed of four electrodes: Two of the electrodes are driven with a current source and the other two electrodes are used for voltage measurements. The two electrode pairs are used for impedance measurements, avoiding interference from effects related to the electrode-tissue interface [100,101]. The tissue dielectric properties are easily evaluated from the measured impedance with knowledge of the sample dimensions. Although the tetrapolar probe method does not require tissue processing and is very sensitive to tissue anisotropies [19,101], it is only suitable for specific low frequencies (in the range of 10^{-6}–100 MHz) [101]. For the tetrapolar probe technique, the electrode configuration should vary according to the interrogated tissue. In order to increase the number of applications, tetrapolar probes may be replaced by spring-loaded multi electrode probes [102]. The multiple surface electrodes permits the setting of a current pattern so that the resulting measured voltage is more sensitive to a local area and less sensitive to other regions. Multi electrode probes can provide improved bioimpedance and anisotropy measurements [102].

3.1.4. Open-ended Coaxial Probe

The coaxial probe technique does not suffer from many of the disadvantages associated with the techniques described above. The open-ended coaxial probe consists of a truncated section of a transmission line. The electromagnetic field propagates along the coaxial line and reflection occurs when the electromagnetic field encounters an impedance mismatch between the probe and the tissue sample. The open-ended coaxial probe measurement set-up and the probe cross-section are schematised in Figure 1. The reflected signals at different frequencies are measured and then converted into complex permittivity values.

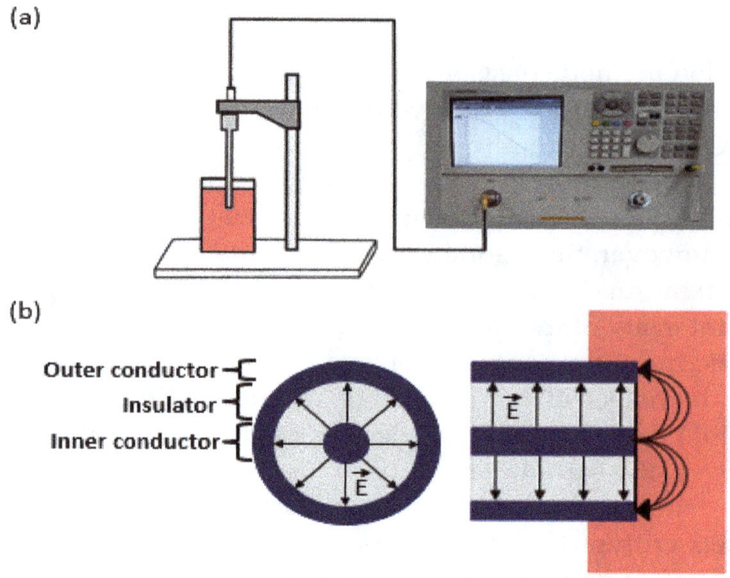

Figure 1. Open-ended coaxial probe technique: (**a**) Schematised measurement set-up, including the Vector Network Analyser (on the right), the cable connecting one port of the VNA to the coaxial probe, the probe bracket, and the liquid sample being measured; (**b**) top and side cross-sections of the coaxial probe, with electric field orientation indicated.

Different methods have been developed to convert the measured reflection coefficient to permittivity [60,103–107]. However, today, this process is generally done automatically by software embedded in the VNA [108]. Therefore, details on the various methods are not discussed in detail here, but more information can be found in [103–107,109–111].

The open-ended coaxial probe has become the most commonly used method to measure the dielectric properties of tissues for several reasons: The method is simple; sample handling is minimal and non-destructive; and both ex vivo and in vivo measurements over a broad frequency range are possible [39,42,43,72,94]. However, the open-ended coaxial method assumes a homogeneous sample that is in good contact with the probe; therefore, air bubbles and uneven sample surfaces can result in inaccurate measurements [95], and heterogeneous samples present a particular challenge. There are also limits to the magnitudes of material properties that can be measured reliably [95]. The limits of what can be measured depend on a number of factors, including the probe design and materials (and, therefore, its impedance), precision of the probe fabrication procedure, calibration procedure (standards used), and the capabilities of the measurement device (i.e., the VNA). Furthermore, what is classified as a "reliable measurement" depends on the experiment and the required accuracy. Although theoretical limits of the measurement set up can be estimated analytically, they are generally estimated experimentally by measuring materials (usually liquids) with different extreme values of relative permittivity and conductivity. Then, the accuracy of the measurement can be estimated in different ranges of complex permittivity and it can be determined if the accuracy is appropriate for the experiment of interest.

Overall, many challenges associated with tissue dielectric property measurements may arise in each of the above measurement techniques, for example, issues related to temperature change and tissue heterogeneity. Since the coaxial probe technique is by far the most commonly used method for tissue measurements [10–12,39–42,44,59,60,62,112,113], it will be examined in more detail in the subsequent sections.

3.2. Evolution of the Coaxial Probe Design and Fabrication

In the 1980s and 1990s, researchers conducting studies on dielectric measurements of biological tissues focused on probe design and fabrication, system development, and systemic error correction techniques [39,40,60–62,73]. The majority of the custom probes were fabricated from 50 Ω semi-rigid coaxial cables [39,40,60–62,94]. Probes were customised depending on the type and size of the tissue sample to be investigated and on the desired frequency range of the dielectric properties study.

Several custom-made probes were made of metal and Teflon [39,40,61,62]. Burdette et al. used a 2.1 mm diameter probe to perform in vivo and ex vivo measurement on animal tissue over the frequency range 0.1–10 GHz. This probe had a flange (i.e., a ground plane) to contain the electromagnetic field at the tip [39]. Kraszewski et al. performed in vivo animal measurements over the frequencies 0.1–12 GHz using a Teflon-filled metal probe with a 3.2 mm external diameter [40]. Gabriel et al. used two Teflon-filled metal probes for in vivo and ex vivo animal studies in order to acquire tissue dielectric properties at both low and high frequencies [42]. The probe used in the low frequency range (10^{-4}–200 MHz) had an external diameter of about 10 mm and the smaller probe, used for dielectric measurements at the frequency range between (0.2–20 GHz), had an external diameter of 2.9 mm [109]. Larger probes require a larger sample size due to the increased sensing volume (i.e., the region of the tissue that is interrogated by the electric field of the probe). In both Burdette et al. and Gabriel et al., the probe tips of the inner and outer conductors were plated with an inert metal, such as gold and platinum, to modify the effect of electrode polarisation, which is a manifestation of chemical reactions between the probe and the electrolytes (water molecules and hydrated ions) in the tissue [39,42]. Specifically, this plating process shifts the electrode polarisation, normally occurring at low frequencies, to even lower frequencies [39,46,109]. Popovic et al. reported that Teflon-filled copper probes, usually used for broadband reflection coefficient measurements, can cause inaccurate measurements because the probe aperture deteriorates easily and mechanical flaws can occur. The effects of small mechanical imperfections at the probe tip were quantified by the measured reflection coefficient and it was found that mechanical flaws at the probe tip can impact measurements by altering the reflection coefficient by up to 30% [114]. Notably, Teflon-filled copper probes do not meet bio-compatibility requirements nor can they be autoclaved (steam sterilised), both of which are required for safe in vivo measurements on human patients [73].

More recently, borosilicate glass-filled, stainless-steel, open-ended coaxial probes were designed and fabricated [73,115]. The use of thermally constant and matched, inert, refractory materials made the probe biocompatible and suitable for high-temperature sterilisation [73].

Over the last decade, a growing number of dielectric studies have been conducted using commercial probes [10,44,84,86]. Modern commercial probes are accurate [115], yet require specific sample dimensions and characteristics. In particular, Keysight probes, including the slim form probe, the performance probe, and the high temperature probe, have been used in most of the recent tissue dielectric studies [12,44,79,86,116]. Out of these, the slim form probe is a common choice for tissue measurements due to its small diameter and the fact that it can be steam-sterilised and, thus, used in vivo. The tissue dielectric measurements performed using these commercial probes are summarised in Table 1.

As the open-ended coaxial probe has been demonstrated to be the most applicable to measuring the dielectric properties of biological tissues, the remainder of this work will focus on the dielectric measurement process using this probe, from system calibration to biological sample preparation and analysis. In the next section, the calibration procedure for open-ended coaxial probes is discussed.

Table 1. Use of the commercial probe in recent works. Studies involving breast tissues are shaded in grey. The others involve liver tissues, apart from the porcine skin study in Karacolak et al. [116]. In the column "Relative permittivity range", the extreme values in relative permittivity are reported from lower to higher frequencies.

Recent Works	Probe	Frequency [GHz]	Tissue Type	Sample Size	Relative Permittivity Range	Conductivity Range [S/m]
Halter et al. (2009) [10]	Slim form with 2.2 mm diameter (in vivo) High temperature with 19 mm flange (ex vivo)	0.1–8.5	Ex vivo and in vivo Breast tumour (human)	5 mm thick	In vivo breast tissue: 95–45 Ex vivo breast tissue: 50–35	In vivo breast tissue: 0.1–10 Ex vivo breast tissue: 0.1–8
Karacolak et al. (2012) [116]	High temperature with 19 mm flange	0.3–3	Ex vivo skin (porcine)	45 × 45 × 4 mm^3	50–36	0.4–2.2
Lopresto et al. (2012) [29]	Slim form with 2.2 mm diameter	2.45	Ex vivo liver tissue (bovine)	20 × 20 × 50 mm^3	44.98–26.11 (temperature incremented from 15 °C to 98.9 °C, then decremented to 39.6 °C)	1.79–1.19 (temperature incremented from 15 °C to 98.9 °C, then decremented to 39.6 °C)
Sabouni et al. (2013) [86]	Performance with 9.5 mm diameter	0.5–20	Ex vivo breast tissue (human)	N/A	Breast tissue: 63–35 Fibroglandular breast tissue: 40–20	Breast tissue: 0.2–32 Fibroglandular breast tissue: 0.2–16.3
Abdilla et al. (2013) [44]	Slim form with 2.2 mm diameter	0.5–50	Ex vivo muscle and liver (bovine, porcine)	60 × 60 × 40 mm^3	Muscle tissue: 58–18 Liver tissue: 51–15	N/A(Loss factor for muscle/liver tissue: 32–10)
Sugitani et al. (2014) [12]	Slim form with 2.2 mm diameter	0.5–20	Ex vivo breast tumour (human)	50–300 mm diameter	Breast tumour tissue: 65–22 Breast fibroglandular tissue: 40–18 Breast fat tissue: 12–6	Breast tumour tissue: 0.1–25 Breast fibroglandular tissue: 0.1–12 Breast fat tissue: 0.1–3
Peyman et al. (2015) [84]	Slim form with 2.2 mm diameter	0.1–5	Ex vivo liver tissue (human)	20 mm thick	Liver normal tissue: 68–43 Liver tumour tissue: 68–32	Liver normal/tumour tissue: 0.7–5
Martellosio et al. (2017) [79]	Slim form with 2.2 mm diameter	0.5–50	Ex vivo breast tumour (human)	6 mm thick volume between 700 mm^3 and 1500 mm^3	Breast normal tissue: 64–3 Breast tumour tissue: 69–9	N/A (Breast normal tissue imaginary part: 41–0.1; Breast tumour tissue imaginary part: 45–4

4. Calibration and Confounders

A standard calibration procedure, involving both the coaxial probe and the VNA, must be performed before recording dielectric measurements [40,60,62,117]. In this section, a description of the calibration process is provided, followed by an in-depth analysis of the related confounders.

4.1. Standard Calibration

In general, coaxial probe measurements use a three load standard calibration procedure for one-port error correction. Any three different standard materials can be used for calibration, as long as the dielectric properties of those standards are well known [117–119]. The choice of standard materials to use may be based on ease of use, availability, or similarity to the materials under test [94,117]. The three most common standards used for coaxial probe calibration are: Open circuit, short circuit, and a broadband load [114,115]. We note that the use of the term "broadband load" here does not indicate a perfectly matched load, but rather, the broadband load can be any liquid with known dielectric properties. The calibration is performed at the reference plane of the probe, while the probe is connected to the VNA. The probe may be connected directly to the VNA or through a phase-stable cable. The calibration procedure aims to find a relation between the measured complex reflection coefficient and the expected one. This procedure allows for all post-calibration measurement data to be corrected [120]. If performed correctly, a good calibration procedure results in reliable measurements. The quality of the calibration depends on the accuracy in the measurements of the three standards and on the level of control over the factors that can affect the process. In the following subsection a list of the calibration steps required to reduce the confounders is reported. In addition, the confounders and methods for their compensation are summarised in Table 2.

Table 2. The standard calibration process: Common errors or confounders that occur for each step in the calibration process, along with the possible correction or compensation techniques. The open circuit, short circuit, and a liquid load material are shown as the three calibration standards.

Calibration Steps	Error or Confounder	Action for Correction or Compensation
Equipment set-up	• Environmental parameter change [95] • Probe contamination [27,37,39,121] • Imperfect connection [39] • Cable movement [43,76,80,115]	• Control environmental parameters [113,122] • Inspect and clean probe [29,41–43] • Check connections [39] • Fixing cable position (if not phase-stable) [29,44,86]
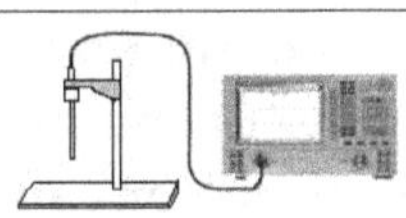 **Open**	• Particles on probe tip [95]	• Cleaning probe [29,41–43] • Checking the Smith Chart [123] to ensure open-circuit impedance is being measured
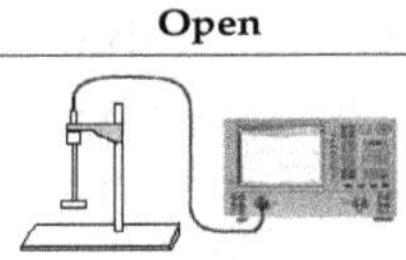 **Short**	• Poor probe-short block contact [95]	• Cleaning short block and probe [95] • Reposition or re-contact short block with probe [95] • Checking the Smith chart [123] to ensure short-circuit impedance is being measured
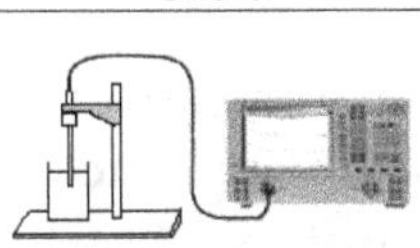 **Load**	• Accuracy of liquid model [94,117] • Liquid temperature [43,94,124,125] • Air bubbles [48,71,126] • Liquid contamination [43] • Probe position in liquid [71]	• Deionised water model has best accuracy [117] • Monitor or control temperature [29,43,44,95,121] • Re-immerse probe in liquid [95] • Limit exposure to air [43] • Place probe distant from beaker sides [71]

4.2. Calibration Procedure and Confounders

4.2.1. Equipment Set-Up and Confounders

Before performing the calibration, environmental parameters, such as temperature, pressure, and humidity, should be controlled or monitored [122,127] because environmental changes may impact measurement results [74]. Furthermore, system components should be checked [39], the probe tip cleaned and verified by visual inspection [29,41–43], and the cable (if not phase-stable) fixed in place [29,44,86] as imperfect connections [39], probe contamination [27,37,39,121], and cable movement [10,27,43,44,76,80,86,95,115] can all result in a poor calibration and, thus, unreliable measurements.

4.2.2. Signal Settings and Confounders

Prior to calibration, the frequency range needs to be selected based on the planned experiment. Subsequently, the number of acquisition frequency points must be defined. Frequency points may be equidistant according to a linear or a logarithmic scale. The use of a logarithmic scale can be advantageous when data is acquired over a larger frequency range as there will be more points taken at the frequency points where the largest change in dielectric properties occurs (due to dispersions) [128]. The signal power and measurement bandwidth must also be selected in the VNA software. The number of points and bandwidth requires a trade-off between the measurement accuracy and speed of data collection.

4.2.3. Measurement of the Three Standards and Confounders

Once the measurement settings are selected, the calibration measurements of the open-circuit, short-circuit, and broadband load can be performed. The common errors and confounders likely to occur during the calibration process are highlighted in Table 2, along with the recommended correction and compensation techniques. As noted in the table, while performing calibration, (when using modern VNAs) visualisation of the complex impedance on the VNA Smith chart is key to identifying the unwanted presence of particles at the probe tip and confirming the quality of the open or short circuit [56,95]. In particular, having a good quality short circuit is vital to a successful calibration [94]. Therefore, proper contact between the short and the probe must be ensured prior to completing the calibration. Other than this, the open and short measurements are relatively straightforward and do not require any additional consideration. In the case that the VNA does not allow visualisation of the Smith chart during calibration, the quality of the calibration can then be verified by performing the validation procedure, as described in Section 5.

Conversely, several confounders can introduce error into the load measurement. Different liquids have been examined as potential load materials. The permittivity of the standard liquid should be selected such that the complex impedance of the load is considerably different from the other two standards [129]. The most typical liquid used as a load is deionised (DI) water [12,27,80,86,116,130]. Polar liquids (for example, ethanol, methanol, and saline) also meet the requirements [129] and exhibit high conductivity and permittivity as a function of frequency. Nyshadham et al. examined the effect of the uncertainty of the models of different standard materials on the uncertainty of the measured permittivity [117]. In this study, different liquids (having different models) were used for calibration and it was verified that DI water has smaller uncertainties in the Debye model than that of other standard liquids (in other words, the dielectric properties of deionised water are the most well-known and well-characterised) [117]. Indeed, the accuracy of the model represents one of the confounders affecting the calibration procedure and the uncertainty of the measured permittivity. Specifically, a quantitative analysis that examined the impact of errors in the model of one of the calibration standards (in this case, acetone) found that model errors of 2% induced a similar magnitude of error into the measured relative permittivity [131]. However, despite the impact of model uncertainties, the best calibration material depends on the measurement scenario as the uncertainty will be lower for materials measured with properties similar to those of the calibration material.

Temperature of the Liquid

During the calibration process, the temperature of the load liquid needs to be maintained and monitored, since dielectric parameters are temperature-dependent [43,94,124,125]. The permittivity of liquids vary by up to 2.2% per degree Celsius [125]. The measurement of deionised water, or any standard liquid, as a calibration load may be performed at room temperature or at any fixed temperature. In the first case, the liquid temperature can be monitored using a thermometer [95]. In the second case, the temperature may be maintained using a water bath [29,43,44,121]. In addition, if the temperature of the liquid is different from the temperature of the probe, it is recommended to wait for the temperature to stabilise before proceeding with the measurement. We note that this information on the liquid temperature also applies to the liquid used in the validation step.

Other Confounders in the Liquid Measurement

Aside from the liquid temperature and model accuracy, other confounders, such as liquid contamination [43], air bubbles between the probe and the liquid [48,71,95,126], and probe position in the liquid-filled beaker [71], have been investigated. These confounders affect the load liquid used during calibration and the liquid used in the validation step equally—indeed, the same types of reference liquids can be used either for calibration or for validation.

In order to avoid any impurity in the water, the beaker filled with liquid should be kept closed [43]. The presence of air bubbles between the probe tip and the standard liquid can result in deviations in the dielectric measurement data by up to 20% due to the fact that the material within the sensing region is then a mixture of air and liquid [126]. A transparent beaker is recommended so that air bubbles can clearly be seen. If bubbles are present, they need to be removed prior to measurement. This may be completed by gently tapping the probe tip on the bottom of the beaker, or lowering the beaker away from the liquid and then re-immersing it on an angle [95]. A soft brush (non-metallic, to avoid scratches) may also be used to remove any bubbles without having to move the probe or the beaker. In addition, the probe should be immersed in the liquid and positioned in the beaker such that the liquid is the only material within the probe sensing volume. Accurate positioning avoids undesirable reflections from the beaker walls. Hagl et al. provided a process for finding the minimum distance between the probe and the beaker sides according to the probe size; these distances also depend on the properties of the liquid material in the beaker and the frequency range of interest [71].

4.3. Confounders Introduced in the System after Calibration

Following the calibration procedure, two additional system confounders can introduce errors in dielectric measurements: VNA drift over time and cable movement, although the movement of a phase-stable cable should not compromise the performance of the system [10,27,43,44,76,80,86,115]. The system drift should be characterised and taken into account in the measured dielectric data [43,44]. This factor can be quantified by taking several measurements on a standard liquid at defined time instants in the period after calibration [43]. When a cable that is not phase-stable is moved, given the difficulty in precisely characterising the systematic error introduced by the cable movement, a new calibration is required. However, low loss and phase-stable cables should be used to minimise the impact of the error of the cable stability on the results [71,76,94]. In some works, the cable was fixed in place (using adhesive tape) to limit the effect of the cable movement in the dielectric data [29,44,86]. An alternative approach may be to replace the cable with a right-angle connector, when the rigid set-up does not overly restrict dielectric data acquisition [128].

After each calibration, it is good practice to first confirm proper calibration by re-measuring one of the calibration standards, commonly the short [44]. Note that re-measuring the properties of materials used during calibration does not guarantee that the system is functioning error-free, it just indicates that the calibration error-correction algorithms were successfully applied. Thus, a measurement of a known liquid, other than the one used in calibration, is also required in order to validate the accuracy of the calibration. Details about the validation procedure and the measurement uncertainty calculation are discussed in the next section.

5. Validation and Measurement Uncertainty

The validation procedure consists of measuring the dielectric properties of a known reference liquid. To ensure that the measurements are accurate in materials with different properties, the validation material should not be the one used during the calibration (i.e., typically not deionised water). Validation enables determination of the quality of the calibration and the monitoring of systematic errors [43,44,75], such as VNA drift and noise due to cable movement [43]. Thus, it is good practice to perform validation immediately following calibration [39,43,71,121,132] and after acquiring a set of tissue dielectric data [76]. The validation should also be completed whenever anomalies are observed in the dielectric data of the investigated material in order to isolate the source of error. For instance, if the same anomalies are observed in the reference liquid dielectric trace, the error is due to changes in the system and a new calibration is needed; if the anomalies are not evident in the liquid trace, the error is sample-related and further investigation is needed to identify the source of the error.

During the validation procedure, monitoring or controlling the temperature of the liquid during the validation process is required, since the dielectric properties of reference liquids are temperature- and frequency-dependent [43,44,132].

Although system validation is a simple procedure, several confounders can introduce errors in the process. The factors that affect the validation quality are similar to those present in the load measurement during the calibration procedure. Thus, details regarding confounders in the liquid dielectric measurement and how they are addressed can be found in the previous section.

In this section, after describing the most common validation liquids, the role of the validation procedure in the calculation of the uncertainty of dielectric data is detailed.

5.1. Validation Liquids: Models, and Their Advantages and Disadvantages

Alcohols and saline are the most common polar reference liquids [39,71,75,76,125,133]. Polar solutions are particularly suitable as validation liquids because they have comparatively high relative permittivity and high dielectric loss at radio and microwave frequencies. Both the relative permittivity and conductivity have a strong frequency dependence, which is a feature of the pronounced molecular dielectric relaxation behaviour [94]. Liquids, in general, are selected for validation purposes as they are homogeneous and are free of many of the confounders affecting solids or semi-solids (e.g., incorrect probe-sample contact, inconsistent probe-sample pressure).

5.1.1. Alcohols

Methanol, ethanol, ethanediol, and butanol are the types of alcohols generally used to characterise the system and calculate the uncertainty in the dielectric measurements [44,71,72,76,117,125,132] prior to tissue measurements. Methanol, ethanol, and butanol, in particular, are used as standard liquids because they represent the high, intermediate, and low dielectric property values, respectively, within the range of those expected for human breast tissues at microwave frequencies [71,72,76,132]. They also have well-established permittivity models [72,76,125,132]. Ethanediol, which has also been modelled in the microwave frequency range [44,132–134], has a static permittivity about half that of pure water [134]. Standard methods for obtaining the known dielectric property values for each of these alcohols have been detailed thoroughly [132].

Although alcohols present properties similar to those of biological tissues at microwave frequencies (0.5–20 GHz), there are some constraints that must be taken into account when using them as reference liquids. For instance, the alcohol models are accurate in restricted frequency ranges and at discrete temperatures only [117,124,132,134,135]. Furthermore, the dielectric properties of alcohols can change during storage and handling. For example, methanol has very low vapour pressure and evaporates rapidly. This can contribute to a decrease in the liquid temperature and, consequently, to a dielectric property change over the course of just a few minutes when exposed to air [72,132]. In order to minimise these effects, the dielectric properties of methanol should be measured almost immediately after it is poured into the measurement beaker [72] and the temperature should be kept constant and monitored. Lastly, since alcohols are inflammable and have an acute inhalation toxicity, working with these liquids requires a safety protocol, such as the use of special fire-proof storage cabinets and handling under a fumehood [132].

5.1.2. Saline

The dielectric properties of different concentrations of NaCl (saline) solutions at various temperatures have been modelled in the microwave frequency range [49,75,136–138]. Specifically, Stogryn provided models in the gigahertz range for computing the complex permittivity of saline as a function of temperature and concentration (between 0.25 M and 0.5 M) in order to allow these liquids to be used as references [136]. More recent models, based on extended experimental data, are now available for solutions having concentrations between 0.001 mol/L and 5 mol/L in the frequency range of 0.10–40 GHz, for any temperature between 0 °C and 60 °C [49,130,133,137,138]. Although alcohol models are, generally, more accurate than saline models, saline solutions are the most convenient reference liquids used [133].

Among all of the saline solutions, 0.1 M NaCl solution is the most commonly used reference liquid to assess the uncertainty in measuring the dielectric properties of biological materials, since it has similar dielectric properties to those of biological tissues [43,44,133]. Furthermore, 0.1 M NaCl is stable in temperature and electrical properties during storage and handling. At room temperature, saline does not evaporate quickly like alcohols. Saline solutions are also straightforward to prepare (hence, commercially-bought solutions are cost-effective) [133] and to use. Saline solutions are also less dangerous than alcohols and, thus, they do not require the use of fire-proof storage cabinets or handling under a fumehood. For 0.1 M NaCl, models that cover relatively wide frequency and temperature ranges are available [133]. However, saline may not be the best choice as a validation liquid when DI water is used as calibration, since these two liquids have very similar dielectric properties in the microwave range. Furthermore, due to poor traceability of the data used to obtain the models in [133] (since the data was acquired with only a single measurement system and a single measurement technique, and then compared to reference data measured under unknown conditions), the saline models are likely not as accurate as the models for alcohols.

To this extent, future studies aimed at improving the reliability and accuracy of saline models have the potential to support dielectric data validation and uncertainty calculations.

5.1.3. Other Liquids

Several other liquids, such as formamide [75,84,134,137], DI water [94,124,132], dimethyl sulphoxide (DMSO) [94,132,139], and acetone [94,132,140], have been used as reference liquids.

Formamide is a polar organic solvent, which has a relative permittivity of approximately 110 at low frequencies that drops down to a high-frequency value of around 7 [134] (when handled at room temperature). The temperature-dependent model for characterising the dielectric properties of formamide across the microwave frequency range was developed by Jordan et al. and, more recently, by Barthel et al. using waveguide interferometry [75,134,135]. The parameters of different models were found at discrete temperatures in the frequency range between 0.2 GHz and 89 GHz. The reliability of the model in Jordan et al. is affected by the limited discrete frequency points used in the dielectric measurements from which the model has been obtained [134]. In both Jordan et al. and Barthel et al., the dielectric models are available only for limited discrete temperatures [134,135]. Also, since formamide is toxic, a custom handling protocol is required.

When it is not used as the broadband load in the calibration procedure, DI water represents an advantageous validation liquid [117,124]. In fact, DI water has dispersive properties similar to those of biological tissues and has been accurately modelled in the microwave frequency range for any temperature between −4.1 °C and 60 °C [124]. DI water also has the advantage of being a stable liquid and does not require special handling.

Dimethyl sulphoxide (DMSO) is a highly polar organic reagent that has a high relaxation frequency. DMSO has relative permittivity values similar to those of muscle tissues. Dielectric models for DMSO have been developed that cover a wide frequency range [139] and different temperatures [132]. DMSO is hygroscopic [94,132] and when it evaporates the liquid temperature increases, causing an increase in relative permittivity values [132]. Therefore, like with many alcohols, care should be taken to keep the liquid in a closed container as much as possible.

Acetone is a polar organic solvent that has intermediate permittivity values, which have been modelled only in the upper microwave frequency range [140]. Acetone requires special handling because it has a boiling point of 56 °C and has the potential to soften some plastics [94,132].

Liquid properties and information about available models and storage/handling procedure related to the most common categories of reference liquids are reported in Table 3. The column "Models" contains the most referenced models, i.e., those which cover the widest frequency range and largest, most continuous temperature interval.

Table 3. Reference liquid properties, available models, and storage and handling procedures (where f = frequency, T = temperature).

Liquid	Models	Storage and Handling
Methanol (alcohol with intermediate permittivity values similar to breast tissue)	Debye model [132]: • f = 0.1–5 GHz • T = [10 °C, 50 °C], 5 °C increments	Inflammable and acute inhalation toxicity. Fire-proof storage cabinets required. Handling in fumehood required.
	Cole-Cole model [134]: • f = 0.01–70 GHz • T = [10 °C, 40 °C], 10 °C increments	Rapid evaporation may occur and should be avoided.
Ethanediol (alcohol with high permittivity values similar to breast glandular tissue)	Cole-Davidson model [132]: • f = 0.1–5 GHz • T = [10 °C, 50 °C], 5 °C increments	Inflammable and acute inhalation toxicity. Fire-proof storage cabinets required. Handling in fumehood required. Ethanediol is hygroscopic and when it evaporates the liquid temperature increases, causing an increase in relative permittivity [132].
Ethanol (alcohol with intermediate permittivity values similar to breast tissue)	Debye-Γ model [132]: • f = 0.1–5 GHz • T = [10 °C, 5 0°C], 5°C increments	Inflammable and acute inhalation toxicity. Fire-proof storage cabinets required. Handling in fumehood required.
Butanol (alcohol with low permittivity values similar to fat tissue)	Double Debye model [132]: • f = 0.1–5 GHz • T = [10°C, 40°C], 5 °C increments	Inflammable and acute inhalation toxicity. Fire-proof storage cabinets required. Handling in fumehood required.
Saline (NaCl) (polar liquid having dielectric properties similar to biological tissues)	Cole-Cole model [133]: • Concentrations = [0.001 mol/l, 5 mol/l] • f = 0.13–20 GHz • T = [5 °C, 35 °C] (any intermediate T)	Storage in sealed containers. No special handling required.
	Cole-Davidson model [49]: • Concentrations = [0.001 mol/l, 1 mol/l] • f = 0.1–40 GHz • T = 17 temperatures in the interval [10 °C, 60 °C]: 10 °C, 20 °C, increments of 2 °C in [24 °C, 50 °C], and 60 °C.	
Formamide (polar organic solvent having wide permittivity spectrum at microwave frequencies)	Cole-Davidson model [135]: • f = 0.2–89 GHz • T = [10 °C, 25 °C], 5 °C increments • T = [25 °C, 65 °C], 10 °C increments	Toxic through inhalation, oral, or skin exposure. Fire-proof storage cabinets required. Handling in fumehood required.
DI water (polar liquid having well-known modelled properties)	Debye model [124]: • f = 1.1–57 GHz • T = [−4.1 °C, 60 °C] (any intermediate T)	Storage in sealed containers. No special handling required.
Dimethyl sulphoxide (DMSO) (highly polar organic reagent having high permittivity)	Debye model [132]: • f = 0.1–5 GHz • T = [10 °C, 50 °C], 5 °C increments Cole-Davidson model [139]: • f = 0.001–40 GHz • T = 25 °C	DMSO is exceptionally hygroscopic and needs to be measured as soon as the container is opened [132].
Acetone (polar organic solvent having intermediate permittivity values)	Static permittivity (since acetone has very high relaxation frequency) [132]: • f = 0.1–5 GHz • T = [10 °C, 50 °C], 5 °C increments	Acetone boiling point is at 56 °C [132].
	Budo model/confined rotator models [140]: • f = 50–310 GHz • T = 20 °C	Special handling is required, since it is a powerful liquid able to soften some plastics [94] and it is inflammable.

5.2. Uncertainty Calculation

It is always good practice to report uncertainty along with measured values. However, in dielectric measurement studies, the definitions used for uncertainty, including how they are calculated and reported, have varied widely.

Today, the uncertainty of measurements is generally calculated according to the guidelines defined by the National Institute of Standard and Technology (NIST) [43,44,75]. Multiple measurements performed on the same material of known dielectric properties enables determination of uncertainty of the measurement system in terms of the repeatability and accuracy. Considering the definition of uncertainty reported in [43,75], the repeatability of the measurement may be expressed quantitatively in terms of the characteristics (e.g., standard deviation) of data repeatedly acquired under the same measurement condition, as defined also in [74]; while the accuracy may be defined as the average percentage difference between the dielectric properties of the acquired data and those of the model [43,44]. These definitions represent practical methods of calculating these parameters. In this way, the repeatability varies between measurements and gives the extent of random errors, while the accuracy is constant across measurements.

The uncertainties in repeatability and accuracy both contribute to the total uncertainty in the dielectric measurements [43,44,74,75]. For example, the combined standard uncertainty may be calculated as the root sum squared of the standard uncertainties [43,75]. In Peyman et al., the standard uncertainties associated with Type A errors (repeatability), Type B errors (in the calibration and measurement of the reference liquids), VNA drift, and cable variations, were estimated and included in the combined standard uncertainty calculation [43]. These uncertainties were determined for 0.1 M NaCl and, undoubtedly, tissue measurements will be impacted by more and/or different uncertainties.

Alternatively, in Gregory et al., uncertainties associated with specific input parameters were thoroughly evaluated by means of Monte Carlo modelling [141]. Notably, this modelling technique also enables estimation of uncertainties in measurement scenarios when there are no suitable reference materials available (e.g., with similar material properties or frequency range) [141].

According to the NIST guidelines, the best practice for expressing uncertainty is to report the mean measured value along with a confidence interval (CI) of 95% [74]. For dielectric measurements, one may wish to present these parameters separately for both the real and imaginary parts of permittivity.

In the next section, techniques related to minimisation or compensation of tissue-related confounders are described.

6. Tissue Sample Preparation and Measurement Procedure

Tissue-related confounders may be the major cause of measurement uncertainty, since the total combined uncertainty for measurements on liquids is relatively small compared to that of tissue measurements [43]. Uncertainties associated with measuring tissue properties seem to be primarily related to the complex structure of biological tissues [39,43,122].

In order to reduce tissue-related confounders, it is useful to plan each set of measurements according to the experimental goal. The first step involves the choice of the target animals (since their age or weight could affect the dielectric properties [43,122,142]) and the sample tissue type. Aside from the source species, the number of samples should be chosen based on the scientific question. The following steps include the analysis of the various tissue-related confounders and the evaluation of different methods that aim to reduce or compensate for these confounders.

In the next subsection, the confounders related to probe choice, sample preparation, and handling are first described. Then, a discussion of the confounders that need to be considered during the measurement procedure is provided.

6.1. Probe Selection Considerations

Open-ended coaxial probes are suitable for use with materials that are liquid or semi-solid [95], homogeneous [95], have flat surfaces [66,95], and have a semi-infinite thickness [39,43,95]. Tissues are generally semi-solid (with the exception of bone), but they are not always homogeneous or have flat surfaces, and tissue samples that are much thicker and larger than the probe tip are not always easy to prepare. Hence, probe selection is affected by three main biological factors: Sample size, heterogeneity, and tissue surface. The desired frequency range of the measurement may also impact the choice of the probe.

6.1.1. Sample Size, Sensing Volume, and Heterogeneity

Dielectric spectroscopy techniques permit the acquisition of the average complex permittivity of the interrogated volume. Thus, the probe should be selected such that the sensing volume only contains the tissue sample of interest and no other material. Since probes with a small diameter have smaller sensing volumes compared to large flanged probes, the sample size has to be taken into account and compared to the sensing volume of the probe [71,72,76].

The sensing volume may be evaluated by performing preliminary experiments with different combinations of materials. To this end, Meaney et al. analysed the dielectric property change in two-layer materials, consisting of saline or DI water with Teflon or acrylic, by varying the thickness of the liquid layer to determine the influence of materials at different depths on the measurement. The experimental results suggested that the dielectric properties are dominantly influenced by the material present within only the first 200–400 microns from the probe tip, and that this depth did not vary significantly across frequency or material properties [80]. This was a key finding as previous studies had assumed a much larger region on the order of several millimetres [11]. While Meaney et al. and Hagl et al. both investigated the depth into a tissue that contributes to the dielectric measurement, they defined the depth parameter differently [71,80]. More recently, Porter et al. demonstrated how different definitions of the sensing depth can impact the determined sensing depth value and highlighted that, for some definitions, the value does depend on the frequency and dielectric properties of the tissues occupying the sensing volume [83]. The work of Porter et al. also confirmed the findings of Meaney et al., in that the experimental results demonstrated that the tissue in contact with the probe has a greater impact on the measured dielectric properties than deeper tissues [82]. Nevertheless, because the sensing volume may be affected by the intrinsic dielectric properties of the investigated sample, further experiments involving the analysis of materials with more complex structures across both radial and axial directions are needed in order to define the sensing volume accurately for complex tissue samples.

Heterogeneity of biological samples is a further factor to consider when choosing a probe, since it is challenging to determine the tissue-specific dielectric properties in an extended heterogeneous volume interrogated by the probe [39,43,76]. To date, the impact of tissue heterogeneity with only simplified configurations has been thoroughly modelled. For example, in Chen et al., it was demonstrated that, for bilayer materials, the permittivity of either layer can be calculated from the reflection coefficient without the need for information on the thickness of the first layer or the probe capacitances [143]. Models for the effective dielectric properties of bilayer materials, in general and in particular for coaxial probes, have also been presented in [107]. These results were also extended to a general multilayer material scenario [107]. Furthermore, Huclova et al. used a numerical three layer skin model to examine how variations in the layer properties (including thickness and permittivity), impact the dielectric measurement across frequency [144]. More complex heterogeneities have yet to be thoroughly investigated or quantified. Specific challenges associated with heterogeneous tissues (aside from their impact on probe selection) are discussed in Section 7.

6.1.2. Tissue Surface Characteristics

In addition to the sample size and heterogeneity, the quality of the tissue surface is another consideration when selecting the appropriate probe to use. Surface irregularities may contribute to inadequate probe-tissue contact and poor repeatability of dielectric measurements [42,43,60]. Characterisation of the tissue surface permits the identification of the tissue area or points that are most suitable for the acquisition of dielectric information [145]. For instance, thick samples and even surfaces are preferable to thin and uneven surfaces in order to ensure good probe contact with the tissue sample [42,60,95]. From the authors' experience, the use of a smaller probe on uneven tissue surfaces results in more reliable measurements, especially if these areas are limited or spatially restricted. Lower uncertainty in the measurements from smaller probes on uneven surfaces may be attributed to smaller forces being applied on smaller surfaces. Indeed, large uneven surfaces require the application of higher forces (and, consequently, higher pressures) to prevent the presence of air gaps between the probe and the tissue. An increased probe-sample pressure may cause fluid accumulation at the probe tip [39,43] or tissue damage [95], both of which can affect the tissue dielectric properties and lead to inaccurate data.

In summary, the probe should be selected not only on the basis of the probe characteristics and specifications (i.e., frequency range, permittivity range, temperature range, mechanical resistance) discussed in Section 3, but also based on the properties of the tissue under investigation. The size of the selected probe has to be consistent with the sample surface, size, and heterogeneity in order to achieve good probe-tissue contact and accurate measurements in a homogeneous region.

After selecting the probe, but before measuring the dielectric properties, it is recommended to carefully plan the tissue preparation and handling procedures in order to reduce tissue-related confounders, such as sample cooling, dehydration, and damage.

6.2. Tissue Preparation and Handling

Tissue measurements can be performed in vivo or ex vivo; the tissue preparation and handling will be different in each case. Often, for reasons of convenience (i.e., patient safety, ethics) or due to difficulties in establishing a good probe-sample contact with in vivo tissues, dielectric measurements of animal and human tissues are performed ex vivo.

6.2.1. In Vivo vs. Ex Vivo Measurements

Several authors have reported on whether or not differences exist in tissue dielectric properties acquired in vivo and ex vivo. These works will be discussed here in chronological order. Initially, Burdette et al. performed in vivo measurements on canine muscle, kidney cortical tissue, and fat tissue, and differences were found between acquired in vivo data and reported ex vivo data [39]. In particular, for in vivo canine fat tissue, the measured permittivity values were a factor of approximately 1.5 to 3 times larger than the in vitro permittivity values acquired previously by other authors [39,52,146]. This difference in dielectric properties was most likely due to differences in water content, in temperature, or actual physiological differences between living and non-living tissues [39]. Next, Kraszewski et al. performed both in vivo and ex vivo dielectric measurements on rat and cat tissues, finding only dielectric changes less than the uncertainty at frequencies between 100 MHz and 8 GHz [40]. Schwartz observed that the permittivity and conductivity of frog heart, in the frequency range 0.2–8 GHz, were higher in vivo than ex vivo, with the difference being attributed to blood perfusion changes [41]. More recently, a variation between in vivo and ex vivo dielectric properties was found by Gabriel et al. and Peyman et al. in skin, spinal cord, skull, long bone, and bone marrow in the microwave frequency range [42,43,66,142]. Similar differences were not observed in other tissues, but might indicate unavoidable contamination of tissues with blood or other body fluids [43]. From the analysis of normal and malignant human liver tissues, O'Rourke et al. found a statistically significant difference between in vivo and ex vivo normal liver tissue, but not between in vivo and ex vivo malignant liver tissue [37]. Furthermore, Halter et al. evaluated the changes of breast cancer dielectric properties between in vivo and ex vivo measurements and found about a 30% drop in the magnitude of the permittivity in tissues analysed 300 min after excision [10]. More recently, Shahzad et al. found that over the 210 min following excision, the relative permittivity of liver tissue, as measured on the surface of the sample, decreased by 32 points [147]. However, this decrease was attributed fully to dehydration of the surface of the tissue sample as dielectric measurements conducted on the interior of the sample did not change considerably over the same time period [147]. The exact magnitude of the change in dielectric properties from time of excision to time of measurement, caused by dehydration and temperature effects, will vary based on the tissue type, the environment that the tissue is stored in, and the tissue handling conditions.

As is clear from the varied results of these studies, there is no consensus on: (i) Whether a difference in the dielectric properties of in vivo and ex vivo tissues exists over the microwave frequency range; and (ii) if a difference does exist, the magnitude and direction of it. Despite these results, the difference between in vivo and ex vivo data in the microwave frequency range is, generally, attributed to the temperature change and tissue dehydration [10,30,39,43,86], and recent studies following best practice in dealing with these confounders suggest no significant difference in the dielectric properties measured from in vivo and ex vivo measurements [84,148]. Therefore, following best measurement practice, it is advantageous to keep the temperature constant during dielectric measurement using a temperature controlled container or a water bath [29,40,43,44,122,127,142] and to minimise dehydration by limiting the time between excision and measurement to a few hours [27,30,40,42,43,62,65,76,78,86,127,142,149–151]. At frequencies lower than 100 MHz, a larger variation between in vivo and ex vivo properties is found. This difference is attributed to physiological parameters, such as blood flow in vessels [27,39,65,86,151], ischemia [10,86,150,151], heart rate [43], arterial pressure [43,86,150], respiration rate [43], and air content in lungs [149], which can affect the permittivity and conductivity values at these frequencies.

In the following subsections, the best-practice steps involved in both in vivo and ex vivo measurements are described: From surgical intervention, to sample access and excision, transportation, handling, and processing. In each step, all potential tissue-related confounders, as well as the different methods used in previous works to compensate for them, are reported.

6.2.2. Surgical Intervention, Sample Access, and Excision

The first step in defining a sample handling procedure involves identifying the surgical methods to be used for tissue access and excision. It is necessary to define a surgical protocol that minimises tissue property modification. The main factors interfering with the dielectric acquisition concern the use of chemicals [39,127], which alter the body physiological condition, the use of tools or techniques [10], which may damage tissues, and the tissue exposure and cooling during the surgical operation [39–41,43,152].

It is useful to test for, and take into account, the effect of anaesthesia or other pharmaceuticals, which are used on animal/human tissues and physiological parameters. For instance, Burdette et al. observed a decrease in body temperature due to anaesthesia [39].

During the surgery, contact with the tissue should be minimised in order to avoid any damage or contamination. For human in vivo studies, the measurement tools need to be sterilised prior to surgery. Normally, steam sterilisation is performed prior to calibration [10,37] and a calibration refresh could be performed in the sterile environment before the in vivo measurements [10]. Furthermore, for in vivo measurements, the temperature tolerance of the probe (that depends on the probe fabrication materials) needs to be taken into account when selecting the sterilisation (or autoclave) procedure. For instance, steam sterilisation is, generally, performed at temperatures within 125 °C, while dry heat sterilisation can be conducted at temperatures up to 190 °C.

Other important confounders to take into consideration in the operating room during in vivo measurements are those related to the tissue exposure to air. Specifically, air contributes to tissue cooling (from body temperature to room temperature) and to tissue dehydration. Different techniques have been adopted in in vivo measurements to prevent tissue cooling and dehydration. For example, Ranck and BeMent performed experiments within a few minutes from the surgical cut used to expose the interior tissues, and used warm saline to wet the measurement region [152]. Schwartz et al. rinsed the tissues and kept them moist with frog physiological solution [41]. Hart and Dunfee applied Ringer's solution with a medicine dropper to the muscle to prevent drying between the measurements [153]. However, these methods to reduce dehydration can impact the dielectric property measurement, since the solutions used have their own dielectric properties that will then contribute to the dielectric measurement of the tissue. Thus, the use of solutions, especially saline, should be avoided. More commonly, tissue dehydration during an in vivo measurement is minimised by reducing the time between the surgical cut performed to expose the tissue and the dielectric measurement, and covering the area of interest with another tissue between measurement times [39,40,43]. This technique does not alter the tissue properties and also minimises tissue cooling. The tissue temperature should be measured frequently, so that any temperature change is taken into account during data analysis.

In previous works, the in vivo tissue temperature was monitored using thermocouple probes [27,29,62] and, more recently, fibre-optic thermometers [29,30]. Infrared thermometers may also be used for tissue temperature monitoring, since they are portable and do not require sample contact [79]. The same sensors can also be used in ex vivo measurements. A further crucial point in in vivo measurements concerns the probe positioning. Typically, in ex vivo scenarios, the probe–tissue contact can be verified by visual inspection; however, this approach can be challenging in a surgical setting. The probe positioning cannot be accurately planned prior to surgery; thus, it is normally decided in the surgical theatre.

6.2.3. Tissue Transportation

When ex vivo measurements are performed, the excised sample may be transported from the operating theatre to a secondary location for measurement, characterisation, or histology (details on histological analysis are presented in Section 7). The time between excision and ex vivo measurements is minimised to prevent tissue dehydration [27,30,40,42,43,62,78,86]. Aside from water content change, care should be taken during tissue transportation to avoid changes in the sample temperature. Since the temperature has a systematic impact on the measured dielectric spectrum of biological tissues, it is usually necessary to transport the tissue in hermetically-sealed, temperature-controlled containers [29,44,76,142].

6.2.4. Tissue Handling

In order to prevent tissue contamination, dehydration, and damage, sample handling prior to the ex vivo measurements should be minimised [39,71,76,142]. The sample temperature can be kept constant during the measurements using a water bath [29,40,43,122,142]. As the temperature setting of the water bath may not be equivalent to the tissue temperature, the tissue temperature should still be verified using an infrared or fibre-optic thermometer [29,30]. In this way, the tissue temperature variation can be taken into account during data analysis. Details on how tissue temperature affects the measured dielectric properties are reported in Section 6.3.3.

If the tissue sample is to be analysed histologically, the measurement points should be marked. Sample marking is necessary to ensure that the histological analysis involves the portion of tissue corresponding to the volume interrogated by the probe. Thus, a good correspondence between the tissue histological and dielectric properties can be found. Further details about the histological characterisation of tissue samples are reported in Section 7. In previous works, acrylic ink [76,79] or pins [10] have been used as sample markers. When ex vivo measurements are performed at the same locations where in vivo measurements were taken, it would be wise to test the effect of the marker on tissue dielectric properties before experimental implementation in order to prevent tissue modification or damage by the marker. Lastly, in order to maintain the integrity of the tissue, the use of additive and preservatives should be avoided until the measurement is completed [127].

Having presented the confounders that should be considered during the planning of the tissue measurement procedure, in the next subsection the actual measurement procedure and the key confounders that affect tissue dielectric property measurements are discussed.

6.3. Procedure for Tissue Measurements

After the equipment set-up, calibration, and validation, the measurements on in vivo or excised tissues can be performed. It is important to note that some confounders cannot be minimised even with careful preplanning. These confounders need to be controlled, monitored, or compensated for during the measurement phase. In order to minimise the effects of the environmental parameters on tissue dielectric properties, it is advantageous to perform measurements in a climate (temperature, pressure, and humidity) controlled room [43,127].

In the following paragraphs the main confounders occurring during the measurement phase, such as measurement region choice, probe-tissue contact, and pressure, as well as tissue sample temperature, are discussed.

6.3.1. Measurement Region Choice Confounders

The confounders mentioned in Section 6.1 (i.e., probe sensing volume, tissue thickness, tissue surface, and sample heterogeneity) need not only be considered in the planning phase, but also need to be controlled and managed in relation to the choice of the measurement region. Additional considerations may also be needed, for instance, in order to prevent undesirable reflections negatively affecting the measured data, Abdilla et al. placed a shorting block under the sample to check for any reflections from the sample boundaries [44].

Confounders intrinsic to the tissue type include: Fibre orientation in anisotropic tissues, presence of blood vessels, and high heterogeneity. It was observed that anisotropic tissues, such as muscles, present different dielectric properties according to the measurement directions along or across the fibre. Specifically, it has been found that in the microwave frequency range (from 200 MHz to 20 GHz) the permittivity values between the two sets of measurements are not substantially different. On the other hand, at lower frequencies (10^{-5}–1 MHz) the fibre direction can change the relative permittivity by 100% [42]. Blood vessels are non-uniformly distributed in tissues and may make up roughly 30% of their volume [144], so the probe position relative to that of blood vessels should be checked by visual inspection [65,151]. In highly heterogeneous and mechanically stiff tissues the uncertainty is generally higher and, in order to minimise the random errors arising from tissue heterogeneity and complexity, it is useful to repeat the measurements at multiple points [43,44,75]. For instance, Peyman et al. stated that as many measurements as possible should be taken on each sample tissue and, in her study conducted in 2005, at least six measurements were taken on each tissue [43]. In most other dielectric studies, three to five measurement locations were, generally, selected on each tissue sample [27,40,44].

6.3.2. Probe-Tissue Contact

Having selected the most suitable measurement region, the probe is placed in contact with the sample. From the authors' experience, in order to reduce the uncertainty due to probe and cable movement, in both ex vivo and in vivo measurements (in in vivo measurements only when the animal size is relatively small), it is convenient to move the sample towards the probe using a lift table until the entire probe aperture makes firm contact with the tissue sample as opposed to moving the probe during the measurement procedure.

Measured reflection coefficient data is extremely sensitive to the probe positioning relative to the sample surface. A high variability in the dielectric properties can be attributed to variability in probe-tissue contact. Thus, a firm contact between the probe and the tissue [76,93] is key. A good quality contact reduces the impact of confounders that increase the measurement uncertainty, such as pressure differences [39,43,80,97,149], air gaps [70,93,95,126], and biological fluid accumulation at the probe tip [39,43]. In most works, these factors have been monitored by a close visual inspection [29,41,43,76,95]. In order to keep the applied pressure constant in ex vivo measurements, weighing scales or force sensors can be placed underneath the sample holder [79]. In fact, the application of a steady pressure contributes to more repeatable measurements [39]. However, in the literature to date, there is no work that quantifies the error in the measured data in terms of the variation of the applied pressure. The authors have performed a number of experiments to quantify the error introduced by probe pressure variations, but observed that the outcome found for one measurement point could not be extended to all the measurement points across the sample. For instance, within the same tissue sample, there can be some differences in terms of sample thickness, tissue mechanical properties, water content, and surface irregularities, which may require the application of different probe pressures on the same sample. Thus, no specific, fixed pressure can be reported for all samples. However, a technique that may be used to obtain a good quality contact is as follows. First, a low pressure is applied to the probe to contact the sample. This low pressure, if too low, can lead to data inconsistencies when repeated measurements are taken at the same point (due to air gaps). If this occurs, a pressure adjustment can be undertaken until measurements at the same location are repeatable. Conversely, the application of high pressure, if too high, can cause tissue compression and can prompt fluid from within the tissue to rise to the tissue surface, or worse, can cause tissue damage [127,149]. In previous works, sample contamination by biological fluids has been reduced by using cotton wipes/swabs [43,99,127,142,152] or suction [43]. However, it should be noted that the suction method is more invasive and has the potential to dehydrate the sample.

6.3.3. Temperature Effects

During dielectric measurements, as discussed in Section 6.2.1, the temperature needs to be controlled and monitored. While different techniques used to monitor or control the temperature have been discussed in earlier sections, in this subsection the effect of temperature on tissue dielectric properties is examined.

In previous studies, the dielectric properties of biological tissues at discrete frequencies and temperatures were measured and, for small temperature variations, they were presented in terms of linear temperature coefficients, which are defined as the percent change in either permittivity or conductivity per degree Celsius [53]. The provided linear temperature coefficients are limited to a number of specific discrete frequencies and temperatures [27,30,62]. Outside of these frequencies and temperatures the impact of temperature on the dielectric properties may no longer be linear [30]. A brief summary of the previously published temperature-dependent dielectric properties data is presented in Lazebnik et al. [30]. In the microwave frequency range, the change in relative permittivity is, at most, 2% per degree Celsius and the change in conductivity is between 1% and 2% per degree Celsius, depending on the tissue and on the frequency and temperature range considered. Generally, the relative permittivity and conductivity trends with temperature differ over frequency. However, the magnitude change in both permittivity and conductivity per degree Celsius tends to be higher at lower frequencies in most biological tissues [27,30,62]. Lazebnik et al. developed a model to characterise the temperature-dependence of liver tissue dielectric properties over the microwave frequency range [30]. In particular, from the liver dielectric measurements, Lazebnik et al. identified different "cross-over" points in the trends of both relative permittivity and conductivity with temperature. In relative permittivity, the cross-over point was found at about 4 GHz. Below the cross-over point, the permittivity decreases slowly as temperature increases and, above the cross-over point, the permittivity increases with temperature. For conductivity, two cross-over points were found: One near 2–3 GHz and the other near 16 GHz. Below the first cross-over point, the conductivity increases slowly as temperature increases. Between the two cross-over points, the trend reverses, and above the second cross-over point, the conductivity again increases as temperature increases. The same trends were also found for water [30].

More recently, temperature coefficients were provided for a wider temperature range (up to 100 °C) at the discrete frequencies of 915 MHz and 2.45 GHz, which are of interest for microwave liver tissue ablation [31,154]. Brace et al. found that linear temperature coefficients across the 5–50 °C range agreed well with the results of Lazebnik et al., with coefficients of −0.22 and −0.18 in relative permittivity for the two frequency points, respectively, and coefficients of 1.29 and −0.2 for conductivity [31]. From 50 °C to 100 °C, both relative permittivity and conductivity were found to decrease by as much as 50%, due to both irreversible damage of the tissues and tissue dehydration [31]. In summary, the temperature coefficients for both permittivity and conductivity depend on tissue-type, on frequency, and on the considered temperature range. Knowledge of these temperature coefficients can be used to compensate for the effect of the temperature change during tissue dielectric measurements.

In this section, the importance of preplanning the measurement procedure was highlighted, the measurement process overviewed, and the main confounders involved in the measurement were described. The most common practices adopted to minimise tissue-related errors are summarised in Figure 2. In the next section, histological analysis of tissue samples is discussed as a method to reduce the confounders related to the intrinsic heterogeneity of biological tissues.

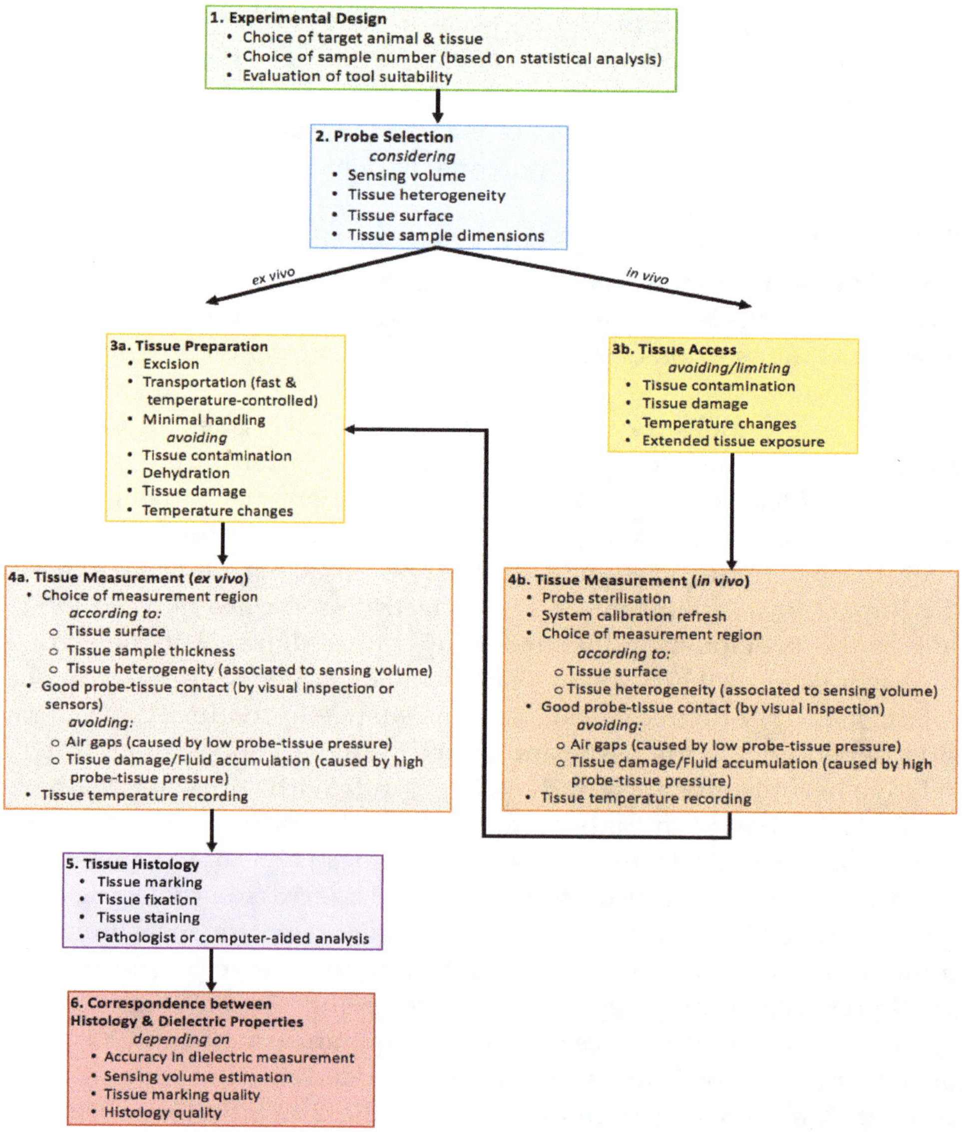

Figure 2. Flow chart of the common steps to minimise tissue-related errors in in vivo and ex vivo measurements.

7. Tissue Sample Histological Analysis

Histology is the study of the microscopic structure of cells and tissues; while histopathology refers to the same, but with diseased tissue [155,156]. There are multiple steps involved in the histological analysis of a tissue sample: The sample must be fixed, embedded in wax, sliced, mounted on slides, stained, and then imaged [157]. Following these steps, the slices are ready to be analysed by a pathologist. The pathologist is able to examine the images and determine: (i) The types of tissues present; (ii) if diseased tissue is present, the disease grade and other characteristics (for example, with breast cancer, the hormone receptor status) [156]; and (iii) the distribution of the tissue types within the sample. Histological analysis is, especially, required after the acquisition of the dielectric properties of a heterogeneous tissue sample in order to determine the tissue types present in the sample and their relative spatial distribution. This is important because the dielectric properties of a sample are determined by those of its constituent tissue types; thus, the histological analysis enables the attribution of measured dielectric properties to the appropriate tissue type.

Many studies performed in the literature involve only homogeneous (or assumed homogeneous) tissues and, thus, the samples do not undergo histological analysis (for example, liver tissue [27,44]). In this section, the focus is on heterogeneous tissue samples. Measuring the dielectric properties of heterogeneous tissues is inherently challenging as spectroscopy has the effect of averaging the dielectric properties throughout the sensing volume that is illuminated by the electromagnetic field [11]. Thus, in the next subsection, confounders that can contribute to any histological analysis are detailed, along with ones that are of specific concern for dielectric measurements of heterogeneous tissues. Finally, histological analysis methods used for attributing dielectric properties to heterogeneous tissues from the literature are overviewed, and the best practice techniques that are known are highlighted.

7.1. Factors Impacting Histological Analysis

The procedures involved with histological preparation of the tissue are applied by pathologists thousands, if not millions, of times per year. In fact, there are more than 14 pathology tests examined per person in the UK each year, and pathological analysis is a part of 70% of all diagnoses [158]. However, the methods are not without flaws. In particular, poor fixation of the sample can lead to changes in the tissue structure [11,157] and uneven levels of staining can result in images that are incomplete or out of focus [157]. Slide digitation can have variations in lighting conditions and magnification that can affect interpretation of the results, particularly when comparing across slices [157]. Each of these issues increases the challenge of interpreting the dielectric measurement of heterogeneous samples based on the histology of tissues samples and makes it especially difficult to compare between studies. Furthermore, the histological interpretation of a slice itself is subjective and variability in results between pathologists are possible [159–161]. Computer-aided diagnosis (CAD) and prognosis (CAP) methods are currently being investigated to create a fully automated analysis that is faster and more consistent than a human-based analysis [157]. An excellent review of challenges associated with histopathological analysis can be found in Veta et al. [157].

7.2. The Link between Heterogeneity, Histology, and Sensing Volume

When performing histology to support interpretation of the tissue content contributing to a dielectric measurement, it is important to include in the histological analysis all of the tissues that are within the sensing volume. However, at the same time, the histological analysis should not include any tissues that are outside of the sensing volume. In this way, only, and exactly, the tissues that have contributed to the measurement are analysed.

As an example, Figure 3 demonstrates the importance of matching the sensing depth with the number and thickness of slices taken into consideration in the histological analysis. If only Slice 1 is analysed, the tissue is found to be composed entirely of homogeneous glandular tissue. If the sensing depth is equal to the thickness of Slice 1, then the measured dielectric properties will be entirely the result of this layer of homogeneous gland tissue. Alternatively, if the sensing depth is equal to, say, the combined thickness of Slices 1 and 2, then the total sensing depth region is occupied by 25% fat tissue and 75% glandular tissue (as Slice 1 is 100% gland, and Slice 2 is 50% gland and 50% fat). Both of these tissue types will contribute to the measured dielectric properties. However, the contribution is not proportional to the tissue type representation (i.e., 25% fat and 75% gland) as the layer closest to the probe has the dominant effect [11,80,81]. Furthermore, not all of a given tissue is occupied fully by cells of that tissue type [12], thus, an additional layer of complication comes into the example based on how to determine what regions are actually "fat" and which are "gland". Obviously, as more slices are involved in the analysis and the tissue becomes more heterogeneous, the more challenging it becomes to conclusively determine the tissue composition breakdown. It is also important to re-emphasise here that the sensing volume is dependent on the tissue content (namely, the tissue dielectric properties), so, ideally, the change in the sensing volume should be taken into account on a sample-to-sample basis, as discussed in Section 6.

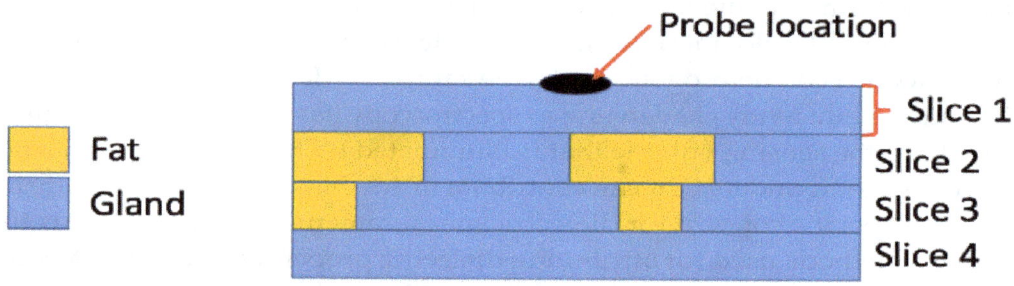

Figure 3. Diagram of sample composition by tissue type (fat—orange, gland—blue). A side view of the sample is shown, with slices marked. The dielectric probe measurement location is denoted with a black oval on the top of Slice 1.

7.3. Histological Analysis Techniques in Dielectric Studies

A limited number of works involving histological analysis for attributing the measured dielectric properties of heterogeneous tissues have been presented in the literature. Of these, some use pathology to categorise tissue samples by type [79,86], while a select few process the tissue for microscopic analysis [10–12,76]. In general, histology for dielectric characterisation is an area that requires further investigation [43]. The most common strategy is to obtain an average estimate of the tissue types present in the sample below the probe [10,11,76]. However, most recently a more quantitative method of counting each cell and corresponding the proportion of tissue with the measured properties has been proposed [12]. These techniques are described and compared in this section. For dielectric property measurements of heterogeneous tissue, breast tissues are by far the most common that have been analysed due to the need for these properties in medical microwave imaging of the breast. As a result, all pathology techniques discussed in this section have all been performed on breast tissues.

In Lazebnik et al., several hundred dielectric measurements were taken from normal and malignant excised breast tissue samples using an open-ended coaxial probe [11,76]. The measurement sites were marked on the tissue samples using a spot of black ink. The authors conducted a histological analysis of each sample based on the tissue composition inside the region of the sensing volume of the probe (3 mm deep $\times$ 7 mm across, for this measurement scenario, as determined in Hagl et al. [71]). In this way, a cross-section of each tissue sample was taken directly below the measurement location (i.e., the ink spot). Digital microscopy images were obtained and visually inspected. The tissue composition within the sensing volume was quantified based on the percentage of each tissue type residing within the slice under consideration. The two-dimensional cross-section was used to obtain an estimate of the tissue composition in the full three-dimensional sensing volume. The percentages of each tissue type (adipose (fat), glandular and fibroconnective tissue, along with benign and malignant tissue) were estimated visually by qualified pathologists [11,76]. A Kappa statistic was used to confirm consistency in the analysis between different pathologists. Several exclusion criteria were applied during the histological process. In particular, samples were eliminated from further consideration if the ink spot was not visible, if the ink had leaked into the tissue, or if the cross-sectional slice was deformed. In this study, nearly half of all samples (49.8%) were excluded based on difficulties during the histological procedure [76].

Following the studies by Lazebnik et al., Halter et al. performed a study that also examined the region under the probe using histological analysis. In Halter et al., the dielectric properties of in vivo and ex vivo breast tissues were measured in the microwave frequency range with open-ended coaxial probes [10]. After the in vivo tissue measurement was recorded, a biopsy clip was embedded in the tissue at the measurement location. The tissue was then excised and sectioned into 5 mm thick pieces. The excised samples were measured again (at the same site as for in vivo, as identified by the clip). Initially, the pathologist examined a 1 cm $\times$ 1 cm square area around the measurement location and, thus, the tissue types were estimated based on a large area. Later, the strategy was improved by inserting two pins covered in ink into the tissue on either side of the depression left by the probe in order to mark the measurement location. The tissue sample was fixed with formalin, stained, and then slides were prepared. The pin holes were then used during the analysis to determine the probed region in which the tissue types were estimated by the pathologist. In this study, details were not provided regarding whether or not samples had to be excluded from consideration due to histological challenges. The pathologist examined the tissue histology within the ~1 cm $\times$ 1 cm region, which was a horizontal slice relative to the probe position (i.e., perpendicular to the plane of the probe axis), unlike the vertical (or parallel) slice used in Lazebnik et al. However, in both cases, the full tissue composition within the sensing volume was estimated based on the given slice. Furthermore, as only one pathologist was involved in the study, a Kappa analysis similar to that in the study by Lazebnik et al. was not needed.

Most recently, in Sugitani et al., excised breast tissue samples were obtained and their complex permittivities measured using an open-ended coaxial probe [12]. The samples contained a combination of tumour tissue, normal fat tissue, and normal stroma (connective) tissue. The work aimed to calculate the effective permittivity of the tumour tissue based on the idea that each sample is an inhomogeneous mixture of cells with different permittivities. It was proposed, and confirmed, that, since the "tumour" tissue is composed of cancer cells mixed in with normal cells, the volume fraction of cancer cells in a sample affects the dielectric properties. In particular, the sample was treated with a hematoxylin-eosin stain and then digital images of each slice of the sample were taken. The slide images were analysed by counting the number of pixels of cancer cells and cells of other tissue types presented. The ratios of each type of tissue cell, relative to all of the cells in the slice, were calculated. The three-dimensional fractional volume of each cell type was calculated based on the two-dimensional slice using Bruggeman's effective medium approximation theory [162]. This method has the advantage of being highly quantifiable—each cell is counted—however, the process is tedious and time-consuming. The work does not mention if any samples had to be discarded or were contaminated during the histological procedures. Furthermore, the sample analysis was not restricted to a specific sensing depth region (sample sizes ranged from 5 cm to 30 cm). A similar study on various types of malignancies was presented in Sugitani et al. [85], for which the pathological procedures were the same as those in Sugitani et al. [12].

Overall, there is no consensus in the literature to date on the best practice for conducting histology in relation to dielectric measurements. Furthermore, there has been no reported comparison of the different histology techniques used in the above-mentioned works, therefore, it is not known if some methods are more accurate than others. However, it is likely that some features from each of the studies lend themselves to obtaining more accurate data, for example, involving multiple pathologists and using Kappa analysis to verify consistency between them (as in the study by Lazebnik et al.) could only add to the study quality.

8. Discussion and Conclusions

Although notable progress has been made in achieving accurate dielectric data, the coaxial probe design still represents a limit for certain types of dielectric experiments. An improved probe design that could allow measurements over a wider spectrum of frequencies and across multiple tissue samples would be useful for future studies. Moreover, during the measurement procedure, the use of appropriate force and position sensors could considerably increase the stability of the measurement system and reduce tissue-related confounders that are strictly dependent on the expertise of the operator conducting the dielectric measurement (i.e., probe-tissue contact and probe-tissue pressure).

Furthermore, interpretation of dielectric data acquired with the open-ended coaxial probe can be improved by quantitatively examining and compensating for tissue-related confounders that cannot be fully eliminated during the measurement procedure. To this extent, dielectric studies have modelled the effect of temperature, tissue dehydration, and animal age on the dielectric measurement of tissues. The quantitative characterisation of tissue-related confounders improves the interpretation of the acquired data and could support the interpretation of dielectric data from historic studies that did not provide information on all confounders. In order to clarify how such a characterisation could be done, a series of examples demonstrating how to determine the total uncertainty in a dielectric measurement are provided below.

This example scenario considers the case of dielectric measurement of mouse liver in the microwave frequency range, as the effect of the time from excision, temperature, and age of the mouse have all been quantified on liver tissue at these frequencies. In this example, it is assumed that the confounders of time from excision (TFE), temperature (T), and age (A), are the only ones impacting the dielectric data. The uncertainties introduced by these confounders are denoted as μ_{TFE}, μ_T, and μ_A, respectively. The relative permittivity of liver has been acquired at room temperature, 3.5 h from excision from a 70 day old mouse. From the literature it is known that at the frequency of 900 MHz, the relative permittivity changes by 0.13% per degree Celsius [30], decreases by about 25% after 3.5 h from excision [147], and decreases by approximately 15% within 70 days of life [142]. This quantitative information needs to be taken into account for the calculation of the combined standard uncertainty according to the NIST guidelines [74,75], which provides μ, the total uncertainty added to dielectric data. A series of hypothetical studies are listed in Table 4, along with the resulting uncertainty. The technique of calculating combined standard uncertainty to achieve a total estimate on the uncertainty introduced in dielectric measurement studies due to tissue-related confounders can and should be applied to all datasets, which lack quantitative information on confounders.

Given the importance of modelling the effect of the confounders for the interpretation and comparison of existing dielectric datasets, further investigation is needed to quantitatively examine the main tissue-related confounders (i.e., temperature, dehydration) on other tissue types and to analyse confounders not yet quantified (i.e., heterogeneity, probe pressure). Such quantitative analysis will not only improve the analysis of new dielectric data, but will also support the interpretation of historical dielectric datasets.

In conclusion, this work has presented the dielectric measurement process with an open-ended coaxial probe and reviewed the most relevant works, with a critical discussion of known equipment- and tissue-related confounders. This work supports the aim of achieving accurate dielectric measurements of biological tissues. As these properties are fundamental to electromagnetic safety studies and medical technology design and improvement, an understanding of the measurement process is of interest to a wide ranging community of scientists and medical professionals.

Table 4. Example calculations of total uncertainty in dielectric data resulting from tissue-related confounders under different measurement scenarios: Uncertainty due to time from excision (μ_{TFE}), due to temperature (μ_T), and due to age (μ_A). μ is the total uncertainty added to dielectric data, calculated as combined standard uncertainty. Uncertainty data is for the relative permittivity of mouse liver at 900 MHz, obtained from the literature. Note that 0.91% is 0.13%/°C · 7°C.

Case Scenarios	μ_T	μ_{TFE}	μ_A	μ
Known TFE, Known age, Unknown T (between 18 °C and 25 °C)	0.91%	N/A	N/A	0.91%
Known T, Known age, Unknown TFE (within 3.5 h)	N/A	25%	N/A	25%
Known T, Known TFE, Unknown age (within 70 days old)	N/A	N/A	15%	15%
Known T, Unknown TFE (within 3.5 h), Unknown age (within 70 days old)	N/A	25%	15%	29.15%
Known TFE, Unknown age (within 70 days old), Unknown T (between 18 °C and 25 °C)	0.91%	N/A	15%	15.02%
Unknown TFE (within 3.5 h), Unknown age (within 70 days old), Unknown T (between 18 °C and 25 °C)	0.91%	25%	15%	29.17%

Author Contributions: Conceptualization, M.O.; Methodology, E.P.; Investigation, A.L.G., I.M., E.P., A.S. and S.S.; Writing-Original Draft Preparation, A.L.G.; Writing-Review & Editing, E.P., I.M., M.O. and M.J.; Supervision, M.O. and E.P.; Project Administration, M.O.; Funding Acquisition, M.O.

Acknowledgments: This work has been developed in the framework of COST Action MiMed (TD1301).

References

1. Formica, D.; Silvestri, S. Biological Effects of Exposure to Magnetic Resonance Imaging: An Overview. *Biomed. Eng. Online* **2004**, *3*, 11. [CrossRef] [PubMed]
2. Martellosio, A.; Pasian, M.; Bozzi, M.; Perregrini, L.; Mazzanti, A. Exposure Limits and Dielectric Contrast for Breast Cancer Tissues: Experimental Results up to 50 GHz. In Proceedings of the 11th European Conference on Antennas and Propagation (EUCAP), Paris, France, 19–24 March 2017; pp. 667–671.
3. Nikolova, N.K. Microwave Imaging for Breast Cancer. *IEEE Microw. Mag.* **2011**, *12*, 78–94. [CrossRef]
4. Pastorino, M. *Microwave Imaging*; John Wiley & Sons: Hoboken, NJ, USA, 2010.
5. Noghanian, S. *Introduction to Microwave Imaging*; Springer: New York, NY, USA, 2014.
6. Zou, Y.; Guo, Z. A Review of Electrical Impedance Techniques for Breast Cancer Detection. *Med. Eng. Phys.* **2003**, *25*, 79–90. [CrossRef]
7. Brown, B. Electrical Impedance Tomography (EIT): A Review. *J. Med. Eng. Technol.* **2003**, *27*, 97–108. [CrossRef] [PubMed]
8. Waldmann, A.D.; Ortola, C.F.; Martinez, M.M.; Vidal, A.; Santos, A.; Marquez, M.P.; Roka, P.L.; Bohm, S.H.; Suarez-Sipmann, F. Position-Dependent Distribution of Lung Ventilation—A Feasability Study. In Proceedings of the 2015 IEEE Sensors Applications Symposium (SAS), Zadar, Croatia, 13–15 April 2015.

9. Avery, J.; Dowrick, T.; Faulkner, M.; Goren, N.; Holder, D. A Versatile and Reproducible Multi-Frequency Electrical Impedance Tomography System. *Sensors* **2017**, *17*, 280. [CrossRef] [PubMed]
10. Halter, R.J.; Zhou, T.; Meaney, P.M.; Hartov, A.; Barth, R.J.; Rosenkranz, K.M.; Wells, W.A.; Kogel, C.A.; Borsic, A.; Rizzo, E.J.; et al. The Correlation of in Vivo and Ex Vivo Tissue Dielectric Properties to Validate Electromagnetic Breast Imaging: Initial Clinical Experience. *Physiol. Meas.* **2009**, *30*, S121–S136. [CrossRef] [PubMed]
11. Lazebnik, M.; McCartney, L.; Popovic, D.; Watkins, C.B.; Lindstrom, M.J.; Harter, J.; Sewall, S.; Magliocco, A.; Booske, J.H.; Okoniewski, M.; et al. A Large-Scale Study of the Ultrawideband Microwave Dielectric Properties of Normal Breast Tissue Obtained from Reduction Surgeries. *Phys. Med. Biol.* **2007**, *52*, 2637–2656. [CrossRef] [PubMed]
12. Sugitani, T.; Kubota, S.; Kuroki, S.; Sogo, K.; Arihiro, K.; Okada, M.; Kadoya, T.; Hide, M.; Oda, M.; Kikkawa, T. Complex Permittivities of Breast Tumor Tissues Obtained from Cancer Surgeries. *Appl. Phys. Lett.* **2014**, *104*, 253702. [CrossRef]
13. Porter, E.; Kirshin, E.; Santorelli, A.; Coates, M.; Popović, M. Time-Domain Multistatic Radar System for Microwave Breast Screening. *IEEE Antennas Wirel. Propag. Lett.* **2013**, *12*, 229–232. [CrossRef]
14. Scapaticci, R.; Bellizzi, G.; Catapano, I.; Crocco, L.; Bucci, O.M. An Effective Procedure for MNP-Enhanced Breast Cancer Microwave Imaging. *IEEE Trans. Biomed. Eng.* **2014**, *61*, 1071–1079. [CrossRef] [PubMed]
15. O'Halloran, M.; Morgan, F.; Flores-Tapia, D.; Byrne, D.; Glavin, M.; Jones, E. Prototype Ultra Wideband Radar System for Bladder Monitoring Applications. *Prog. Electromagn. Res. C* **2012**, *33*, 17–28. [CrossRef]
16. Arunachalam, K.; MacCarini, P.; De Luca, V.; Tognolatti, P.; Bardati, F.; Snow, B.; Stauffer, P. Detection of Vesicoureteral Reflux Using Microwave Radiometrysystem Characterization with Tissue Phantoms. *IEEE Trans. Biomed. Eng.* **2011**, *58*, 1629–1636. [CrossRef] [PubMed]
17. Ireland, D.; Bialkowski, M.E. Microwave Head Imaging for Stroke Detection. *Prog. Electromagn. Res. M* **2011**, *21*, 163–175. [CrossRef]
18. Persson, M.; Fhager, A.; Trefna, H.D.; Yu, Y.; McKelvey, T.; Pegenius, G.; Karlsson, J.E.; Elam, M. Microwave-Based Stroke Diagnosis Making Global Prehospital Thrombolytic Treatment Possible. *IEEE Trans. Biomed. Eng.* **2014**, *61*, 2806–2817. [CrossRef] [PubMed]
19. Dowrick, T.; Blochet, C.; Holder, D. In Vivo Bioimpedance Measurement of Healthy and Ischaemic Rat Brain: Implications for Stroke Imaging Using Electrical Impedance Tomography. *Physiol. Meas.* **2015**, *36*, 1273–1282. [CrossRef] [PubMed]
20. Scapaticci, R.; Bucci, O.M.; Catapano, I.; Crocco, L. Differential Microwave Imaging for Brain Stroke Followup. *Int. J. Antennas Propag.* **2014**. [CrossRef]
21. Datta, N.R.; Ordóñez, S.G.; Gaipl, U.S.; Paulides, M.M.; Crezee, H.; Gellermann, J.; Marder, D.; Puric, E.; Bodis, S. Local Hyperthermia Combined with Radiotherapy And-/or Chemotherapy: Recent Advances and Promises for the Future. *Cancer Treat. Rev.* **2015**, *41*, 742–753. [CrossRef] [PubMed]
22. Issels, R.D.; Lindner, L.H.; Ghadjar, P.; Reichardt, P.; Hohenberger, P.; Verweij, J.; Abdel-Rahman, S.; Daugaard, S.; Salat, C.; Vujaskovic, Z.; et al. 13LBA Improved Overall Survival by Adding Regional Hyperthermia to Neo-Adjuvant Chemotherapy in Patients with Localized High-Risk Soft Tissue Sarcoma (HR-STS): Long-Term Outcomes of the EORTC 62961/ESHO Randomized Phase III Study. *Eur. J. Cancer* **2015**, *51*, S716. [CrossRef]
23. Wessalowski, R.; Schneider, D.T.; Mils, O.; Friemann, V.; Kyrillopoulou, O.; Schaper, J.; Matuschek, C.; Rothe, K.; Leuschner, I.; Willers, R.; et al. Regional Deep Hyperthermia for Salvage Treatment of Children and Adolescents with Refractory or Recurrent Non-Testicular Malignant Germ-Cell Tumours: An Open-Label, Non-Randomised, Single-Institution, Phase 2 Study. *Lancet Oncol.* **2013**, *14*, 843–852. [CrossRef]
24. Ekstrand, V.; Wiksell, H.; Schultz, I.; Sandstedt, B.; Rotstein, S.; Eriksson, A. Influence of Electrical and Thermal Properties on RF Ablation of Breast Cancer: Is the Tumour Preferentially Heated? *Biomed. Eng. Online* **2005**, *4*. [CrossRef] [PubMed]
25. Bargellini, I.; Bozzi, E.; Cioni, R.; Parentini, B.; Bartolozzi, C. Radiofrequency Ablation of Lung Tumours. *Insights Imaging* **2011**, *2*, 567–576. [CrossRef] [PubMed]

26. Curley, S.A.; Marra, P.; Beaty, K.; Ellis, L.M.; Vauthey, J.N.; Abdalla, E.K.; Scaife, C.; Raut, C.; Wolff, R.; Choi, H.; et al. Early and Late Complications after Radiofrequency Ablation of Malignant Liver Tumors in 608 Patients. *Ann. Surg.* **2004**, *239*, 450–458. [CrossRef] [PubMed]
27. Stauffer, P.R.; Rossetto, F.; Prakash, M.; Neuman, D.G.; Lee, T. Phantom and Animal Tissues for Modelling the Electrical Properties of Human Liver. *Int. J. Hyperth.* **2003**, *19*, 89–101. [CrossRef]
28. Yang, D.; Converse, M.; Mahvi, D.; Webster, J. Measurement and Analysis of Tissue Temperature during Microwave Liver Ablation. *IEEE Trans. Biomed. Eng.* **2007**, *54*, 150–155. [CrossRef] [PubMed]
29. Lopresto, V.; Pinto, R.; Lovisolo, G.; Cavagnaro, M. Changes in the Dielectric Properties of Ex Vivo Bovine Liver during Microwave Thermal Ablation at 2.45 GHz. *Phys. Med. Biol.* **2012**, *57*, 2309–2327. [CrossRef] [PubMed]
30. Lazebnik, M.; Converse, M.; Booske, J.H.; Hagness, S.C. Ultrawideband Temperature-Dependent Dielectric Properties of Animal Liver Tissue in the Microwave Frequency Range. *Phys. Med. Biol.* **2006**, *51*, 1941–1955. [CrossRef] [PubMed]
31. Brace, C.L. Temperature-Dependent Dielectric Properties of Liver Tissue Measured during Thermal Ablation: Toward an Improved Numerical Model. In Proceedings of the IEEE Engineering in Medicine and Biology Society, Vancouver, BC, Canada, 20–25 August 2008; pp. 230–233.
32. Wust, P.; Hildebrandt, B.; Sreenivasa, G.; Rau, B.; Gellermann, J.; Riess, H.; Felix, R.; Schlag, P.M. Hyperthermia in Combined Treatment of Cancer. *Lancet Oncol.* **2002**, *3*, 487–497. [CrossRef]
33. Ahmed, M.; Brace, C.L.; Lee, F.T.; Goldberg, S.N. Principles of and Advances in Percutaneous Ablation. *Radiology* **2011**, *258*, 351–369. [CrossRef] [PubMed]
34. Dupuy, D.E. Image-Guided Thermal Ablation of Lung Malignancies. *Radiology* **2011**, *260*, 633–655. [CrossRef] [PubMed]
35. Ji, Z.; Brace, C.L. Expanded Modeling of Temperature-Dependent Dielectric Properties for Microwave Thermal Ablation. *Phys. Med. Biol.* **2011**, *56*, 5249–5264. [CrossRef] [PubMed]
36. Cavagnaro, M.; Pinto, R.; Lopresto, V. Numerical Models to Evaluate the Temperature Increase Induced by Ex Vivo Microwave Thermal Ablation. *Phys. Med. Biol.* **2015**, *60*, 3287–3311. [CrossRef] [PubMed]
37. O'Rourke, A.P.; Lazebnik, M.; Bertram, J.M.; Converse, M.C.; Hagness, S.C.; Webster, J.G.; Mahvi, D.M. Dielectric Properties of Human Normal, Malignant and Cirrhotic Liver Tissue: In Vivo and Ex Vivo Measurements from 0.5 to 20 GHz Using a Precision Open-Ended Coaxial Probe. *Phys. Med. Biol.* **2007**, *52*, 4707–4719. [CrossRef] [PubMed]
38. Stuchly, M.A.; Athey, T.W.; Samaras, G.M.; Taylor, G.E. Measurement of Radio Frequency Permittivity of Biological Tissues with an Open-Ended Coaxial Line: Part II—Experimental Results. *IEEE Trans. Microw. Theory Tech.* **1982**, *30*, 87–92. [CrossRef]
39. Burdette, E.; Cain, F.; Seals, J. In Vivo Probe Measurement Technique for Determining Dielectric Properties at VHF through Microwave Frequencies. *IEEE Trans. Microw. Theory Tech.* **1980**, *28*, 414–427. [CrossRef]
40. Kraszewski, A.; Stuchly, M.A.; Stuchly, S.S.; Smith, A.M. In Vivo and in Vitro Dielectric Properties of Animal Tissues at Radio Frequencies. *Bioelectromagnetics* **1982**, *3*, 421–432. [CrossRef] [PubMed]
41. Schwartz, J.L.; Mealing, G.A. Dielectric Properties of Frog Tissues in Vivo and in Vitro. *Phys. Med. Biol.* **1985**, *30*, 117–124. [CrossRef] [PubMed]
42. Gabriel, S.; Lau, R.W.; Gabriel, C. The Dielectric Properties of Biological Tissues: II. Measurements in the Frequency Range 10 Hz to 20 GHz. *Phys. Med. Biol.* **1996**, *41*, 2251–2269. [CrossRef] [PubMed]
43. Peyman, A.; Holden, S.; Gabriel, C. *Mobile Telecommunications and Health Research Programme: Dielectric Properties of Tissues at Microwave Frequencies*; Microwave Consultants Limited: London, UK, 2005.
44. Abdilla, L.; Sammut, C.; Mangion, L. Dielectric Properties of Muscle and Liver from 500 MHz–40 GHz. *Electromagn. Biol. Med.* **2013**, *32*, 244–252. [CrossRef] [PubMed]
45. Schwan, H.P.; Foster, K.R. RF Field Interactions with Biological Systems: Electrical Properties and Biophysical Mechanisms. *Proc. IEEE* **1980**, *68*, 104–113. [CrossRef]
46. Foster, K.; Schwan, H. Dielectric Properties of Tissues and Biological Materials: A Critical Review. *Crit. Rev. Biomed. Eng.* **1989**, *17*, 25–104. [PubMed]
47. Gabriel, S.; Lau, R.W.; Gabriel, C. The Dielectric Properties of Biological Tissues: III. Parametric Models for the Dielectric Spectrum of Tissues. *Phys. Med. Biol.* **1996**, *41*, 2271–2293. [CrossRef] [PubMed]
48. Gregory, A.; Clarke, R.; Hodgetts, T.; Symm, G. *RF and Microwave Dielectric Measurements upon Layered Materials Using Coaxial Sensors*; NPL Report MAT 13; National Physical Laboratory: Teddington, UK, 2008.

49. Gulich, R.; Köhler, M.; Lunkenheimer, P.; Loidl, A. Dielectric Spectroscopy on Aqueous Electrolytic Solutions. *Radiat. Environ. Biophys.* **2009**, *48*, 107–114. [CrossRef] [PubMed]
50. England, T.S.; Sharples, N.A.A. Dielectric Properties of the Human Body in the Microwave Region of the Spectrum. *Nature* **1949**, *163*, 487–488. [CrossRef] [PubMed]
51. Cook, H.F. The Dielectric Behaviour of Some Types of Human Tissues at Microwave Frequencies. *Br. J. Appl. Phys.* **1951**, *2*, 295–300. [CrossRef]
52. Schwan, H.P. Electrical Properties of Tissue and Cell Suspensions. *Adv. Biol. Med. Phys.* **1957**, *5*, 147–209. [CrossRef] [PubMed]
53. Schwan, H.P.; Li, K. Capacity and Conductivity of Body Tissues at Ultrahigh Frequencies. *Proc. IRE* **1953**, *41*, 1735–1740. [CrossRef]
54. Stuchly, M.A.; Stuchly, S.S. Dielectric Properties of Biological Substances—Tabulated. *J. Microw. Power* **1980**, *15*, 19–25. [CrossRef]
55. Burdette, E.C.; Friederich, P.G.; Seaman, R.L.; Larsen, L.E. In Situ Permittivity of Canine Brain: Regional Variations and Postmortem Changes. *IEEE Trans. Microw. Theory Tech.* **1986**, *34*, 38–50. [CrossRef]
56. Smith, S.R.; Foster, K.R. Dielectric Properties of Low-Water-Content Tissues. *Phys. Med. Biol.* **1985**, *30*, 965–973. [CrossRef] [PubMed]
57. Zhadobov, M.; Augustine, R.; Sauleau, R.; Alekseev, S.; Di Paola, A.; Le Quément, C.; Mahamoud, Y.S.; Le Dréan, Y. Complex Permittivity of Representative Biological Solutions in the 2–67 GHz Range. *Bioelectromagnetics* **2012**, *33*, 346–355. [CrossRef] [PubMed]
58. Di Meo, S.; Martellosio, A.; Pasian, M.; Bozzi, M.; Perregrini, L.; Mazzanti, A.; Svelto, F.; Summers, P.; Renne, G.; Preda, L.; et al. Experimental Validation of the Dielectric Permittivity of Breast Cancer Tissues up to 50 GHz. In Proceedings of the IEEE MTT-S International Microwave Workshop Advanced Materials and Processes for RF and THz Applications (IMWS-AMP), Pavia, Italy, 20–22 September 2017; pp. 20–22.
59. Stuchly, M.A.; Stuchly, S.S. Coaxial Line Reflection Methods for Measuring Dielectric Properties of Biological Substances at Radio and Microwave Frequencies-A Review. *IEEE Trans. Instrum. Meas.* **1980**, *29*, 176–183. [CrossRef]
60. Athey, T.W.; Stuchly, M.A.; Stuchly, S.S. Measurement of Radio Frequency Permittivity of Biological Tissues with an Open-Ended Coaxial Line: Part I. *IEEE Trans. Microw. Theory Tech.* **1982**, *30*, 82–86. [CrossRef]
61. Gabriel, C.; Grant, E.H.; Young, I.R. Use of Time Domain Spectroscopy for Measuring Dielectric Properties with a Coaxial Probe. *J. Phys. E* **1986**, *19*, 843–846. [CrossRef]
62. Foster, K.R.; Schepps, J.L.; Stoy, R.D.; Schwan, H.P. Dielectric Properties of Brain Tissue between 0.01 and 10 GHz. *Phys. Med. Biol.* **1979**, *24*, 1177–1187. [CrossRef] [PubMed]
63. Surowiec, A.; Stuchly, S.S.; Eidus, L.; Swarup, A. In Vitro Dielectric Properties of Human Tissues at Radiofrequencies. *Phys. Med. Biol.* **1987**, *32*, 615. [CrossRef] [PubMed]
64. Pethig, R. Dielectric Properties of Biological Materials: Biophysical and Medical Applications. *IEEE Trans. Electr. Insul.* **1984**, *EI-19*, 453–474. [CrossRef]
65. Schepps, J.L.; Foster, K.R. The UHF and Microwave Dielectric Properties of Normal and Tumour Tissues: Variation in Dielectric Properties with Tissue Water Content. *Phys. Med. Biol.* **1980**, *25*, 1149. [CrossRef] [PubMed]
66. Gabriel, C.; Gabriel, S.; Corthout, E. The Dielectric Properties of Biological Tissues: I. Literature Survey. *Phys. Med. Biol.* **1996**, *41*, 2231–2249. [CrossRef] [PubMed]
67. Gabriel, C. *Compilation of the Dielectric Properties of Body Tissues at RF and Microwave Frequencies*; Report N.AL/OE-TR-1996-0037; Occupational and Environmental Health Directorate, Radiofrequency Radiation Division: Brooks Air Force Base, TX, USA, 1996.
68. Federal Communications Commission. *Tissue Dielectric Properties*; FCC: Washington, DC, USA, 2008. Available online: https://www.fcc.gov/general/body-tissue-dielectric-parameters (accessed on 30 October 2017).
69. Andreuccetti, D.; Fossi, R.; Petrucci, C. *An Internet Resource for the Calculation of the Dielectric Properties of Body Tissues in the Frequency Range 10 Hz–100 GHz*; IFAC-CNR: Florence, Italy, 1997; Available online: http://niremf.ifac.cnr.it/tissprop/ (accessed on 4 June 2018).
70. Alanen, E.; Lahtinen, T.; Nuutinen, J. Variational Formulation of Open-Ended Coaxial Line in Contact with Layered Biological Medium. *IEEE Trans. Biomed. Eng.* **1998**, *45*, 1241–1248. [CrossRef] [PubMed]

71. Hagl, D.; Popovic, D.; Hagness, S.C.; Booske, J.H.; Okoniewski, M. Sensing Volume of Open-Ended Coaxial Probes for Dielectric Characterization of Breast Tissue at Microwave Frequencies. *IEEE Trans. Microw. Theory Tech.* **2003**, *51*, 1194–1206. [CrossRef]
72. Popovic, D.; Okoniewski, M.; Hagl, D.; Booske, J.H.; Hagness, S.C. Volume Sensing Properties of Open Ended Coaxial Probes for Dielectric Spectroscopy of Breast Tissue. In Proceedings of the IEEE Antennas and Propagation Society, Boston, MA, USA, 8–13 July 2001; pp. 254–257.
73. Popovic, D.; McCartney, L.; Beasley, C.; Lazebnik, M.; Okoniewski, M.; Hagness, S.C.; Booske, J.H. Precision Open-Ended Coaxial Probes for in Vivo and Ex Vivo Dielectric Spectroscopy of Biological Tissues at Microwave Frequencies. *IEEE Trans. Microw. Theory Tech.* **2005**, *53*, 1713–1721. [CrossRef]
74. Taylor, B.N.; Kuyatt, C.E. *Guidelines for Evaluating and Expressing the Uncertainty of NIST Measurement Results*; NIST Technical Note 1297; US Department of Commerce, Technology Administration, National Institute of Standards and Technology: Gaithersburg, MD, USA, 1994.
75. Gabriel, C.; Peyman, A. Dielectric Measurement: Error Analysis and Assessment of Uncertainty. *Phys. Med. Biol.* **2006**, *51*, 6033–6046. [CrossRef] [PubMed]
76. Lazebnik, M.; Popovic, D.; McCartney, L.; Watkins, C.B.; Lindstrom, M.J.; Harter, J.; Sewall, S.; Ogilvie, T.; Magliocco, A.; Breslin, T.M.; et al. A Large-Scale Study of the Ultrawideband Microwave Dielectric Properties of Normal, Benign and Malignant Breast Tissues Obtained from Cancer Surgeries. *Phys. Med. Biol.* **2007**, *52*, 6093–6115. [CrossRef] [PubMed]
77. Chaudhary, S.S.; Mishra, R.K.; Swarup, A.; Thomas, J.M. Dielectric Properties of Normal & Malignant Human Breast Tissues at Radiowave & Microwave Frequencies. *Indian J. Biochem. Biophys.* **1984**, *21*, 76–79. [PubMed]
78. Joines, W.T.; Zhang, Y.; Li, C.; Jirtle, R.L. The Measured Electrical Properties of Normal and Malignant Human Tissues from 50 to 900 MHz. *Med. Phys.* **1994**, *21*, 547–550. [CrossRef] [PubMed]
79. Martellosio, A.; Pasian, M.; Bozzi, M.; Perregrini, L.; Mazzanti, A.; Svelto, F.; Summers, P.E.; Renne, G.; Preda, L.; Bellomi, M. Dielectric Properties Characterization from 0.5 to 50 GHz of Breast Cancer Tissues. *IEEE Trans. Microw. Theory Tech.* **2017**, *65*, 998–1011. [CrossRef]
80. Meaney, P.M.; Gregory, A.; Epstein, N.; Paulsen, K.D. Microwave Open-Ended Coaxial Dielectric Probe: Interpretation of the Sensing Volume Re-Visited. *BMC Med. Phys.* **2014**, *14*, 1–11. [CrossRef] [PubMed]
81. Meaney, P.M.; Gregory, A.P.; Seppälä, J.; Lahtinen, T. Open-Ended Coaxial Dielectric Probe Effective Penetration Depth Determination. *IEEE Trans. Microw. Theory Tech.* **2016**, *64*, 915–923. [CrossRef] [PubMed]
82. Porter, E.; La Gioia, A.; Santorelli, A.; O'Halloran, M. Modeling of the Dielectric Properties of Biological Tissues within the Histology Region. *IEEE Trans. Dielectr. Electr. Insul.* **2017**, *24*, 3290–3301. [CrossRef]
83. Porter, E.; O'Halloran, M. Investigation of Histology Region in Dielectric Measurements of Heterogeneous Tissues. *IEEE Trans. Dielectr. Electr. Insul.* **2017**, *65*, 5541–5552. [CrossRef]
84. Peyman, A.; Kos, B.; Djokić, M.; Trotovšek, B.; Limbaeck-Stokin, C.; Serša, G.; Miklavčič, D. Variation in Dielectric Properties Due to Pathological Changes in Human Liver. *Bioelectromagnetics* **2015**, *36*, 603–612. [CrossRef] [PubMed]
85. Sugitani, T.; Arihiro, K.; Kikkawa, T. Comparative Study on Dielectric Constants and Conductivities of Invasive Ductal Carcinoma Tissues. *IEEE Eng. Med. Biol. Soc.* **2015**, 4387–4390. [CrossRef]
86. Sabouni, A.; Hahn, C.; Noghanian, S.; Sauter, E.; Weiland, T. Study of the Effects of Changing Physiological Conditions on Dielectric Properties of Breast Tissues. *ISRN Biomed. Imaging* **2013**, *2013*, 894153. [CrossRef]
87. Reinecke, T.; Hagemeier, L.; Schulte, V.; Klintschar, M.; Zimmermann, S. Quantification of Edema in Human Brain Tissue by Determination of Electromagnetic Parameters. In Proceedings of the IEEE Sensors, Baltimore, MD, USA, 3–6 November 2013; pp. 1–4.
88. Nicolson, A.; Ross, G.F. Measurement of the Intrinsic Properties of Materials by Time-Domain Techniques. *IEEE Trans. Instrum. Meas.* **1970**, *19*, 377–382. [CrossRef]
89. Weir, W.B. Automatic Measurement of Complex Dielectric Constant and Permeability. *Proc. IEEE* **1974**, *62*, 33–36. [CrossRef]
90. Baker-Jarvis, J.; Vanzura, E.J.; Kissick, W.A. Improved Technique for Determining Complex Permittivity with the Transmission/Reflection Method. *IEEE Trans. Microw. Theory Tech.* **1990**, *38*, 1096–1103. [CrossRef]
91. Kim, S.; Baker-Jarvis, J. An Approximate Approach To Determining the Permittivity and Permeability near $\lambda/2$ Resonances in Transmission/Reflection Measurements. *Prog. Electromagn. Res. B* **2014**, *58*, 95–109. [CrossRef]

92. Boughriet, A.H.; Legrand, C.; Chapoton, A. Noniterative Stable Transmission/Reflection Method for Low-Loss Material Complex Permittivity Determination. *IEEE Trans. Microw. Theory Tech.* **1997**, *45*, 52–57. [CrossRef]
93. Baker-Jarvis, J.; Janezic, M.; Domich, P.; Geyer, R. Analysis of an Open-Ended Coaxial Probe with Lift-off for Non Destructive Testing. *IEEE Trans. Instrum. Meas.* **1994**, *43*, 1–8. [CrossRef]
94. Gregory, A.; Clarke, R. A Review of RF and Microwave Techniques for Dielectric Measurements on Polar Liquids. *IEEE Trans. Dielectr. Electr. Insul.* **2006**, *13*, 727–743. [CrossRef]
95. Agilent. *Basics of Measuring the Dielectric Properties of Materials*; Agilent Technologies: Santa Clara, CA, USA, 2005.
96. Land, D.V.; Campbell, A.M. A Quick Accurate Method for Measuring the Microwave Dielectric Properties of Small Tissue Samples. *Phys. Med. Biol.* **1992**, *37*, 183. [CrossRef] [PubMed]
97. Campbell, A.; Land, D.V. Dielectric Properties of Female Human Breast Tissue Measured in Vitro at 3.2 GHz. *Phys. Med. Biol.* **1992**, *37*, 193–210. [CrossRef] [PubMed]
98. Peng, Z.; Hwang, J.Y.; Andriese, M. Maximum Sample Volume for Permittivity Measurements by Cavity Perturbation Technique. *IEEE Trans. Instrum. Meas.* **2014**, *63*, 450–455. [CrossRef]
99. Campbell, A. Measurements and Analysis of the Microwave Dielectric Properties of Tissues. *J. Appl. Phys.* **1990**, *22*, 95.
100. Ramos, A.; Bertemes-Filho, P. Numerical Sensitivity Modeling for the Detection of Skin Tumors by Using Tetrapolar Probe. *Electromagn. Biol. Med.* **2011**, *30*, 235–245. [CrossRef] [PubMed]
101. Raghavan, K.; Porterfield, J.E.; Kottam, A.T.G.; Feldman, M.D.; Escobedo, D.; Valvano, J.W.; Pearce, J.A. Electrical Conductivity and Permittivity of Murine Myocardium. *IEEE Trans. Biomed. Eng.* **2009**, *56*, 2044–2053. [CrossRef] [PubMed]
102. Karki, B.; Wi, H.; McEwan, A.; Kwon, H.; Oh, T.I.; Woo, E.J.; Seo, J.K. Evaluation of a Multi-Electrode Bioimpedance Spectroscopy Tensor Probe to Detect the Anisotropic Conductivity Spectra of Biological Tissues. *Meas. Sci. Technol.* **2014**, *25*, 075702. [CrossRef]
103. Misra, D.K. A Quasi-Static Analysis of Open-Ended Coaxial Lines. *IEEE Trans. Microw. Theory Tech.* **1987**, *35*, 925–928. [CrossRef]
104. Grant, J.P.; Clarke, R.N.; Symm, G.T.; Spyron, N.M. A Critical Study of the Open-Ended Coaxial-Line Sensor Technique for RF and Microwave Complex Permittivity Measurements. *J. Phys. E Sci. Instrum.* **1989**, *22*, 757–770. [CrossRef]
105. Jenkins, S.; Preece, A.W.; Hodgetts, T.E.; Symm, G.T.; Warham, A.G.P.; Clarke, R.N. Comparison of Three Numerical Treatments for the Open-Ended Coaxial Line Sensor. *Electron. Lett.* **1990**, *26*, 234–236. [CrossRef]
106. Misra, D. On the Measurement of the Complex Permittivity of Materials by an Open-Ended Coaxial Probe. *IEEE Microw. Guid. Wave Lett.* **1995**, *5*, 161–163. [CrossRef]
107. Perez Cesaretti, M.D. General Effective Medium Model for the Complex Permittivity Extraction with an Open-Ended Coaxial Probe in Presence of a Multilayer Material under Test. Ph.D. Thesis, University of Bologna, Bologna, Italy, 2012.
108. Keysight Technologies. *Keysight E5063A ENA Series Network Analyzer*; Keysight Technologies: Santa Clara, CA, USA, 2015.
109. Gabriel, C.; Chan, T.Y.; Grant, E.H. Admittance Models for Open Ended Coaxial Probes and Their Place in Dielectric Spectroscopy. *Phys. Med. Biol.* **1994**, *39*, 2183–2200. [CrossRef] [PubMed]
110. Berube, D.; Ghannouchi, F.M.; Savard, P. A Comparative Study of Four Open-Ended Coaxial Probe Models for Permittivity Measurements of Lossy Dielectric/Biological Materials at Microwave Frequencies. *IEEE Trans. Microw. Theory Tech.* **1996**, *44*, 1928–1934. [CrossRef]
111. Zajíček, R.; Oppl, L.; Vrba, J. Broadband Measurement of Complex Permitivity Using Reflection Method and Coaxial Probes. *Radioengineering* **2008**, *17*, 14–19.
112. Schwan, H.P.; Foster, K.R. Microwave Dielectric Properties of Tissue. Some Comments on the Rotational Mobility of Tissue Water. *Biophys. J.* **1977**, *17*, 193–197. [CrossRef]
113. Peyman, A. Dielectric Properties of Tissues; Variation with Structure and Composition. In Proceedings of the International Conference on Electromagnetics in Advanced Applications (ICEAA), Torino, Italy, 14–18 September 2009; pp. 863–864.
114. Popovic, D.; Okoniewski, M. Effects of Mechanical Flaws in Open-Ended Coaxial Probes for Dielectric Spectroscopy. *IEEE Microw. Wirel. Components Lett.* **2002**, *12*, 401–403. [CrossRef]

115. Keysight. N1501A Dielectric Probe Kit 10 MHz to 50 GHz: Technical Overview. 2015. Available online: http://www.Keysight.Com/En/Pd-2492144-Pn-N1501A/Dielectric-Probe-Kit (accessed on 30 October 2017).
116. Karacolak, T.; Cooper, R.; Unlu, E.S.; Topsakal, E. Dielectric Properties of Porcine Skin Tissue and in Vivo Testing of Implantable Antennas Using Pigs as Model Animals. *IEEE Antennas Wirel. Propag. Lett.* **2012**, *11*, 1686–1689. [CrossRef]
117. Nyshadham, A.; Sibbald, C.L.; Stuchly, S.S. Permittivity Measurements Using Open-Ended Sensors and Reference Liquid Calibration—An Uncertainty Analysis. *IEEE Trans. Microw. Theory Tech.* **1992**, *40*, 305–314. [CrossRef]
118. Marsland, T.P.; Evans, S. Dielectric Measurements with an Open-Ended Coaxial Probe. *IEE Proc. H Microw. Antennas Propag.* **1987**, *134*, 341–349. [CrossRef]
119. Piuzzi, E.; Merla, C.; Cannazza, G.; Zambotti, A.; Apollonio, F.; Cataldo, A.; D'Atanasio, P.; De Benedetto, E.; Liberti, M. A Comparative Analysis between Customized and Commercial Systems for Complex Permittivity Measurements on Liquid Samples at Microwave Frequencies. *IEEE Trans. Instrum. Meas.* **2013**, *62*, 1034–1046. [CrossRef]
120. Packard, H. Automating the HP 8410B Microwave Network Analyzer. *Appl. Note* **1980**, *221*, 1–25.
121. Bobowski, J.S.; Johnson, T. Permittivity Measurements of Biological Samples by an Open-Ended Coaxial Line. *Prog. Electromagn. Res.* **2012**, *40*, 159–183. [CrossRef]
122. Peyman, A.; Holden, S.J.; Watts, S.; Perrott, R.; Gabriel, C. Dielectric Properties of Porcine Cerebrospinal Tissues at Microwave Frequencies: In Vivo, in Vitro and Systematic Variation with Age. *Phys. Med. Biol.* **2007**, *52*, 2229–2245. [CrossRef] [PubMed]
123. Smith, P.H. Transmission Line Calculator. *Electronics* **1939**, *12*, 29–31.
124. Kaatze, U. Complex Permittivity of Water as a Function of Frequency and Temperature. *J. Chem. Eng. Data* **1989**, *34*, 371–374. [CrossRef]
125. Anderson, J.M.; Sibbald, C.L.; Stuchly, S.S. Dielectric Measurements Using a Rational Function Model. *IEEE Trans. Microw. Theory Tech.* **1994**, *42*, 199–204. [CrossRef]
126. De Langhe, P.; Blomme, K.; Martens, L.; De Zutter, D. Measurement of Low-Permittivity Materials Based on a Spectral-Domain Analysis for the Open-Ended Coaxial Probe. *IEEE Trans. Instrum. Meas.* **1993**, *42*, 879–886. [CrossRef]
127. Peyman, A.; Gabriel, C.; Grant, E.H.; Vermeeren, G.; Martens, L. Variation of the Dielectric Properties of Tissues with Age: The Effect on the Values of SAR in Children When Exposed to Walkie-Talkie Devices. *Phys. Med. Biol.* **2009**, *54*, 227–241. [CrossRef] [PubMed]
128. Salahuddin, S.; Porter, E.; Meaney, P.M.; O'Halloran, M. Effect of Logarithmic and Linear Frequency Scales on Parametric Modelling of Tissue Dielectric Data. *Biomed. Phys. Eng. Express* **2017**, *3*, 1–11. [CrossRef] [PubMed]
129. Kraszewski, A.; Stuchly, M.A.; Stuchly, S.S. ANA Calibration Method for Measurements of Dielectric Properties. *IEEE Trans. Instrum. Meas.* **1983**, *32*, 385–387. [CrossRef]
130. Buchner, R.; Hefter, G.T.; May, M.P. Dielectric Relaxation of Aqueous NaCl Solutions. *J. Phys. Chem.* **1999**, *103*, 1–9. [CrossRef]
131. Wei, Y.Z.; Sridhar, S. Radiation-Corrected Open-Ended Coax Line Technique for Dielectric Measurements of Liquids up to 20 GHZ. *IEEE Trans. Microw. Theory Tech.* **1991**, *39*, 526–531. [CrossRef]
132. Gregory, A.P.; Clarke, R.N. *Tables of the Complex Permittivity of Dielectric Reference Liquids at Frequencies up to 5 GHz*; NPL Report MAT 23; National Physical Laboratory: Teddington, UK, 2012.
133. Peyman, A.; Gabriel, C.; Grant, E.H. Complex Permittivity of Sodium Chloride Solutions at Microwave Frequencies. *Bioelectromagnetics* **2007**, *28*, 264–274. [CrossRef] [PubMed]
134. Jordan, B.P.; Sheppard, R.J.; Szwarnowski, S. The Dielectric Properties of Formamide, Ethanediol and Methanol. *J. Phys. D Appl. Phys.* **1978**, *11*, 695–701. [CrossRef]
135. Barthel, J.; Buchner, R. High Frequency Permittivity and Its Use in the Investigation of Solution Properties. *Pure Appl. Chem.* **1991**, *63*, 1473–1482. [CrossRef]
136. Stogryn, A. Equations for Calculating the Dielectric Constant of Saline Water. *IEEE Trans. Microw. Theory Tech.* **1971**, *19*, 733–736. [CrossRef]
137. Nortemann, K.; Hilland, J.; Kaatze, U. Dielectric Properties of Aqueous NaCl Solutions at Microwave Frequencies. *J. Phys. Chem. A* **1997**, *101*, 6864–6869. [CrossRef]

138. Lamkaouchi, K.; Balana, A.; Delbos, G.; Ellison, W.J. Permittivity Measurements of Lossy Liquids in the Range 26-110 GHz. *Meas. Sci. Technol.* **2003**, *14*, 444–450. [CrossRef]
139. Kaatze, U.; Pottel, R.; Schaefer, M. Dielectric Spectrum of Dimethyl Sulfoxide/Water Mixtures as a Function of Composition. *J. Phys. Chem.* **1989**, *93*, 5623–5627. [CrossRef]
140. Vij, J.K.; Grochulski, T.; Kocot, A.; Hufnagel, F. Complex Permittivity Measurements of Acetone in the Frequency Region 50–310 GHz. *Mol. Phys.* **1991**, *72*, 353–361. [CrossRef]
141. Gregory, A.P.; Clarke, R.N. Dielectric Metrology with Coaxial Sensors. *Meas. Sci. Technol.* **2007**, *18*, 1372–1386. [CrossRef]
142. Peyman, A.; Rezazadeh, A.; Gabriel, C. Changes in the Dielectric Properties of Rat Tissue as a Function of Age at Microwave Frequencies. *Phys. Med. Biol.* **2001**, *46*, 1617–1629. [CrossRef] [PubMed]
143. Chen, G.; Li, K.; Ji, Z. Bilayered Dielectric Measurement With an Open-Ended Coaxial Probe. *IEEE Trans. Microw. Theory Tech.* **1994**, *42*, 966–971. [CrossRef]
144. Huclova, S.; Baumann, D.; Talary, M.; Fröhlich, J. Sensitivity and Specificity Analysis of Fringing-Field Dielectric Spectroscopy Applied to a Multi-Layer System Modelling the Human Skin. *Phys. Med. Biol.* **2011**, *56*, 7777–7793. [CrossRef] [PubMed]
145. Meaney, P.M.; Golnabi, A.; Fanning, M.W.; Geimer, S.D.; Paulsen, K.D. Dielectric Volume Measurements for Biomedical Applications. In Proceedings of the 13th International Symposium on Antenna Technology and Applied Electromagnetics and the Canadian Radio Sciences Meeting, Toronto, ON, Canada, 15–18 February 2009.
146. Johnson, C.C.; Guy, A.W. Nonionizing Electromagnetic Wave Effects in Biological Materials and Systems. *Proc. IEEE* **1972**, *60*, 692–718. [CrossRef]
147. Shahzad, A.; Sonja, K.; Jones, M.; Dwyer, R.M.; O'Halloran, M. Investigation of the Effect of Dehydration on Tissue Dielectric Properties in Ex Vivo Measurements. *Biomed. Phys. Eng. Express* **2017**, *3*, 1–9. [CrossRef]
148. Farrugia, L.; Wismayer, P.S.; Mangion, L.Z.; Sammut, C.V. Accurate in Vivo Dielectric Properties of Liver from 500 MHz to 40 GHz and Their Correlation to Ex Vivo Measurements. *Electromagn. Biol. Med.* **2016**, *8378*, 1–9. [CrossRef]
149. Nopp, P.; Rapp, E.; Pfützner, H.; Nakesch, H.; Ruhsam, C. Dielectric Properties of Lung Tissue as a Function of Air Content. *Phys. Med. Biol.* **1993**, *38*, 699–716. [CrossRef] [PubMed]
150. Gabriel, C.; Peyman, A.; Grant, E.H. Electrical Conductivity of Tissue at Frequencies below 1 MHz. *Phys. Med. Biol.* **2009**, *54*, 4863–4878. [CrossRef] [PubMed]
151. Haemmerich, D.; Ozkan, R.; Tungjitkusolmun, S.; Tsai, J.Z.; Mahvi, D.; Staelin, S.T.; Webster, J.G. Changes in Electrical Resistivity of Swine Liver after Occlusion and Postmortem. *Med. Biol. Eng. Comput.* **2002**, *40*, 29–33. [CrossRef] [PubMed]
152. Ranck, J.B.; Bement, S.L. The Specific Impedance of the Dorsal Columns of Cat: An Anisotropic Medium. *Exp. Neurol.* **1965**, *11*, 451–463. [CrossRef]
153. Hart, F.X.; Dunfee, W.R. In Vivo Measurement of the Low-Frequency Dielectric Spectra of Frog Skeletal Muscle. *Phys. Med. Biol.* **1993**, *38*, 1099–1112. [CrossRef] [PubMed]
154. Lopresto, V.; Pinto, R.; Farina, L.; Cavagnaro, M. Treatment Planning in Microwave Thermal Ablation: Clinical Gaps and Recent Research Advances. *Int. J. Hyperth.* **2017**, *33*, 83–100. [CrossRef] [PubMed]
155. Young, B.; Woodford, P.; O'Dowd, G. *Wheater's Functional Histology: A Text and Colour Atlas*, 6th ed.; Elsevier Health Sciences: London, UK, 2013.
156. Cross, S.S. Grading and Scoring in Histopathology. *Histopathology* **1998**, *33*, 99–106. [CrossRef] [PubMed]
157. Veta, M.; Pluim, J.P.W.; Van Diest, P.J.; Viergever, M.A. Breast Cancer Histopathology Image Analysis: A Review. *IEEE Trans. Biomed. Eng.* **2014**, *61*, 1400–1411. [CrossRef] [PubMed]
158. National Health Service (NHS). *Pathology*; National Health Service (NHS): London, UK, 2016.
159. Verkooijen, H.M.; Peterse, J.L.; Schipper, M.E.I.; Buskens, E.; Hendriks, J.H.C.L.; Pijnappel, R.M.; Peeters, P.H.M.; Borel Rinkes, I.H.M.; Mali, W.P.T.M.; Holland, R. Interobserver Variability between General and Expert Pathologists during the Histopathological Assessment of Large-Core Needle and Open Biopsies of Non-Palpable Breast Lesions. *Eur. J. Cancer* **2003**, *39*, 2187–2191. [CrossRef]
160. Gomes, D.S.; Porto, S.S.; Balabram, D.; Gobbi, H. Inter-Observer Variability between General Pathologists and a Specialist in Breast Pathology in the Diagnosis of Lobular Neoplasia, Columnar Cell Lesions, Atypical Ductal Hyperplasia and Ductal Carcinoma in Situ of the Breast. *Diagn. Pathol.* **2014**, *9*, 121. [CrossRef] [PubMed]

161. Gage, J.C.; Schiffman, M.; Hunt, W.C.; Joste, N.; Ghosh, A.; Wentzensen, N.; Wheeler, C.M. Cervical Histopathology Variability among Laboratories: A Population-Based Statewide Investigation. *Am. J. Clin. Pathol.* **2013**, *139*, 330–335. [CrossRef] [PubMed]
162. Bruggeman, D.A.G. Berechnung Verschiedener Physikalischer Konstanten von Heterogenen Substanzen. 1. Dielektizitatskonstanten Und Leitfahigkeiten Der Mischkorper Aus Isotropen Substanzen. *Ann. Phys.* **1935**, *24*, 636–679. [CrossRef]

7

Impact of Information Loss on Reconstruction Quality in Microwave Tomography for Medical Imaging

Zhenzhuang Miao, Panagiotis Kosmas * and Syed Ahsan

Faculty of Natural and Mathematical Sciences, King's College London, Strand, London WC2R 2LS, UK; zhenzhuang.miao@kcl.ac.uk (Z.M.); syed.s.ahsan@kcl.ac.uk (S.A.)

* Correspondence: panagiotis.kosmas@kcl.ac.uk

Abstract: This paper studies how limited information in data acquired by a wideband microwave tomography (MWT) system can affect the quality of reconstructed images. Limitations can arise from experimental errors, mismatch between the system and its model in the imaging algorithm, or losses in the immersion and coupling medium which are required to moderate this mismatch. We also present a strategy for improving reconstruction performance by discarding data that is dominated by experimental errors. The approach relies on recording transmitted signals in a wide frequency range, and then correlating the data in different frequencies. We apply this method to our wideband MWT prototype, which has been developed in our previous work. Using this system, we present results from simulated and experimental data which demonstrate the practical value of the frequency selection approach. We also propose a K-neighbour method to identify low quality data in a robust manner. The resulting enhancement in imaging quality suggests that this approach can be useful for various medical imaging scenarios, provided that data from multiple frequencies can be acquired and used in the reconstruction process.

Keywords: microwave tomography; medical imaging; reconstruction

---

1. Introduction

Microwave tomography (MWT) is emerging as a promising method for medical imaging [1], as it is capable of producing quantitative diagnostic images by estimating the distribution of dielectric properties in a tissue region. This requires solving an electromagnetic (EM) inverse scattering problem using, for example, conjugate gradient techniques [2,3] and algorithms based on the Gauss-Newton (GN) [4] or distorted Born iterative method (DBIM) [5,6]. EM inverse scattering algorithms typically require a forward solver to model experimental data acquisition; therefore, MWT prototypes [7–11] must be carefully designed to reduce the error between this forward model and the actual experiment.

In our previous work [12,13], we presented a novel DBIM approach which applied the two-step iterative shrinkage/thresholding algorithm (TwIST) to solve the ill-posed linear system at each DBIM iteration. The TwIST algorithm uses two previous iterates [14] to compute the update of the linear solver at each DBIM iteration. This can lead to faster convergence and more accurate reconstructions compared to conventional adaptive thresholding methods [15]. Our work first showed that the TwIST algorithm can increase robustness relative to one-step iterative methods by optimising a set of flexible parameters [12]. Subsequently, we presented a set of additional optimisation strategies, which can improve significantly the quality of reconstructions in microwave breast imaging [13]. Recently, we deployed the DBIM-TwIST algorithm with an in-house wideband microwave tomography system to reconstruct cylindrical targets filled with water inside a background medium of 90% glycerol-water mixture [16].

MWT algorithms are challenged by various sources of error which are inevitable in experimental systems and cannot be accounted for in the forward model employed by any EM inverse scattering algorithm. These include, for example, antenna fabrication and soldering errors which result in non-identical array elements, EM coupling not only by the antennas but also their coaxial cables, and EM interference by the environment due to imperfect shielding of the measurement system. In addition to these, signal contributions from surface waves and multiple reflections can also obscure the signal due to the object of interest. We note that information loss is also caused by signal attenuation due to the coupling liquid; although this can be accounted for in the inversion, increased losses in the immersion-coupling liquid can have a deteriorating effect upon the reconstruction quality [13]. Designing a wideband measurement system that can diminish these errors and information loss is of course impossible, but developing a strategy to discard frequencies for which data is dominated by errors can improve reconstruction quality. To this end, we propose applying a correlation function to select frequencies with highly-correlated data. Our results demonstrate that this is a simple but effective way to improve reconstruction quality and avoid convergence into wrong solutions.

The remainder of this paper is structured as follows. Section 2 provides a summary of the hardware and software features of our MWT prototype, which sets the context for the challenges and methods presented in this work. It also discusses how information loss is caused in MWT, and illustrates its strong impact on image quality, even if data is produced by numerical simulations without any experimental errors. Finally the section proposes a simple strategy to reduce reconstructions errors by applying a correlation metric to select highly correlated data and discard outliers which can be due to numerical modeling or experimental errors. Results in Section 3 present reconstructions from simulated and experimental data which demonstrate the benefit of this approach for improving image quality. Finally, Section 4 provides a short summary and discussion of our findings with some further observations.

2. Materials and Methods

2.1. Overview of Our MWT System

2.1.1. Experimental System

Our MWT system was fully presented in [16], and is reviewed in Figure 1. The setup consists of two concentric cylindrical tanks with 100 and 200 mm diameters. A target of 16 mm diameter can be placed inside the inner tank to emulate the discontinuity in the homogeneous background medium. We have surrounded the outer periphery of the larger tank with an absorber covered with a metallic shield. Our eight-antenna configuration forms a circular ring of 130 mm diameter inside the outer acrylic tank. Vertical and horizontal mounts allow us to control the antenna positions with good precision.

The system's antenna has been designed to operate inside various dielectrics, with a reflection coefficient below -10 dB almost within the whole range of 1.0–3.0 GHz, and a voltage standing ratio (VSWR) below 2.0. The antenna's small size (12×15 mm^2) can reduce unwanted multipath signals, while its monopole-resembling operation allows it to be easily modelled by our imaging algorithm, relative to more complex antenna designs. For cases of simple cylindrical targets with high dielectric contrast, the system operates well with a 90% glycerol-water mixture as immersion liquid. In particular, 90% glycerol-water has shown to widen the antenna operation and reduce multipath signals without attenuating signal transmission levels below the noise floor. Although the reflection coefficient of the antenna is below -10 dB in the whole range 1.0–3.0 GHz, our initial reconstruction results are more accurate around 1.5–2.0 GHz, where the antenna operates more efficiently inside 90% glycerol-water.

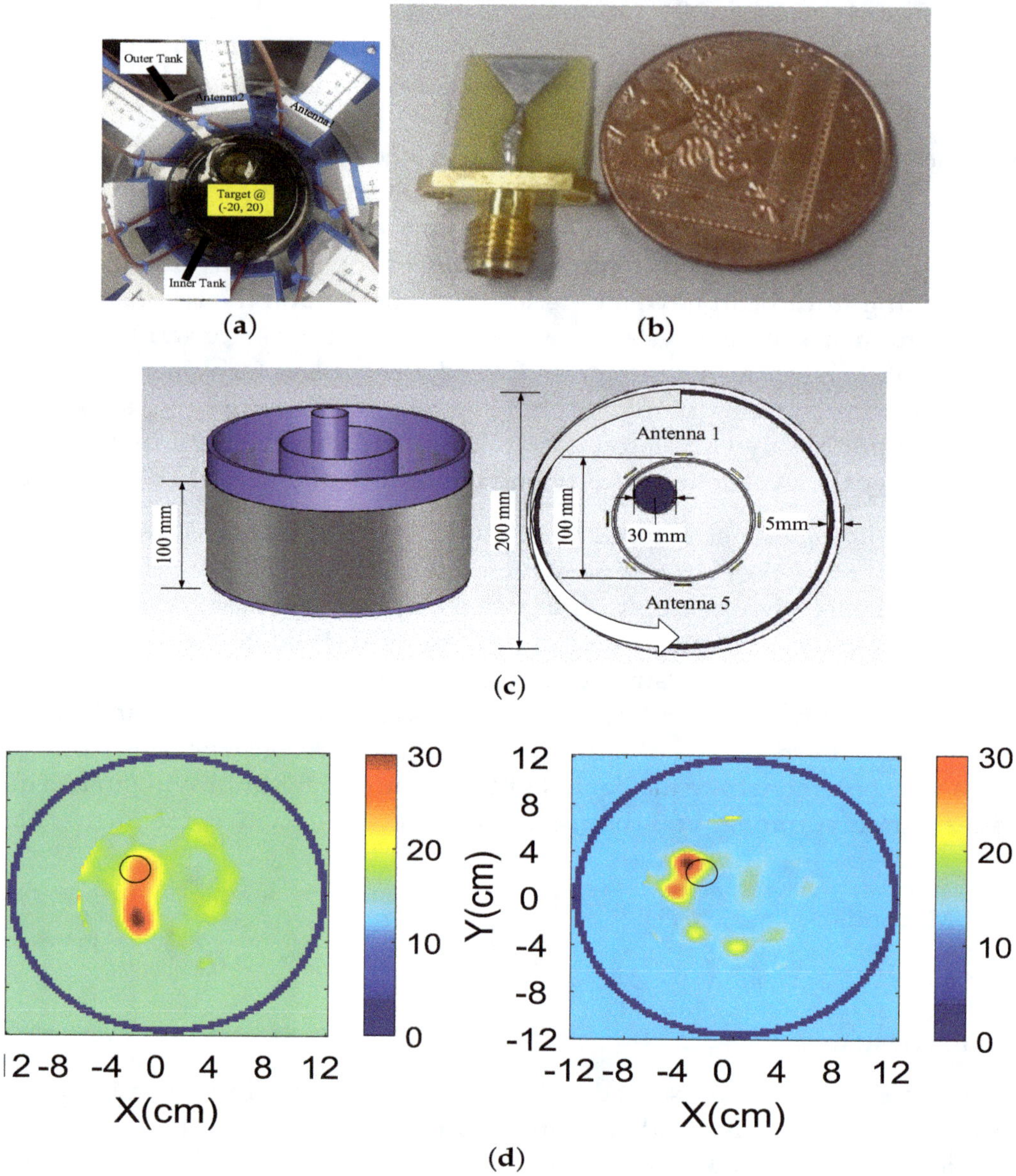

Figure 1. Overview of our employed microwave tomography (MWT) system. (**a**,**b**) Photos of the experimental measurement prototype and the antenna element; (**c**) Schematic of the MWT system with the cylindrical target inside the tank; (**d**) Reconstructed dielectric constant ϵ' for a cylindrical target filled with water, using experimental data at: (left) 1.0 GHz, and (right) 1.5 GHz.

2.1.2. The DBIM-TwiST Algorithm

The DBIM is an iterative inverse scattering algorithm which is commonly used to estimate the spatial distribution of dielectric properties within a region V [17]. Under the Born approximation, a linear integral equation at each iteration can be discretized for all transmit-receive pairs as,

$$\boldsymbol{A}(\omega)\boldsymbol{o} = \boldsymbol{b}(\omega) \tag{1}$$

where $\boldsymbol{A}(\omega)$ is an M-by-K propagation matrix, with M the number of transmit-receive pairs in the antenna array and K the number of elements in the discretisation in the reconstruction range V. The K-by-1 vector $\boldsymbol{o}$ contains the unknown dielectric properties contrast for the K voxels in V, while $b(\omega)$ is the M-by-1 vector of the scattered fields recorded at the recievers. The TwIST algorithm [14] can be introduced by considering the linear system described by (1) at each DBIM iteration as an inverse problem where the goal is to estimate an unknown original image vector x from an observation vector y, described by the linear equation $Ax = y$. Many approaches to this *Linear Inverse Problem* (LIP) define a solution $\hat{x}$ as a minimizer of a convex objective function $f : \chi \rightarrow R = [-\infty, +\infty]$, given by

$$f(x) = \frac{1}{2}||y - Ax||_2^2 + \lambda\Phi(x) \tag{2}$$

where $\Phi(x)$ is a regularization function for the convex optimization problem, $\lambda \in [0, +\infty]$ is a weighting parameter, and $|| \cdot ||_p = \sqrt{(\sum_n | \cdot |^p)}$. The two-step iterative shrinkage thresholding (TwIST) algorithm algorithm relies on splitting the matrix to structure a two-step iterative equation [14] as,

$$\begin{aligned} x_{t+1} &= (1-\alpha)x_{t-1} + (\alpha - \beta)x_t + \beta\Gamma_\lambda(x_t) \\ \Gamma_\lambda(x) &= \Psi_\lambda(x + A^T(y - Ax)) \end{aligned} \tag{3}$$

where α and β are the parameters of the TwIST algorithm, and Ψ_λ is the denoising function corresponding to the regularization function Φ. The designation "two-step" stems from the fact that the next estimate x_{t+1} depends on both the current solution x_t and the previous solution x_{t-1}, rather than only on x_t, as in conventional iterative shrinkage thresholding algorithms.

Our previous work has tested this algorithm extensively in microwave breast imaging simulations based on phantoms from the UW-Madison repository. We first presented a methodology to increase robustness by optimising the parameters of the TwIST algorithm in [12]. We also proposed to combine multiple frequency information to enhance resolution, and to use a Pareto-curve regularization method in cases of very strong noise. Finally, we argued that reconstructions of these numerical breast phantoms can be improved significantly by a two-step process which estimates the average breast properties prior to reconstructing the full breast structure [13]. After being tested extensively with numerical breast phantoms, the algorithm was also applied to data from our measurement system [16], which was acquired experimentally or was generated by simulating the full system and experiment using the CST Microwave Studio EM solver. An example of reconstructed images from experimental data presented in [16] is shown in Figure 1d. Information loss due to various factors inevitably affects the reconstruction quality, producing for example ghost targets as in the bottom row plots. The remainder of this paper will focus on investigating and dealing with this issue in more detail.

2.2. *Information Loss in MWT Reconstructions*

2.2.1. Simulation Models

We choose to first use simulation data to better understand the impact of information loss which is not due to random errors such as radio frequency interference, effects of cable movements, etc. To this end, we have simulated our experiment in CST Microwave Studio based on the computer-aided design (CAD) model of Figure 1c. Data from these simulations includes signal contributions that are not modeled by our forward solver, such as antenna coupling, surface waves, three-dimensional (3-D) propagation and scattering effects, etc. Our forward solver uses a two-dimensional (2-D) finite-difference time-domain (FDTD) model through the cross-section of the 3-D CST model where the printed monopoles are centered, with line sources at the same planar positions as the eight antennas of the 3-D model. To benchmark performance, we have also reconstructed data from this FDTD model, which is perfectly matched with the forward solver of our algorithm (i.e., an "inverse-crime" problem).

As performance for 90% glycerol-water mixture has already been studied in [16], we have focused on three other types of immersion liquids: Triton X-100, which exhibits low losses and has also been proposed for mimicking breast tissues [18], 92% corn syrup mixture with 8% water (not very lossy) [19], and 80% glycerine mixture with 20% water (very lossy) [4]. We derived first-order Debye parameters for these background media in the 1.0–3.0 GHz range by curve-fitting data from experimental measurements of their dielectric properties, which were acquired using the dielectric probe kit by Keysight. The resulting parameters are shown in Table 1. In addition to these immersion/coupling liquids, we used pure water to fill the cylinder representing the target. As the target size is small, we approximated water as non-dispersive material in our simulation models.

To study the impact of information loss on the signal scattered from the target of interest, we have simulated cases with and without the target using the aforementioned CST and FDTD models. We have compared these two datasets by plotting the transmitted signals recorded by the antenna array using a relative location ordering, in which the receiver is counted relative to the current transmitter anti-clockwise. The advantage of this receiver ordering scheme is that we can compare signal data (amplitude or phase) at different receivers due to the same transmit antenna in one figure. An example is shown in Figure 2, which is associated with "Antenna 1" transmitting and the remaining seven receiving.

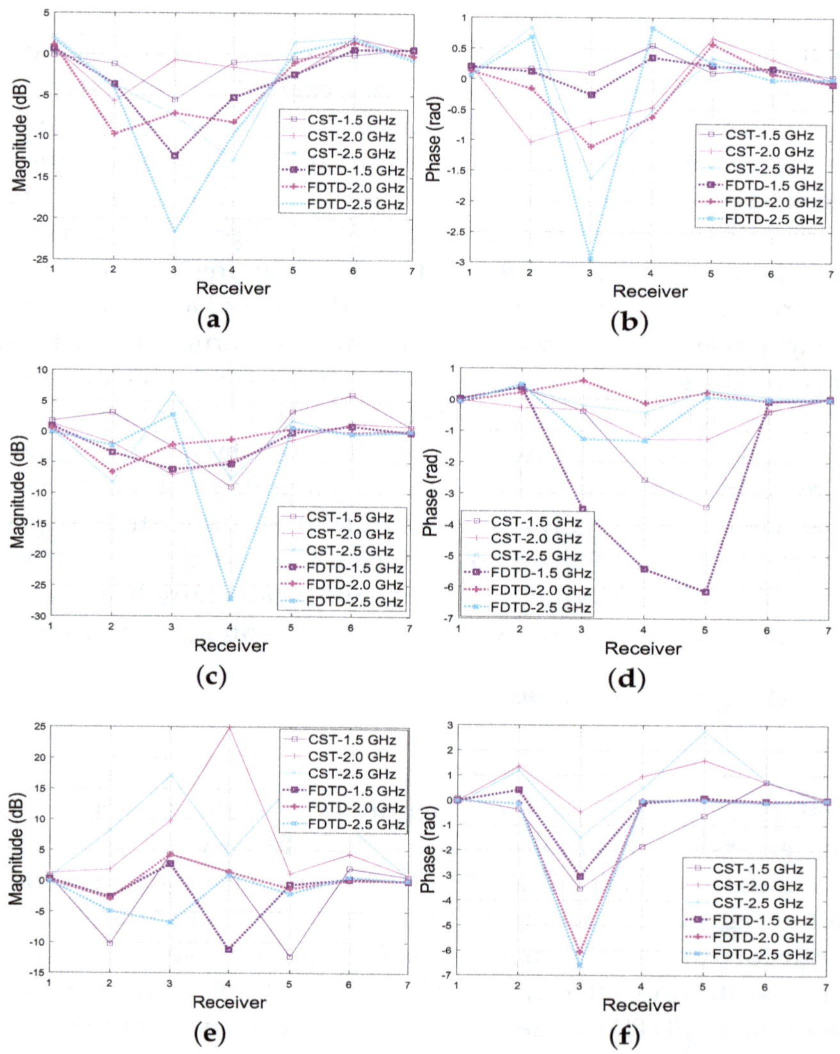

Figure 2. Amplitude (in dB) and phase differences due to the water-filled cylindrical target, recorded at each receiver for the first antenna used as transmitter, and for different background media. (**a**,**b**) Triton X-100; (**c**,**d**) 92% Corn syrup; (**e**,**f**) 80% Glycerine. The plots compare results from simulations of the physical experiment in CST Microwave Studio, using the computer-aided design (CAD) model of Figure 1c, with a 2-D simplified finite-difference time-domain (FDTD) model, which is also used as a forward solver in our imaging algorithm.

Plots Figure 2a,b show a similar trend between the 3-D CST and 2-D FDTD models for Triton-X-100 at 1.5 GHz. This suggests that the 2-D FDTD model is a good approximation of the experimental prototype for this dataset. The inflection points of these v-shape plots at Receiver 3 rightly suggest a target location between Antennas 1 and 4. However, there are also clear differences at 2.5 GHz in Figure 2a and at 2.0 GHz in Figure 2b. This means that the mismatch between the two models becomes more significant for higher frequencies where signal losses increase and the antenna is less efficient. In Figure 2c–f, higher signal losses for the more lossy corn and glycerine mixtures result not only in an increased mismatch between the CST and FDTD models, but also in irretrievable loss of signal information from the target. For 80% glycerine–water, in particular, there seems to be very little correlation between the received signals and the target location which suggests that reconstructing the target using these frequencies is almost hopeless.

Table 1. Debye parameters for the considered immersion liquids (derived by experimental measurements and data fitting in the range 1.0–3.0 GHz.

Medium	ϵ_∞	$\Delta\epsilon$	σ_s	τ
Triton	3.512	2.582	0.0655	5.3505×10^{-11}
80% Glycerine	4.75	30	0.3779	1.2346×10^{-10}
92% Corn syrup	4.124	12.01	0.3405	1.6667×10^{-10}
Cylinder	3.5	0	0.055	0
Pure Water	78	0	1.59	0

2.2.2. Calibration

In microwave imaging experiments, measured data will inevitably include random noise such as environmental noise, thermal noise, coupling due to cable movement, and machine noise. The impact of these errors can be reduced by applying denoising techniques directly to the measured data, or as regularisation in the reconstruction process. A method to calibrate measured and simulated datasets is also required to deal with errors due to differences between the physical experiment and its numerical model used in the imaging algorithm. This calibration step is also necessary if CST-simulated data is used as the "measured data", as the CST model of Figure 1c is very different from its 2-D FDTD version used by our imaging algorithm.

To this end, we apply a simple calibration step based on "tank-only" signals measured and simulated in the absence of the target. The calibrated data used in the first iteration of our algorithm can be calculated as,

$$\begin{aligned} \Gamma_{E_{meas}} &= |E^{inh}_{meas}|_{dB} + \Delta\Gamma_{dB} \\ \Phi_{E_{meas}} &= \Phi(E^{inh}_{meas}) + \Delta\Phi \end{aligned} \quad (4)$$

where $\Delta\Gamma_{dB}$ and $\Delta\Phi$ are given by,

$$\begin{aligned} \Delta\Gamma_{dB} &= |E^{hom}_{cal}|_{dB} - |E^{hom}_{meas}|_{dB} \\ \Delta\Phi &= \Phi(E^{hom}_{cal}) - \Phi(E^{hom}_{meas}). \end{aligned} \quad (5)$$

In these equations, Γ denotes the magnitude of the received signals in the frequency domain, and Φ denotes the corresponding phase. E^{hom}_{cal} is generated by running the FDTD forward solver for an empty tank filled with any of the background media modeled by the Debye parameters of Table 1. E^{hom}_{meas} is the signal measured by the corresponding "tank-only" experiment, while E^{inh}_{meas} is the signal measured with the target. As mentioned previously, the notation "measured" can also correspond to data produced by the 3-D CST model that simulates the physical experiment.

2.2.3. Representative Reconstruction Results

To confirm our predictions on the impact of information loss on reconstruction quality, we have applied our DBIM-TwIST algorithm to data from the CST and FDTD simulation models analysed in Section 2.2.1. Depending on whether the data comes from the 3-D CST or the 2-D FDTD model, we implement a 3-D/2-D or 2-D/2-D reconstruction approach, respectively (our imaging algorithm always uses a 2-D forward solver). The DBIM-TwIST algorithm and a frequency hopping approach are employed in the range 1.5–2.7 GHz with a 100 MHz step. The algorithm is initialised by filling the tank with the known background medium dielectric properties.

The resulting reconstructed images are shown in Figures 3 and 4. These plots present estimated ϵ' and ϵ'' distributions, which are calculated from the Debye models at 1.5 GHz. The target is detected for both datasets when low loss Triton X-100 is used as the background medium. Performance degrades significantly for the other two media, even for the FDTD-generated dataset. This degradation is correlated with inconsistencies in the transmitted signals observed in Figure 2. These results motivate our proposed strategy to evaluate the data produced by our MWT system and select a set of optimal frequencies for our imaging algorithm. To this end, we propose a frequency selection method based on correlation analysis, which is presented in the next section.

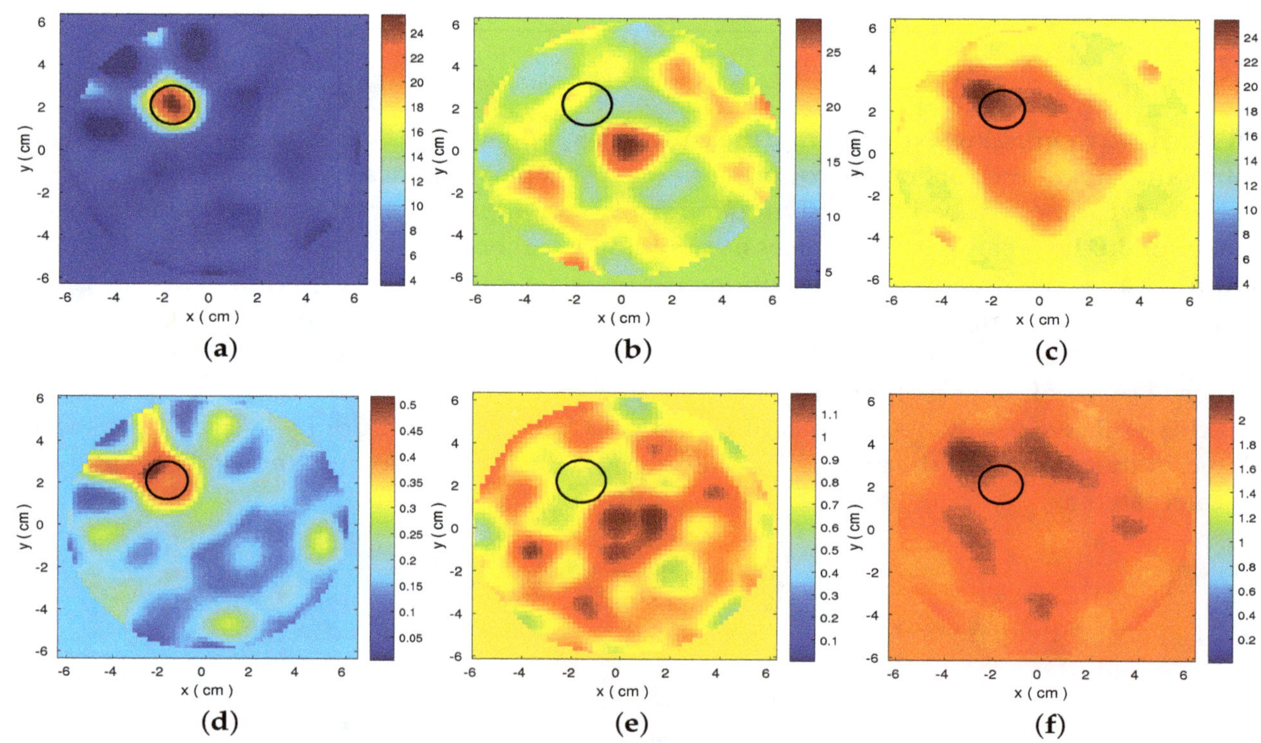

Figure 3. 2-D reconstructed complex permittivity distributions from 3-D CST simulated data for the three different background media considered, using a frequency hopping approach in the range 1.5–2.7 GHz. Top images reconstruct the real part ϵ' for (**a**) Triton X-100; (**b**) 90% corn syrup; and (**c**) 80% glycerine, and the bottom images correspond to ϵ'' for (**d**) Triton X-100; (**e**) 90% corn syrup; and (**f**) 80% glycerine.

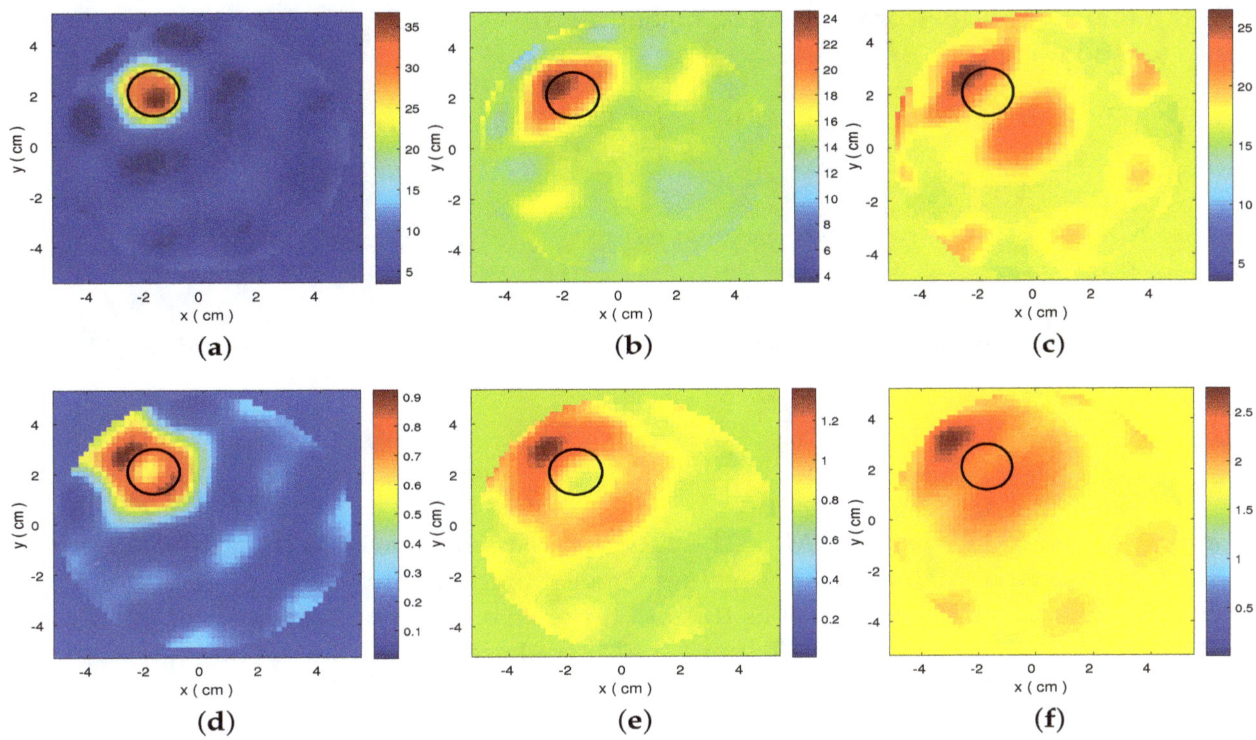

Figure 4. Same as Figure 3 for data produced by the 2-D FDTD model that is also used as forward solver in our imaging algorithm. Top images reconstruct the real part ϵ' for (**a**) Triton X-100; (**b**) 90% corn syrup; and (**c**) 80% glycerine; and the bottom images correspond to ϵ'' for (**d**) Triton X-100; (**e**) 90% corn syrup; and (**f**) 80% glycerine.

2.3. *Improving Reconstructions by Frequency Selection*

Plots such as those in Figure 2 offer a way to compare the relative measured magnitude between adjacent frequencies across the range of operation for the MWT system. Taking into account that signals measured by a MWT system should carry similar information at adjacent frequencies [20], we can relate data quality in a frequency range with a high correlation of measured data between adjacent frequencies. This concept has been applied successfully to other disciplines [21,22], but it has never been presented, to the best of the authors' knowledge, in the context of microwave or other imaging modalities. This comparative information can be used to discard low quality data, for example by selecting frequencies for which the amplitude plots in dB are not highly correlated with each other. To this end, our approach aims to provide a simple but systematic method of discarding low quality data by classifying frequencies with similar trends into a "high-correlation group", and the rest into "moderate" and "low-correlation" groups. We note that we have focused only on correlation maps of the transmitted signals' magnitudes (in dB) , to take advantage of the approximate linear magnitude change vs. frequency which can be observed in MWT measurements [20].

A simple metric for this purpose is the Pearson's correlation coefficient for variables X and Y, which is defined as,

$$\rho(X,Y) = \frac{cov(X,Y)}{\sigma_X \sigma_Y} \tag{6}$$

where cov is the covariance, and σ_X and σ_Y denote the standard deviation of X and Y respectively. For an array of N antennas measuring at M frequencies, we can define the variable $F_m^n (m = 1, 2, \ldots M)$ representing a series of received magnitudes $[R^n(m,i), i = 1, 2, \ldots N-1]$ for all $N-1$ receivers regarding the n_{th} transmitter at the m_{th} frequency,

$$F_m^n = [R^n_{(m,1)}, R^n_{(m,2)}, \ldots, R^n_{(m,N-1)}]^T \tag{7}$$

We can then obtain the correlation coefficient matrix $\boldsymbol{P}^n$ for the n_{th} transmitter by combining Equations (6) and (7),

$$\boldsymbol{P}^n = \begin{bmatrix} \rho(F_1^n, F_1^n) & \rho(F_1^n, F_2^n) & \dots & \rho(F_1^n, F_M^n) \\ \rho(F_2^n, F_1^n) & \rho(F_2^n, F_2^n) & \dots & \rho(F_2^n, F_M^n) \\ \vdots & \vdots & \vdots & \vdots \\ \rho(F_M^n, F_1^n) & \rho(F_M^n, F_2^n) & \dots & \rho(F_M^n, F_M^n) \end{bmatrix} \tag{8}$$

We can also calculate an aggregate cross-correlation matrix by averaging P^n over all transmitters as,

$$\bar{\boldsymbol{P}} = \frac{1}{N} \sum_{n=1}^{N} \boldsymbol{P}^n \tag{9}$$

For our MWT system, we chose $M = 21$ frequencies equally spaced in the 1.0–3.0 GHz range.

A conformation that high correlation values suggest high quality data is presented in Figure 5a, which corresponds to the same dataset as this of Figure 2a,b. The dataset was generated using the simple 2-D FDTD model with low-loss Triton X-100 as background medium. The contributions from the signal scattered from the cylindrical target are highly correlated for this simple model, as shown in Figure 5b for 1.3–1.7 GHz. This is captured well by the correlation map of the relative signal magnitude differences ("target"-"empty") in dB shown in Figure 5a, which shows cross-correlation values of 0.85 or higher.

We can use the same approach using Equation (9), which provides a single average matrix to select frequencies with the highest correlation across all receivers. An example is illustrated in Figure 6 for the more challenging case of 3-D CST-produced data in 90% corn syrup presented in Figure 2c,d. For this more lossy background medium, the overall correlation values are lower than the 2-D FDTD Triton X-100 model considered in the previous case of Figure 5. Similar to that case, the map in Figure 6a can assist in selecting the higher correlation "sub-bands" to consider in the reconstruction process. This approach can improve reconstruction performance, as demonstrated in Section 3.

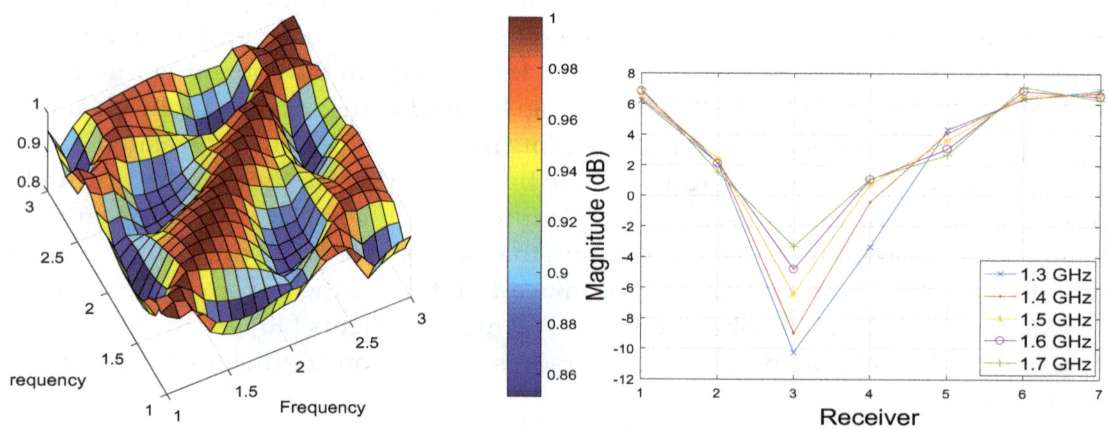

(a) (b)

Figure 5. (**a**) Cross-correlation calculation using Equation (8) for Transmitter 1 and 2-D FDTD data in Triton X-100 (the dataset in Figure 2a,b). These correlations were calculated on relative signal ("target"-"empty") magnitudes in dB (**b**) Example of a "sub-band" with highly-correlated data selected from the map in (**a**).

3. Results

3.1. Application to Simulated Data

To illustrate how our proposed frequency selection method can be used to improve reconstructions, we consider the case of 3-D CST-produced data in 90% corn syrup, with the cross-correlation map shown in Figure 6. The map is used to identify frequencies of low correlation against all other frequencies, such as 1.2 or 1.3 GHz, which can be removed from the reconstruction process. The plot in Figure 6b confirms that the scattered signals at 1.3 GHz differ from those of neighbouring frequencies. The cross-correlation map also suggests two "sub-bands" of high correlation as representatives of low (1.5–1.8 GHz) and high (2.5–2.8 GHz) frequency ranges, confirmed by the plots in Figure 6b. The reconstructed images using these two sub-bands are shown in Figure 7. In comparison with the results in Figure 3b,e, these images estimate more accurately the target location.

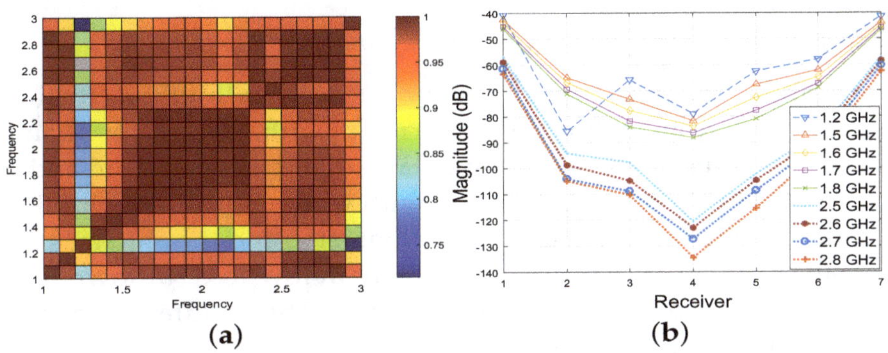

Figure 6. (**a**) Average cross-correlation map in Equation (9) using 3-D CST data in 90% corn syrup (the dataset in Figure 2c,d); (**b**) Example of amplitude plots for Transmitter 1 in two "sub-bands" of highly-correlated data selected from the map in (**a**), and how they differ from an "outlier" at 1.2 GHz.

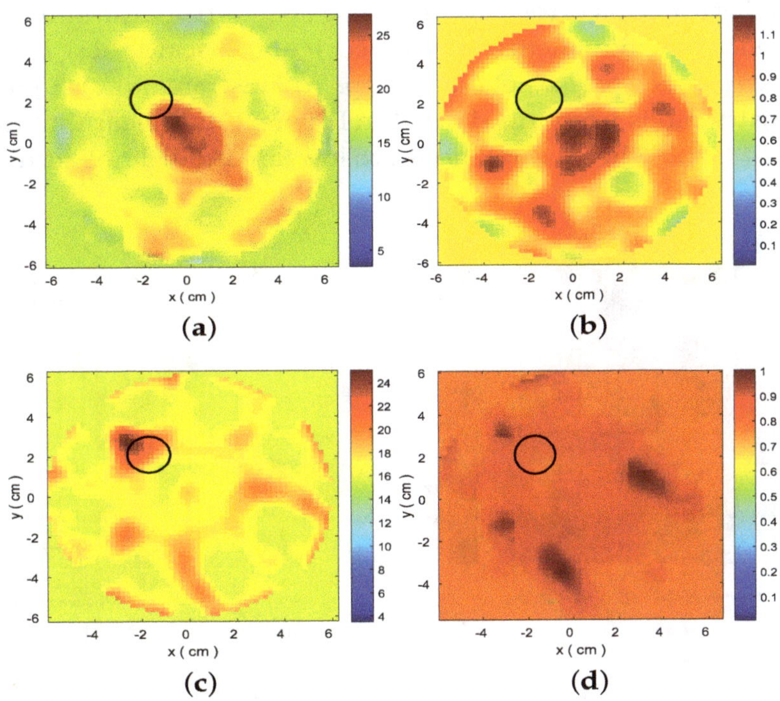

Figure 7. 2-D reconstructed complex permittivity distributions from 3-D CST data in 90% corn syrup, using our frequency selection approach illustrated in Figure 6. Resulting distributions of (**a**) ϵ' and (**b**) ϵ'' by frequency hopping in 1.5–1.8 GHz; and (**c**) ϵ' and (**d**) ϵ'' by frequency hopping in 2.5–2.8 GHz.

Despite this improvement, errors are still present in these images. This is because high cross-correlation values do not necessarily guarantee accurate reconstructions in related frequencies, as they may be the result of systematic errors in the data acquisition process. Our method, however, can be used to identify low cross-correlation values as outliers dominated by random measurement errors. These frequencies can be excluded from the reconstruction process, as in the case of 1.2 GHz for the example of Figure 6b. We note that we considered cross-correlation of total received signals (i.e., data with target) rather than relative received signals , i.e., magnitude differences with and without the target in dB, which can be equally used. The "relative signal" approach was used, for example, in Figure 5. These two different correlation maps should provide common but also complementary information. In particular, relative signal correlations will be more sensitive to small signals differences due to the target. Total signal correlations will be higher on average and less sensitive to the target, but can detect more safely frequencies where measurements are dominated by error, such as the "outlier" of 1.2 GHz in Figure 6b.

3.2. *Application to Experimental Data from a Two-Layer Cylindrical Phantom*

We demonstrate the impact of our frequency selection method further in this section, by considering measured data from an imaging experiment with a two-layer phantom. The two-layer phantom geometry is as in Figure 1, where the inner tank diameter is 100 mm and the diameter of the target container is 31 mm. The target is again filled with water, but safflower oil is used in the inner tank. The eight-antenna array forms a ring of 130 mm diameter, and the antennas are immersed in 90% corn syrup. As the transmitted waves propagate mostly in low-loss safflower oil, the loss in signal information in this case is mostly due to experimental errors. This is different to the previous one-layer model simulations, which resulted in significant signal attenuation inside the lossy corn-syrup or glycerol-water immersion liquids.

Figure 8a presents cross-correlations calculations using Equations (8) and (9) from relative received signals, similar to the previous section. The map shows low correlation values for frequencies up to 1.4 GHz, where the antenna is less efficient and radiation from the antenna cables can become an important experimental error. This error was of course absent from the simulations of the previous sections, but our frequency selection method can detect it and discard these low frequencies from our dataset based on observing this cross-correlations map. To illustrate our argument further, we present single-frequency reconstructions from this dataset in Figure 9. It is clear that from these images that reconstructions up to 1.4 GHz, where correlations are low, are indeed not accurate.

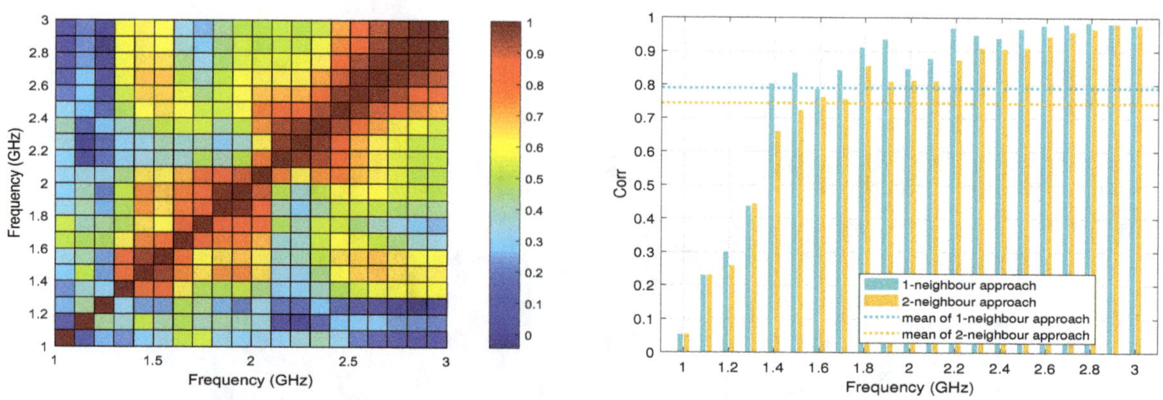

(a) (b)

Figure 8. (**a**) Average cross-correlation map using Equation (9) for all transmitters and experimental data in a two-layer phantom with 90% corn syrup as immersion, and safflower oil surrounding the target; (**b**) Example of using the 1-neighbour and 2-neighbour approach to assess the correlations of the map in (**a**) through calculating moving averages of correlation coefficients.

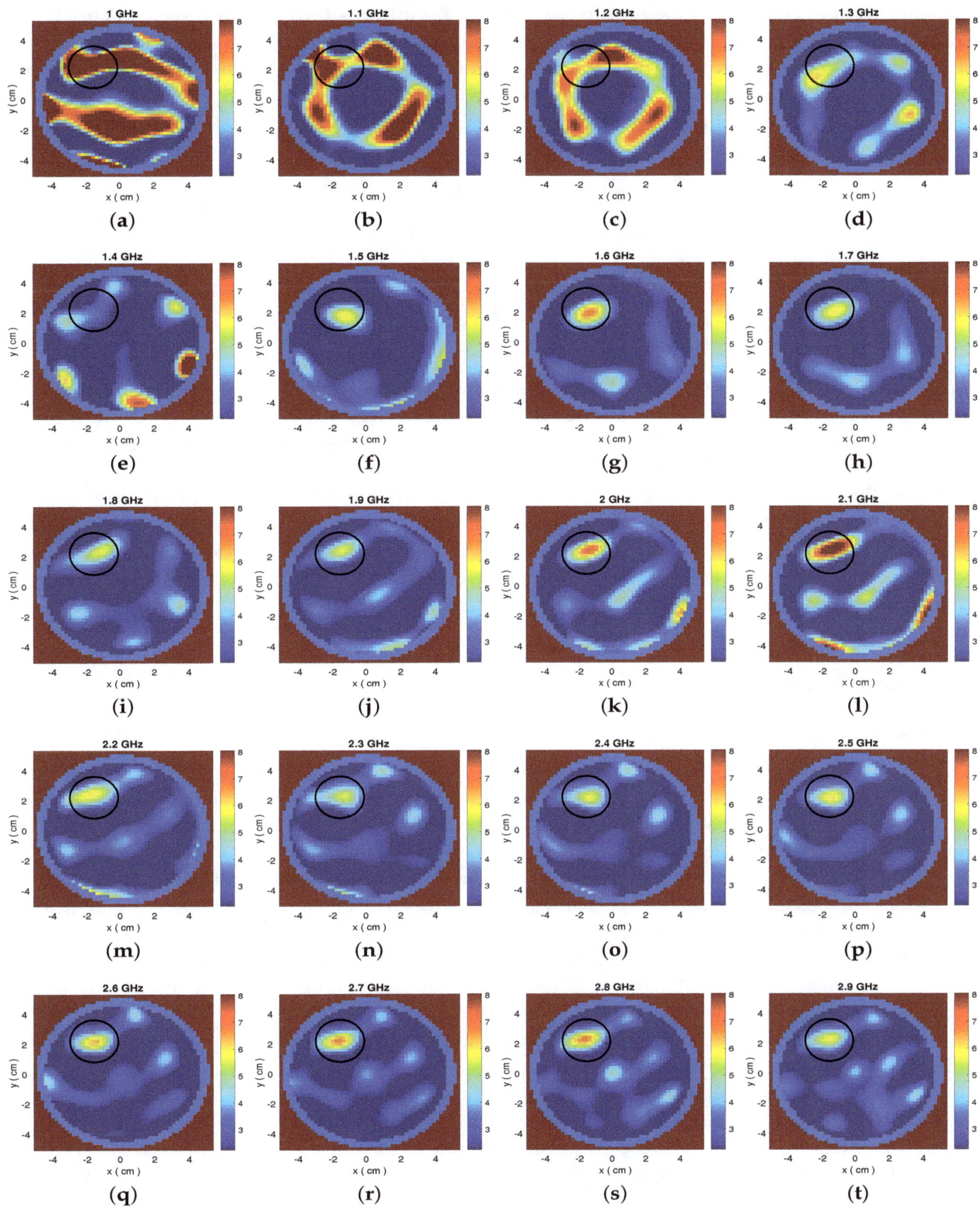

Figure 9. (**a–t**): Single-frequency reconstructions of the Debye parameter ϵ_∞ from 1.0 to 2.9 GHz using the experimental dataset from our two-layer cylindrical system.

Relying on correlation maps for discarding frequencies may not be always straightforward. Therefore, we propose here a selection process which relies on the observation that signal magnitudes at adjacent frequencies should be highly correlated. Taking this into account, we can consider the average value of correlation coefficients at K-neighbour frequencies [21] as a metric for the degree (low or high) of data quality at a given frequency. For example, we can use a 1-neighbour frequency approach to obtain the correlation average at 1.5 GHz by an arithmetic mean of $\rho(F_{1.5GHz}, F_{1.4GHz})$ and $\rho(F_{1.5GHz}, F_{1.6GHz})$. The explicit definition of this K-neighbour approach for N sampling frequencies $[f_1, f_2, ..., f_N]$ is [21],

$$Q_K(f_i) = \begin{cases} \rho(1,2) & i = 1 \\ \sum_{m=1}^{2i-1} \rho(i,m) & 1 < i \leq K \\ \sum_{m=i-K}^{i+K} \rho(i,m) & K < i \leq N-K \\ \sum_{m=2i-N}^{N} \rho(i,m) & N-K < i < N \\ \rho(N-1,N) & i = N \end{cases} \quad \textbf{s.t.} \quad K \leq N/2 \tag{10}$$

where ρ has been defined in (8), and Q_K denotes the average correlation at K-neighbour frequencies. This function Q_K is designed to smooth out fluctuations between adjacent frequencies and provide longer-term trends. In practice, the value of K will depend on the sampling frequency step and the calculated correlation map.

After this smoothing process, we can set a threshold by calculating the mean of $Q_K(f_i), i = 1, 2, \ldots N$. The frequencies for which the corresponding $Q_K(f_i)$ is below this threshold will then correspond to a "low degree" of data quality, and will be discarded in the reconstruction process. Figure 8b presents an example of the 1-neighbour and 2-neighbour approaches based on the correlation map in Figure 8a. Based on their corresponding thresholds, the 1-neighbour approach would discard frequencies 1.0, 1.1, 1.2, 1.3 and 1.6 GHz, while the 2-neighbour approach would discard frequencies from 1.0 to 1.5 GHz. As expected, using more samples for averaging (higher K) improves the selection performance.

4. Discussion

This paper argued the impact of information loss on microwave tomography by presenting reconstructions of a simple imaging problem (a cylindrical target inside another cylinder filled with a background medium) from a wide range of datasets. We showed that reconstruction quality can deteriorate significantly even in "inverse crime" scenarios where the models for the forward and inverse solver are identical (Figure 4). This will occur in situations where signals propagate inside quite lossy media such as corn syrup or glycerol water mixtures, which can attenuate the signal scattered from the target to levels that could not be recovered from our imaging algorithm. We must note that, in addition to loss, failure to reconstruct the target in these "inverse-crime" cases may be due to a "higher degree of non-linearity" that a shorter wavelength experiences when propagating inside corn syrup or glycerol water mixtures, where the dielectric constant is also high.

Beyond numerical simulations, we considered experimental data from a case where signal loss was less significant, but experimental errors dominated low-frequency data. For both of these imaging scenarios, we presented a simple cross-correlation method that can be used to select "high-quality" data. We used this technique to select frequencies with high correlation values, and demonstrated that it can improve reconstruction results significantly. The method relies on simple calculations from data that is readily available (numerically or experimentally), and can therefore be useful as a pre-processing step in imaging algorithms used by practical experimental systems. The same rationale could also be used to create correlation maps focusing on other system parameters; for example, one could correlate receiver data at a fixed frequency to exclude certain antenna elements (rather than frequencies) which may be dominated by experimental errors.

Finally, me must emphasize that this analysis is by no means a complete assessment of our MWT system performance. For example, it does not include an error metric to quantify the accuracy of reconstructions, or a more thorough investigation of the impact of working frequency, number of antennas, and immersion liquid on system performance. These matters will be investigated further in our future work which aims first to build a new prototype which can improve the quality of our measured data. In this respect, the cross-correlation methodology presented in this paper can be used as an easy tool to evaluate (and improve) a MWT measurement system without having to face additional challenges introduced by the inversion process.

Author Contributions: Conceptualization, Z.M. and P.K.; Methodology, Z.M., S.A. and P.K.; Software, Z.M.; Validation, Z.M. and S.A.; Resources, P.K.; Writing—Original Draft Preparation, P.K., Z.M. and S.A.; Supervision, P.K.; Project Administration, P.K.; Funding Acquisition, P.K.

Acknowledgments: This work has been developed in the framework of COST Action TD1301, MiMed. The authors would like to thank Francesca Vipiana and Jorge Tobon for hosting Ahsan (via a MiMed Short Terms Scientific Mission) in their lab, and sharing their valuable expertise in microwave imaging experiments. The authors would also like to thank Paul Meaney for hosting Miao (via a MiMed Short Terms Scientific Mission) at Dartmouth College, and and training him in experimental microwave imaging.

References

1. Semenov, S. Microwave tomography: Review of the progress towards clinical applications. *Philos. Trans. A Math. Phys. Eng. Sci.* **2009**, *367*, 3021–3042. [CrossRef] [PubMed]
2. Gilmore, C.; Abubakar, A.; Hu, W. Microwave biomedical data inversion using the finite-difference contrast source inversion method. *IEEE Trans. Antennas Propag.* **2009**, *57*, 1528–1538. [CrossRef]
3. Scapaticci, R.; Catapano, I.; Crocco, L. Wavelet-based adaptive multiresolution inversion for quantitative microwave imaging of breast tissues. *IEEE Trans. Antennas Propag.* **2012**, *60*, 3717–3726. [CrossRef]
4. Meaney, P.M.; Fanning, M.W.; Raynolds, T.; Fox, C.J.; Fang, Q.; Kogel, C.A.; Poplack, S.P.; Paulsen, K.D. Initial clinical experience with microwave breast imaging in women with normal mammography. *Acad. Radiol.* **2007**, *14*, 207–218. [CrossRef] [PubMed]
5. Shea, J.D.; Kosmas, P.; Hagness, S.C.; Van Veen, B.D. Three-dimensional microwave imaging of realistic numerical breast phantoms via a multiple-frequency inverse scattering technique. *Med. Phys.* **2010**, *37*, 4210–4226. [CrossRef] [PubMed]
6. Kosmas, P.; Shea, J.D.; Van Veen, B.D.; Hagness, S.C. Three-dimensional microwave imaging of realistic breast phantoms via an inexact Gauss-Newton algorithm. In Proceedings of the 2008 IEEE Antennas and Propagation Society International Symposium, San Diego, CA, USA, 5–11 July 2008; pp. 1–4.
7. Meaney, P.M.; Fanning, M.W.; Li, D.; Poplack, S.P.; Paulsen, K.D. A clinical prototype for active microwave imaging of the breast. *IEEE Trans. Microw. Theory Tech.* **2000**, *48*, 1841–1853.
8. Semenov, S.Y.; Svenson, R.H.; Boulyshev, A.E.; Souvorov, A.E.; Borisov, V.Y.; Sizov, Y.; Starostin, A.N.; Dezern, K.R.; Tatsis, G.P.; Baranov, V.Y. Microwave tomography: Two-dimensional system for biological imaging. *IEEE Trans. Biomed. Eng.* **1996**, *43*, 869–877. [CrossRef] [PubMed]
9. Gilmore, C.; Mojabi, P.; Zakaria, A.; Ostadrahimi, M.; Kaye, C.; Noghanian, S.; Shafai, L.; Pistorius, S.; LoVetri, J. A wideband microwave tomography system with a novel frequency selection procedure. *IEEE Trans. Biomed. Eng.* **2010**, *57*, 894–904. [CrossRef] [PubMed]
10. Yu, C.; Yuan, M.; Stang, J.; Bresslour, E.; George, R.T.; Ybarra, G.A.; Joines, W.T.; Liu, Q.H. Active microwave imaging II: 3-D system prototype and image reconstruction from experimental data. *IEEE Trans. Microw. Theory Tech.* **2008**, *56*, 991–1000.
11. Zeng, X.; Fhager, A.; He, Z.; Persson, M.; Linner, P.; Zirath, H. Development of a time domain microwave system for medical diagnostics. *IEEE Trans. Instrum. Meas.* **2014**, *63*, 2931–2939. [CrossRef]
12. Miao, Z.; Kosmas, P. Microwave breast imaging based on an optimized two-step iterative shrinkage/thresholding method. In Proceedings of the 2015 9th European Conference of Antennas and Propag (EuCAP), Lisbon, Portugal, 13–17 April 2015; pp. 1–4.

13. Miao, Z.; Kosmas, P. Multiple-frequency DBIM-TwIST algorithm for microwave breast imaging. *IEEE Trans. Antennas Propag.* **2017**, *65*, 2507–2516. [CrossRef]
14. Bioucas-Dias, J.; Figueiredo, M. A new TwIST: Two-Step iterative shrinkage/thresholding algorithms for image restoration. *IEEE Trans. Image Process.* **2007**, *16*, 2992–3004. [CrossRef] [PubMed]
15. Azghani, M.; Kosmas, P.; Marvasti, M. Microwave medical imaging based on sparsity and an iterative method with adaptive thresholding. *IEEE Trans. Med. Imag.* **2015**, *34*, 357–365. [CrossRef] [PubMed]
16. Ahsan, S.; Guo, Z.; Miao, Z.; Sotiriou, I.; Koutsoupidou, M.; Kallos, T.G.P.; Kosmas, P. Design and experimental validation of a wideband microwave tomography system employing the DBIM-TwIST algorithm. *Sensors* under preparation.
17. Chew, W.; Lin, J. A frequency-hopping approach for microwave imaging of large inhomogeneous bodies. *Microwave Guided Wave Lett.* **1995**, *5*, 439–441. [CrossRef]
18. Stefania, R.; Loreto, D.D.; Mario, B.O.; Ilaria, C.; Lorenzo, C.; Rosaria, S.M.; Rita, M. Dielectric characterization study of liquid-based materials for mimicking breast tissues. *Microwave Opt. Technol. Lett.* **2011**, *53*, 1276–1280.
19. Bindu, G.; Lonappan, A.; Thomas, V.; Aanandan, C.K.; Mathew, K.T. Dielectric studies of corn syrup for applications in microwave breast imaging. *Prog. Electromagn. Res.* **2006**, *59*, 175–186. [CrossRef]
20. Meaney, P.M.; Paulsen, K.D.; Pogue, B.W.; Miga, M.I. Microwave image reconstruction utilizing log-magnitude and unwrapped phase to improve high-contrast object recovery. *IEEE Trans. Med. Imaging* **2001**, *20*, 104–116. [CrossRef] [PubMed]
21. Masson, L.; McNeill, G.; Tomany, J.; Simpson, J.; Peace, H.; Wei, L.; Grubb, D.; Bolton-Smith, C. Statistical approaches for assessing the relative validity of a food-frequency questionnaire: Use of correlation coefficients and the kappa statistic. *Public Health Nutr.* **2003**, *6*, 313–321. [CrossRef] [PubMed]
22. Jolliffe, I.T. Discarding variables in a principal component analysis. I: Artificial data. *J. R. Stat. Soc. Ser. C Appl. Stat.* **1972**, *21*, 160–173. [CrossRef]

8

Radio-Frequency and Microwave Techniques for Non-Invasive Measurement of Blood Glucose Levels

Tuba Yilmaz [1], Robert Foster [2] and Yang Hao [3,*]

1 Department of Electronics and Communication Engineering, Istanbul Technical University, 34469 Istanbul, Turkey; tuba.yilmaz@itu.edu.tr

2 Department of Electronic, Electrical and Systems Engineering, University of Birmingham, Birmingham B15 2TT, UK; r.n.foster@ieee.org

3 School of Electronic Engineering and Computer Science, Queen Mary University of London, London E1 4NS, UK

* Correspondence: y.hao@qmul.ac.uk

Abstract: This paper reviews non-invasive blood glucose measurements via dielectric spectroscopy at microwave frequencies presented in the literature. The intent is to clarify the key challenges that must be overcome if this approach is to work, to suggest some possible ways towards addressing these challenges and to contribute towards prevention of unnecessary 'reinvention of the wheel'.

Keywords: blood glucose levels; non-invasive measurement; glucose-dependent dielectric properties; RF sensing; microwave resonators; microwave spectroscopy; dielectric spectroscopy; on-body antennas

---

1. Introduction

The prevalence of Type 2 diabetes has been rapidly increasing through the latter half of the twentieth and into the twenty-first century. It has been associated with changes in life style during that period, including increasing adoption of unhealthy dietary habits and limited daily activity. In 2014, the prevalence of diabetes among adults older than 18 years globally had increased to 8.5%, from 4.7% in 1980 [1]. Mortality resulting directly from diabetes was estimated to be 1.6 million in 2015. Diabetes is a chronic condition and must be managed well to prevent complications of the disease, including (but not limited to) cardiovascular disease, blindness, kidney failure, increased risk of stroke and lower limb amputation [2].

A large number of techniques have been considered for non-invasive glucose monitoring, including the analysis of sweat, urine (e.g., [3]), tears (e.g., [4]), and saliva (see the recent review in [2]), breath analysis (relating blood glucose levels to acetone, which is produced during ketosis [5–8]), as well as various spectroscopic methods, with limited or no success to date [2,9,10]. Furthermore, few of these techniques are suitable for continuous monitoring (particularly those requiring samples of saliva, urine and breath), although potentially still of use for non-invasive validation, or even calibration, of other wearable sensors.

Currently, blood glucose levels are mostly monitored with ambulatory monitoring devices, where a drop of blood has to be drawn via a lancet and placed onto a chemically pre-treated strip inserted in a device [2]. When the blood is dropped onto the strip, the glucose creates a low-level current. The monitoring device quantifies the blood glucose level via the intensity of the current. These ambulatory devices suffer from error rates as high as 20% for older devices and 15% for devices meeting the current International Standards Organisation standard for blood-glucose monitoring systems [10,11]. Furthermore, these devices measure the capillary blood glucose levels (since the blood sample is usually drawn from finger tips, or sub-cutaneous measurements using 'needle-patches' placed on the torso for more modern 'continuous monitoring' systems) and it is known that the capillary blood glucose levels lags behind the actual glucose levels (e.g., [2,10]). The main disadvantage of the current ambulatory monitoring devices are the invasiveness, after the relatively recent development of commercial 'continuous monitoring' systems (such as Dexcom's G6 system, Abbott's FreeStyle Flash/Libre system and Medtronic's Guardian systems, some of which have sensor lifetimes up to 14 days [10]). Off-the-shelf monitoring devices have a number of practical obstacles, however, for example, the blood glucose levels is known to be affected from the sanitation of the measurement site, it is advised that the measurement site should be washed with warm water to increase the circulation, the patient is vulnerable to infections, the tissue becomes increasingly deformed at the measurement site over time and the cost of the measurement. Therefore, there is a need for new technologies that can offer reliable and continuous measurements while being unobtrusive to the patient and reducing costs. It is worth noting that blood glucose monitoring would also be of interest for non-diabetic people, such as astronauts, elite athletes and security personnel.

One such technique that has captured the attention of researchers is the RF/microwave sensing of blood glucose levels. Within the last decade, with the development of wireless technologies, an increased interest in the interaction of electromagnetic waves and biological tissues has emerged. With the motivation of designing medical diagnostic and therapeutic devices, many studies focussed on characterization of dielectric property profiles of biological tissues and anomalies, with applications including burn or wound monitoring and detection of cancerous tissue (for example, [12–14]). The possibility of using radio-frequency (RF) or microwave sensing for blood glucose level characterization has also been investigated during this period (in fact, such technologies have been investigated throughout the twenty-first century at least, including various unsuccessful attempts at commercialisation; an interesting perspective on research into non-invasive glucose monitoring can be found in [10]). In this paper, we review the studies conducted to investigate the interaction of electromagnetic waves with glucose molecules, covering frequencies between approximately 1 kHz and 100 GHz, with a focus on 'microwave' frequencies (which we take to mean 0.1–20 GHz in this paper). We will mostly use the term 'microwave spectroscopy' to describe this technique, but will also use dielectric spectroscopy interchangeably (although the latter is the more general). A related term, impedance spectroscopy, is used at low radio frequencies (below about 1 MHz), where it is more convenient to represent the material properties as resistances, capacitances and inductances. As these are related directly to the complex permittivity (and complex permeability, where relevant), we will mostly avoid this terminology to avoid confusion.

The paper is organized as follows: we begin by examining the glucose-dependent properties of human tissues, with the intent being to highlight the first major obstacle to non-invasive monitoring via microwave spectroscopy, sensitivity. We also briefly discuss the second major issue, selectivity, or how to attribute measured changes in dielectric properties to changes in blood glucose. We then review the various frequencies used in the literature and discuss how the operating frequency might be chosen in the light of the sensitivity and selectivity issues. A survey of resonators and antennas used in the literature follows, with some comments based on the frequency and mode of operation and the sensitivity and selectivity issues. We conclude with a brief discussion of possible ways to meet the sensitivity and selectivity challenges.

2. Glucose Dependent Dielectric Properties

The dielectric properties of a material govern the wave behaviour in that medium. Therefore, the dielectric properties of a medium are one of the primary design parameters of RF/microwave structures. The growth of, first, mobile (cellular) communications, followed by body-centric communications (including various wearable and implantable communications devices), together with the possibility of using such devices for physiological monitoring, has encouraged a great deal of interest in how the human body affects electromagnetic waves, whether for health and safe exposure, maintaining links between a cellular phone and base station or maintaining links between that same phone and a Bluetooth headset [15]. To provide the necessary database, the dielectric properties of biological tissues, including those with biological anomalies, have been extensively reported in the literature [16–19]. Since the success of microwave diagnostics and treatment applications depend on the dielectric property discrepancy between the normal and abnormal tissues (e.g., [13,14]), the evaluation of the dielectric properties is critical. Recently, the possible application of microwaves for non-invasive and continuous blood glucose monitoring has motivated many researchers to investigate the glucose-dependent dielectric properties of blood and other liquids. To this end, dielectric properties of blood plasma, blood, saline solutions and deionized water have been reported in the literature. The remainder of this section summarizes the reported literature on glucose-dependent dielectric properties. We first provide a brief primer on terminology.

The permittivity is a complex quantity, with the imaginary part representing the loss, which includes heating and conductive effects. Key terms include:

- permittivity—a bulk (that is, volume-average) material property quantifying the ability of the medium to store electrical energy;
- electric constant—also called the vacuum permittivity or permittivity of free space, this is the permittivity for an ideal vacuum and a physical constant;
- relative permittivity—the permittivity of a medium normalised by the electric constant (this is often applied to the real part of the normalised permittivity only);
- dielectric loss factor—another name for the imaginary part of the permittivity (often referring to the imaginary part of the normalised permittivity);
- effective permittivity—the permittivity of a composite (heterogeneous) material (for example, a layered structure, where each homogeneous layer has different properties) represented as an equivalent homogeneous medium (this could be used for the relative effective permittivity, which should be evident from context);
- loss tangent—a means of representing the loss in a dielectric as the ratio of imaginary to real parts (usually denoted '$\tan(\delta)$');
- conductivity—the ability to transfer charge, which is a loss mechanism for dielectrics;
- phantom—a digital or physical object that allows the parameter of interest to be changed in a controlled manner;
- tissue-mimicking material—a material designed to have the same dielectric properties as the tissue of interest, for use in physical phantoms;
- Q factor—a term used to quantify the performance of resonators, where greater Q-factors imply stronger resonances and more narrow bandwidths. A distinction is made between the ideal ('unloaded') performance and the 'measured' ('loaded') performance;
- resonant frequency—strictly, this is the frequency at which the input impedance of a resonator is purely real (resistive); in practice, this can be used for the frequency of a maximum (transmit-mode) or minimum (reflect-mode) of the resonator response. Changes in the dielectric properties 'loading' the resonator can affect some or all the resonant frequency, the bandwidth at resonance and the magnitude of the resonance (maximum or minimum) in detectable amounts.

2.1. *Measurements Performed with Biological Tissues*

In [20], glucose levels of blood plasma, collected from ten adults with ages ranging from 18 to 40 years, were changed in-vitro by adding 5% dextrose solution to the plasma to achieve values between 0 mg/dL to 16,000 mg/dL. The blood glucose concentration was changed by doubling the previous level; that is, first the plasma glucose levels were increased from 0 mg/dL to 250 mg/dL, then from 250 mg/dL to 500 mg/dL, etc. The dielectric properties of the blood plasmas were measured for each glucose level between 0.5 GHz and 20 GHz. A meaningful change was observed when the glucose levels were increased from 2000 mg/dL to 4000 mg/dL. The dielectric properties were measured with Agilent's Open-ended Coaxial Dielectric Probe Kit [21]. As a continuation of this study, the Cole–Cole equation was fit to the collected dielectric property data [22]. The Cole–Cole equation is a mathematical expression that has been utilized in the literature to model dielectric property behaviour with a minimum number of variables. In [18], the four-pole Cole–Cole equation was utilized to model the dielectric properties of biological tissues; however, it was concluded in more recent studies that a single-pole Cole–Cole equation is adequate to model dielectric property behaviour of biological tissues over an ultra-wide frequency range. The single-pole equation is [23]:

$$\hat{\varepsilon}(\omega) = \varepsilon_\infty + \frac{\varepsilon_s - \varepsilon_\infty}{1 + (j\omega\tau)^{(1-\alpha)}} + \frac{\sigma_i}{j\omega\varepsilon_0} \tag{1}$$

where ε_∞ is the relative permittivity at field frequencies, ε_s is the static permittivity, τ is the relaxation time for a dispersion region, α represents the broad distribution of the relaxation time constant and σ_i is the ionic conductivity. The difference $\varepsilon_s - \varepsilon_\infty$ is denoted as $\Delta\varepsilon$ and the effective permittivity $\hat{\varepsilon}$ is a function of frequency $f = \omega/2\pi$.

In [22], after fitting the Cole–Cole parameters to blood plasmas with different glucose concentrations, the Cole–Cole parameters were represented as polynomial equations to depict the glucose-dependent change of dielectric properties. These polynomial equations for the Cole–Cole parameters are used in this work with the intention to demonstrate quantitatively the dielectric property behaviour of tissues when changing the glucose level. The polynomial equation is a quadratic, of the form:

$$u(\chi) = a_n\chi^2 + b_n\chi + c_n \tag{2}$$

with u a dummy variable representing a given parameter and χ representing the glucose concentration. Coefficients a_n, b_n and c_n are given in [22] for each Cole–Cole model parameter. The polynomials with numerical coefficients are also given below:

$$\varepsilon_\infty(\chi) = 0.99 \times 10^{-2} \times \chi^2 + 0.47 \times 10^{-1} \times \chi + 2.3 \tag{3}$$

$$\Delta\varepsilon(\chi) = 0.93 \times 10^{-2} \times \chi^2 - 0.21 \times \chi + 71.0 \tag{4}$$

$$\tau(\chi) = 0.12 \times 10^{-2} \times \chi^2 + 0.23 \times \chi + 8.7 \tag{5}$$

$$\sigma_i(\chi) = 0.63 * 10^{-2} * \chi^2 - 0.14 * \chi + 2.0 \tag{6}$$

The Cole–Cole equations are plotted using the polynomials and coefficients for glucose concentrations of 72 mg/dL, 216 mg/dL, 330 mg/dL and 600 mg/dL (equivalently, 4 mmol/L, 12 mmol/L, 18.3 mmol/L and 33.3 mmol/L, respectively). Figure 1a,b show the change in relative permittivity and conductivity, respectively. This range of glucose concentrations was chosen based on the following: first, the blood glucose of a healthy human changes between 72 mg/dL to 216 mg/dL; second, a glucose level of 330 mg/dL was reported in [24] for a diabetic patient and is here used as a realistic value that must be detectable; and the maximum glucose level that can be measured by the current commercial ambulatory monitoring devices [25], 600 mg/dL. It can be seen that both relative permittivity and conductivity decrease as the glucose concentration increases from 72 mg/dL to 600 mg/dL. More importantly, however, it is evident that the sensitivity of the dielectric properties to realistic values is extremely small, being around 0.2 units for the relative permittivity and 0.1 S/m for the conductivity. The decrease in relative permittivity with the increase in blood glucose levels is slightly greater than the decrease in conductivity, but monitoring of both parameters may still be required. Furthermore, highly sensitive sensors will be required to detect small changes if continuous monitoring is desired, especially when including the effects of system noise and other factors that also affect the tissue dielectric properties. Although [22] presents a model to represent the glucose-dependent dielectric properties, the Cole–Cole parameter fittings show that ε_ϵ increases with the increase in glucose levels. This is not consistent with the measurement results and the fitting provided for the $\Delta\epsilon$. Nevertheless, to the best of the authors' knowledge, both the approach and utilization of blood plasma provides the most realistic insight to the glucose-dependent dielectric property change.

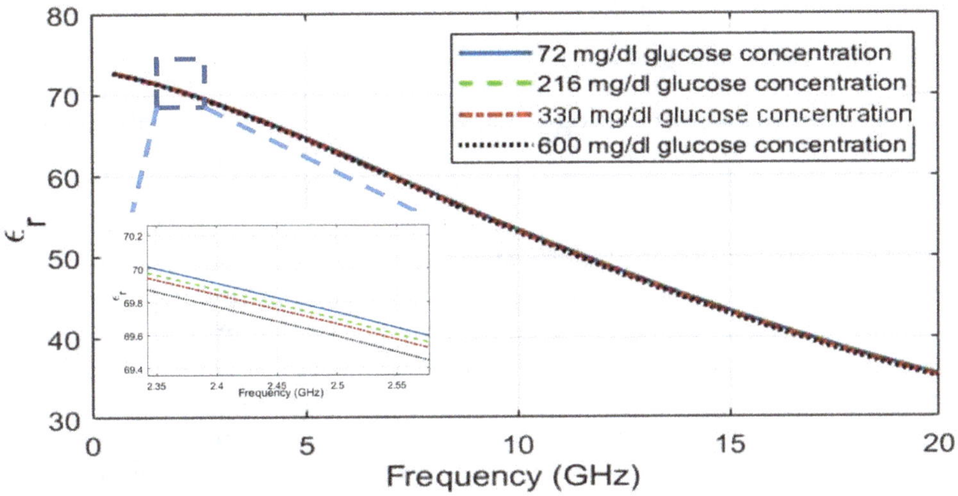

(a)

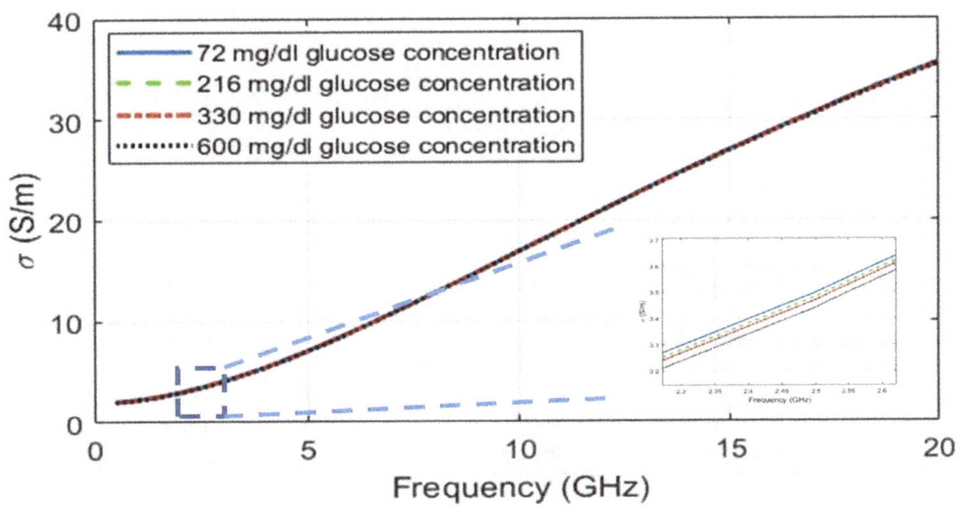

(b)

Figure 1. Dielectric properties of blood plasma with glucose variations graphed with Cole–Cole parameters polynomials given in [22]: (**a**) relative permittivity ϵ_r; (**b**) conductivity σ.

In another study [24], blood samples were collected from twenty patients (two per patient), where eight of the patients were diabetic and twelve of the patients were non-diabetic. One blood sample per volunteer was placed in a vial containing Ethylenediaminetetraacetic acid, utilized to prevent blood clots forming in the withdrawn sample; the other samples were kept without additives. The volume of each blood sample was 3 mL. The blood samples were then transferred to 5-mL dishes and the dielectric properties of the samples in the dish containers measured with Agilent's high temperature dielectric probe kit [21]. The blood glucose levels of the collected blood samples varied between 79 mg/dL to 330 mg/dL. A modified two pole Cole–Cole model was fit to the collected dielectric property measurements. It was concluded that the relative permittivity of blood drops five units between 80 mg/dL and 140 mg/dL. It should be noted that the measurement results were noisy and this could be due to the small sample size. The sensing volume of the probe could be larger than the sample thickness. Also, the number of measurements was not given in detail in the reported study.

2.2. Measurements Performed with Phantom Materials

Performing measurements using biological tissues is necessary for obtaining realistic results, but carries legal, ethical and financial implications. In addition, the complexity of real tissues can make the task of interpreting measurements challenging. The use of phantoms in place of tissues is common, particularly in the earlier stages of research and product development, to minimise these issue, although in vivo studies will always be required at some stage. In one study [26], tissue-mimicking phantoms replicating the dielectric properties of blood and other tissues were fabricated with oil-in-gelatin dispersion phantoms to quantify the realistic glucose-dependent dielectric properties. Oil-in-gelatine dispersion phantoms are used in the literature to imitate the dielectric properties of all biological tissues [27]. Such phantoms mainly include deionized water, gelatin, oil, a surfactant (e.g., dishwasher detergent) and salt (NaCl). The gelatin helps to solidify the phantom, deionized water is both used for dissolving the gelatine and increasing the dielectric properties. The surfactant is used increase the homogeneity when mixing the oil and other ingredients. Oil has very low dielectric properties and thus, decreases the dielectric properties of the mixture; finally, NaCl is utilized for increasing the conductivity of the phantom. Most (all) human body tissues can be obtained by using the same base recipe; however, the amounts of the ingredients have to be adjusted to obtain the desired tissue dielectric properties. For high water-content tissues, the amount of oil should be reduced and the reverse is true for low water-content tissues. Examples of the recipes for fat-, skin-, muscle- and blood-mimicking materials are given in Table 1 [26].

Table 1. Recipes of Tissue-Mimicking Materials including low, intermediate and high water-content tissues from 300 MHz to 20 GHz [26] (food colouring is used to distinguish the materials).

Ingredient (g)	Wet Skin	Fat	Blood	Muscle
Deionized Water	230.0	57.4	230.0	230.0
Gelatine	34.1	15.0	34.1	34.1
NaCl	1.4	0.0	1.2	1.2
Oil	75.0	329.6	15.0	35.0
$detergent_1$	40.0	0.0	40.0	40.0
$detergent_2$	0.0	10.0	0.0	0.0
food colouring	1.3	0.0	0.0	1.3

After characterizing the blood-mimicking material, different amounts of powdered dextrose was added to four blood-mimicking phantom materials. Note that the dextrose is the naturally available form of glucose in the blood and it can either be obtained in powder form or dissolved in water. The amount of dextrose added to the phantoms is equivalent to the blood glucose levels between 0 mg/dL and

216 mg/dL. This captured the realistic dielectric property change, since the blood glucose levels of a healthy person varies between 72 mg/dL and 216 mg/dL. The phantoms were prepared and left overnight to solidify. Next, the dielectric properties of the phantoms were measured with Agilent's high temperature open-ended coaxial dielectric probe kit. The measurements were repeated twenty times for each phantom and the median values of the measurements were taken as the dielectric properties of the phantom materials. This process was important, since the commercially available open-ended coaxial probes suffer from high measurement error rates, 5% for off-the-shelf open-ended coaxial probes [21]. According to the authors' experience, the reported error rate may increase depending on the equipment wear off, cable type, calibration quality and cable/probe movements. Considering that the change of blood glucose levels does not result in high dielectric contrast, the accuracy of the dielectric property measurements becomes critical to quantify the glucose-dependent dielectric property change.

A one-pole Cole–Cole equation, given by (1), was fit to the measured dielectric properties to quantify the glucose-dependent dielectric property change [26]. The accuracy of the fitting was checked by calculating the Euclidean distance, given in Equation (7). The accuracy of the fitting is also critical to minimize error that would hinder accurate detection of the dielectric property change due to a change in glucose levels.

$$e = \frac{1}{N}\sum_{i=1}^{N}\left[\left(\frac{\varepsilon'_{\omega_i} - \hat{\varepsilon}'_{\omega_i}}{median\left[\varepsilon'_{\hat{\omega}_i}\right]}\right)^2 + \left(\frac{\varepsilon''_{\omega_i} - \hat{\varepsilon}''_{\omega_i}}{median\left[\varepsilon''_{\hat{\omega}_i}\right]}\right)^2\right] \quad (7)$$

where ε'_{ω_i} and ε''_{ω_i} are the measured real and imaginary parts of the permittivity, $\hat{\varepsilon}'_{\omega_i}$ and $\hat{\varepsilon}''_{\omega_i}$ are the equivalent fitted dielectric properties and N is the number of points used within the measurement frequency range.

When the fitted Cole–Cole parameters were analysed, it was seen that the $\Delta\epsilon$ parameter decreased with the increase in the dextrose levels in the blood-mimicking phantoms. This is consistent with the previously reported results, where it was concluded that the increase in dextrose levels decreases the permittivity of the blood plasma [20]. The change in $\Delta\epsilon$ parameter is shown in Figure 2; it can be seen that ϵ parameter changed by one unit when the dextrose levels increased from 0 mg/dL to 216 mg/dL. This again emphasises how the sensitivity of the measurement system will be critical in successfully tracking changes in blood glucose level, particularly in continuous measurement scenarios.

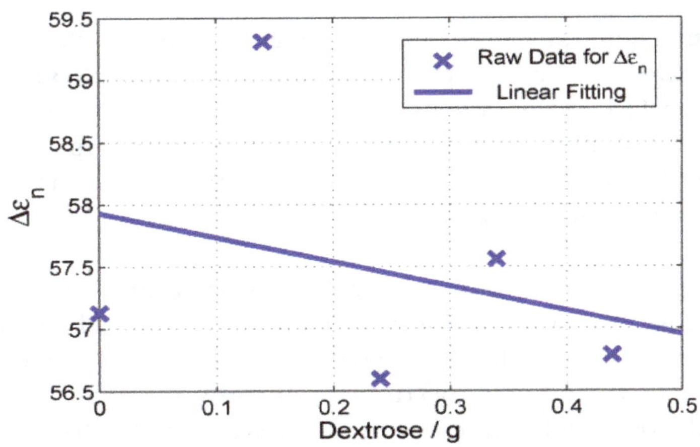

Figure 2. Glucose-dependent change in $\Delta\epsilon$ parameter collected from the blood-mimicking phantoms with glucose levels ranging from 0 mg/dL to 216 mg/dL, reported in [26].

The authors of [28] also used recipes for blood mimicking phantom materials (proposed in [29]). The phantoms were composed with water, salt, flour and sugar [28]. The recipe for the blood-mimicking material required 66.9%, 0.8%, 25.0%, and 7.3% by weight for water, salt, flour, and sugar, respectively [28]. A change of glucose level was emulated by adding varying amounts of sugar. In particular, the results from real blood samples (Section 2.1) were used to predict the equivalent amount of sugar to use in the phantom recipe (in place of the amount specified in the provided phantom recipe [28]). Reasonable agreement at the higher frequencies used (approximately 2.2–6 GHz) were observed between the blood measurements and phantoms fabricated for all sugar amounts (two phantoms were made for each amount of sugar), with greater divergence at the lower frequencies.

Most of the reported work in the literature was performed to characterize the glucose-dependent dielectric property change with broadband measurement techniques; namely, open-ended coaxial probes. Although the technique offers a number of advantages, including minimal sample preparation requirements and broadband measurement capabilities, it suffers from greater measurement errors. Therefore, a more narrow-band resonator technique was employed in [30] to retrieve the dielectric properties of phantom materials made using flour, water and sugar (note that these phantoms were not blood mimicking material, but were used to represent the lossy medium of the human body). With the proposed analytical method, highly accurate permittivity results were obtained, despite the fact that the resonator was not fully optimised for this task. The loss in the phantom (human body) acts to increase the bandwidth of the resonator, increasing the noise included with the measurement and reducing sensitivity. An extremely narrow-band (high Q-factor) resonator may give even greater sensitivity, also improving accuracy. Importantly, the methodology employed [30] gave accurate results despite the limitations of the narrow-band resonator employed.

2.3. Measurements Performed with De-Ionized Water

In an attempt to simplify the sample preparation, some research groups approximate blood with water. In some studies, this was justified by the fact that the blood plasma is a high water-content tissue and, since the mineral percentages in blood plasma are very low, the minerals can be ignored. Others argued that a 'physiological solution' (0.9% NaCl solution) tends to imitate blood and can thus, be used as a base for measuring the change in dielectric properties with respect to change in glucose levels. The rest simply investigated the glucose-dependent dielectric properties of de-ionized water, since it is free of other interactions and this helps with quantifying the effect of only glucose to dielectric properties.

In [31], blood-simulating solutions were obtained by adding 10, 20, 30, 40 and 50 percent-by- weight table sugar into the de-ionized water. The dielectric properties of the solutions were measured from 200 MHz to 5 GHz. As expected, the permittivity of the solutions decreased with the increase in sugar levels, whereas the conductivity increased. Essentially, this work shows the macro trends in dielectric property behaviour with respect to changes in sugar levels. However, this may not represent the dielectric property behaviour for realistic glucose levels.

In [32], the dielectric properties of physiological solutions and de-ionized water were measured, having seven different glucose amounts varying from 0 mol/L to 6 mol/L at 1 mol/L increments (that is, from 0 mg/dL to 108,000 mg/dL with 18,000 mg/dL increments). As noted earlier, the normal range of glucose is between 72 mg/dL and 216 mg/dL for a healthy person. A Type 2 diabetes patient can experience higher blood glucose levels. Ambulatory devices are unable to measure glucose levels above 600 mg/dL [25]. If the blood glucose levels are above 600 mg/dL, the patient is at high risk of experiencing hyperosmolar hyperglycaemic state (HHS). Therefore, an increase of 18,000 mg/dL is much higher than the realistic glucose level changes. Also, this study does not specify the type of glucose used to obtain the mixtures. The reported measurement results confirm that the increase in the glucose levels decreases the relative permittivity of the mixture at lower frequencies. However, it concludes that, at higher frequencies, the increase in glucose levels increases the relative permittivity of the mixture. For conductivity, it was concluded that the increase in glucose levels has an effect on conductivity and this effect is frequency-dependent; also, the amount of change in conductivity is smaller when compared to relative permittivity. It should also be noted that the reported measurements were performed with Agilent's open-ended coaxial performance probe between 500 MHz and 67 GHz. The technical specifications indicate that the probe is reliably operational between 500 MHz and 50 GHz [21]. Therefore, the reported measurements above 50 GHz are higher than the recommended operation range of the probe. Unlike other reported studies, the measurements presented in [32] were performed at 37 °C (that is, at human body temperature). It was concluded that the sensitivity of both relative permittivity and conductivity values to the glucose was between 0.01% to 0.02% per mmol glucose change in one litre of blood-mimicking material. Considering that the relative permittivity of blood in the 2.45 GHz license-exempt Industrial, Scientific and Medical (ISM) band is 58.2 units [17,18], the relative permittivity change will be 0.05 units if the blood glucose is increased from 72 mg/dL to 216 mg/dL.

The dielectric properties of glucose–water solutions were used to model the glucose-dependent dielectric property change at 25 °C in [33–35], with glucose concentrations between 0 mg/dL and 16,000 mg/dL. The measurements were performed with an in-house fabricated open-ended coaxial probe and an in-house algorithm. The dielectric properties were retrieved using artificial neural networks that fit the Debye model to the measurements for each glucose concentration. The Debye model is very similar to the Cole–Cole model; in the Debye model, the α parameter in Equation (1) is zero and the ionic conductivity is also ignored ($\sigma_i = 0$). The Debye parameters were then again expressed as polynomials with variables representing the change in glucose levels, with the same basic polynomial model given in Equation (2) used. The coefficients of the polynomials are given in Table 2 for ε_∞, ε_s and τ.

Table 2. Polynomial coefficients fitted to the Debye parameters [33]. Reproduced with permission from Turgul V., Kale I., Sensors and Actuators A: Physical, Elsevier, 2018.

u	a_n	b_n	c_n
ε_∞	-8.214×10^{-8}	2.148×10^{-3}	8.722
ε_s	2.318×10^{-9}	-2.793×10^{-4}	81.015
τ	-8.370×10^{-9}	5.150×10^{-4}	8.776

The approach used in [22] was modified for the Debye parameters and adopted in this study to characterize the glucose-dependent dielectric properties of de-ionized water. Equation (2) and the Debye parameter coefficients are used to obtain Figure 3, depicting the dielectric property change as the glucose levels increase from 72 mg/dL to 600 mg/dL. As seen from the magnified plots inset in the figures, the relative permittivity of the de-ionized water decreases with the increase in glucose concentration, while the conductivity of the deionized water increases. In fact, the observed behaviour of the conductivity changes when the frequency is increased above 9 GHz. The conductivity of the mixture started to decrease with the increase in glucose concentration. Although the trend in relative permittivity agrees with the earlier publications, the trend in conductivity is different when compared to other reported work. As explained earlier, the broadband dielectric property measurement techniques are prone to errors. Since the change in conductivity is expected to be even smaller than the change in permittivity, the conductivity change due to glucose concentration might have been lost.

The dielectric properties at four different frequencies (0.5 GHz, 2.5 GHz, 5.0 GHz and 10.00 GHz) are listed in Table 3, generated using the dielectric property graphs given in Figures 1 and 3. These frequencies were chosen since 500 MHz is close to the Medical Device Radiocommunications Service (MedRadio) and Wireless Medical Telemetry Service (WMTS) bands [36,37], 2.5 GHz and 5.0 GHz are close to license-exempt ISM bands in common use for wearable devices and 10 GHz represents the glucose-dependent dielectric behaviour at higher frequencies.

The conductivity of blood plasma is higher than the conductivity of the deionized water at frequencies lower than 10 GHz. This could be due to sodium and other minerals present in the blood plasma. The change in conductivity is very small at all frequencies. Figure 3b does suggest that the conductivity change between 18–20 GHz is greater than other frequencies. It should be noted, however, that measurements at higher frequencies require special equipment and this change might merely due to the greater measurement/fitting errors at higher frequencies. The relative permittivity change is somewhat greater than the conductivity change and seems to be greatest at 10 GHz, among the frequencies shown in Table 3.

This quantitative comparison of models from the literature serves to confirm that the dielectric property changes due to changes in glucose levels are very small. The relative permittivity displays a consistent trend: an increase in glucose level corresponds to a decrease in the relative permittivity of blood plasma and other blood mimicking materials.

Since the glucose-dependent relative permittivity change is very small, there is a need to develop structures that are sensitive to dielectric property change and algorithms that can sense the glucose-dependent change among other factors that may affect the dielectric properties of the biological tissue.

In [38], an impedance analyser was utilized in the frequency range of 1 kHz to 1 MHz. Two sets of measurements were performed. The first used aqueous solutions of glucose, with concentrations from 0 mmol/L (0 mg/dL) to 225 mmol/L (4050 mg/dL), at steps of 25 mmol/L (450 mg/dL); hence, this set of measurements did not address the sensitivity issue. It was observed that both the permittivity and conductivity of the glucose solutions were decreasing with the increase in the glucose concentrations [38]. Similar to other studies, the dielectric properties were modelled with the three pole Cole–Cole equation, while the changes in Cole–Cole parameters with respect to change in glucose concentration was modelled with polynomials.

The change in the $\Delta\varepsilon_1$ plotted to demonstrate that the $\varepsilon_s - \varepsilon_{inf}$ is decreasing with the increase in glucose concentration [38]. The second set of measurements examined the effect of changes in blood volume during the cardiac cycle and used the bio-impedance parameter directly, rather than extracting permittivity and conductivity [38]. These are discussed further in Section 3.2.

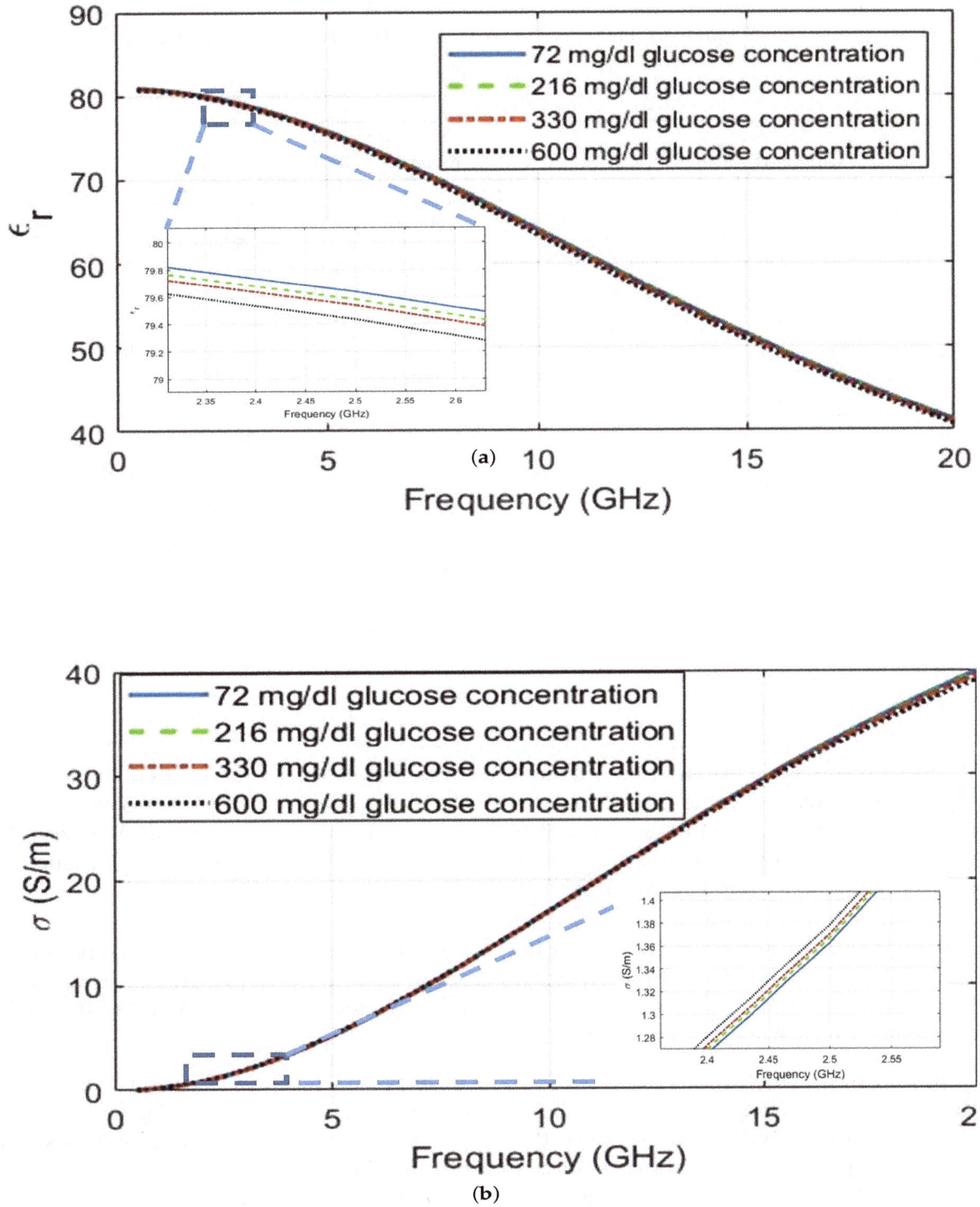

Figure 3. Dielectric properties of water with glucose variations graphed with Debye parameters polynomials given in [33]: (**a**) relative permittivity; (**b**) conductivity.

Table 3. Dielectric property change of blood plasma (BP) and water–glucose with respect to glucose concentration at 0.5, 2.5, 5.0 and 10 GHz based on the Cole–Cole and Debye parameter polynomials given in [22,33]. (*d-water*—de-ionised water)

Glucose Concentration (mg/dL)	Frequency (GHz)	ε_r BP [22]	ε_r *d-water* [33]	σ BP [22] (S/m)	σ *d-water* [33] (S/m)
72	0.50	72.75	80.94	2.065	5.55×10^{-2}
219		72.73	80.9	2.046	5.57×10^{-2}
330		72.71	80.87	2.030	5.58×10^{-2}
600		72.66	80.79	1.995	5.62×10^{-2}
72	2.50	69.74	79.64	3.498	13.62×10^{-1}
219		69.70	79.58	3.482	13.67×10^{-1}
330		69.67	79.54	3.470	13.70×10^{-1}
600		69.59	79.43	3.441	13.78×10^{-1}
72	5.00	64.62	75.86	7.078	51.59×10^{-1}
219		64.56	75.76	7.069	51.71×10^{-1}
330		64.51	75.69	7.062	51.80×10^{-1}
600		64.39	75.51	7.046	52.01×10^{-1}
72	10.00	53.24	64.07	16.91	17.00
219		53.14	63.90	16.91	17.00
330		53.07	63.76	16.91	16.99
600		52.88	63.44	16.90	16.97

2.4. Discussion

It is clear, from the qualitative review and quantitative examples given, that the application of dielectric spectroscopy for glucose detection is both possible (as seen by the in vitro experiments) and extremely challenging, due to the small magnitude changes in permittivity associated with the small changes in glucose encountered in realistic scenarios. The next section discusses the issues around selection of the operating frequency and bandwidth.

A few comments must be made here regarding the selectivity issue. All the studies reported on above have examined the behaviour of the dielectric properties under the controlled change of sugar level and our discussion has focussed on the sensitivity issue. In reality, these properties will be affected by other inter-related factors, such as:

- temperature—much of the above research was conducted at standard laboratory temperature and there is little-to-no research available on the combined effect of temperature and glucose-level changes on the dielectric properties. Furthermore, the effect of temperature on various tissues is known to be frequency-dependent with complex behaviour [39];
- perfusion—the volume of blood in the measured region during the measurement period will obviously affect the data and this volume will change with temperature, pulse rate, activity level and clothing (for example, tight sleeves or watch bands can restrict the flow of blood);
- sensor positioning and motion—different locations on the body have been considered for sensor placement (such as the ear lobe, the wrist, the thumb and the torso, as discussed in Sections 3.2 and 4), either for convenience of testing, comfort for continuous-monitoring scenarios, or for tissue properties at that location (e.g., the ear lobe has a relatively thin skin layer and no bone or muscle). Small motions of the test subject can induce errors in the measurement (e.g., introduction of a small air gap between sensor and skin), potentially even for static test scenarios. For the ideal of continuous monitoring, any

sensor must be robust to motion-induced artefacts from small changes in sensor position, as well as related issues (e.g., activity level, contamination of the test site from sweat, dirt and other materials);

- other biological activity—tissues are dynamic inhomogeneous materials, with many bio-chemical and bio-physical process occurring. Examples that may affect the dielectric properties include (but are not limited to) changes in the levels of blood gases (particularly oxygen and carbon dioxide), urea, lactic acid (affected by activity level), as well as changes induced by injury or infection.

Amperometric glucose-sensing, such as used with minimally invasive needle-type bio-sensors, use specific enzymes and filtering membranes to provide selectivity, sensitivity and sensor longevity [2]. A major challenge for non-invasive spectroscopic detection methods is to achieve the selectivity necessary to properly attribute dielectric changes to blood glucose changes.

Another aspect that must be considered is the subject-specific variation in tissues. In particular, there can be significant variation across the population in tissue thickness for various locations on the body, possibly correlating across one or more of gender, age, ethnicity and affluence (and its impact on physical health and fitness), among other factors. Any system that could not accommodate such variation into its model for extracting the dielectric properties would be restricted in application at best. Those systems attempting to penetrate furthest into the body will need to account for variation in muscle and fat tissues, plus other internal tissues (dependent on the location of the device on the body); all systems must account for skin thickness variation. To illustrate this issue, we summarise some key points of a recent paper on measuring the dielectric properties of skin (not aimed at glucose monitoring [12]).

As described in [12] and elsewhere (e.g., [26,40]), there are at least five different ways of modelling skin (ignoring voxelized phantoms from MRI scans). The skin can be considered as a single homogeneous layer in its simplest form, with one effective permittivity. This can be perfectly acceptable and accurate, electromagnetically speaking, depending on the application. Increasing complexity comes by sub-dividing the skin into constituent layers, with the most complex in use being a four-layer model, consisting of the [12]:

- stratum corneum (the outermost and driest layer);
- viable epidermis;
- dermis;
- subcutaneous fat layer.

Intermediate-complexity models come from merging one or more of these layers into homogeneous effective media. (Some also may argue against including the fat layer; from an electromagnetic perspective, there is no particular problem with this, so long as the effective medium averages the constituent media correctly.) The stratum corneum is approximately 20 μm thick, but can be thicker, dependent on body location (and likely varying between subjects to some extent) [12]. The epidermis is normally between 0.06–0.1 mm thick and the dermis is between 1.2–2.8 mm thick [12]. It is noted that a blood layer may be added for glucose-monitoring applications. Furthermore, resonators will typically include at least one dielectric layer in their construction, which must be included in models appropriately.

The models and the effect of the various layers, were investigated numerically between 26.5 GHz and 40 GHz, using models of open-ended coaxial probes and open-ended waveguide (two common probes used in material characterisation) [12]. Further measurements were made at several body locations on three test subjects [12]. The important sources of both modelling and measurement errors were also investigated. Accuracies of up to 85% and 95% were reported for relative permittivity and relative dielectric loss factor, respectively [12].

In addition to this, it has been shown that non-invasive blood glucose sensing at finger-tips is affected by layer thickness and even the presence of small air-gaps caused by finger-prints [41,42]. A shift in resonant frequency of around 20 MHz was observed due to these air-gaps [41] and potentially as much as 100 MHz, depending on fingerprint depth [42]. Given that the air-gaps will differ depending on how the finger is placed on the sensor [41,42], in addition to the effect of pressure on the tissues in the finger tip, it is clear that this effect must be carefully considered, given that frequency shifts as low as 8 MHz [43] could be produced by changes in glucose concentrations, at least for resonators with relatively low Q-factors.

It is also worth noting that the models discussed above assume planar layers of uniform thickness in most instances. The effect of pressure (e.g., of a finger pressed on a sensor, or a smart watch strap on the wrist) will be to reduce the thickness of at least some of the layers in a non-uniform manner, in addition to affecting the flow of blood and interstitial fluid through the tissues.

3. Frequency of Choice

3.1. An Empirical Approach

Different frequencies have been utilized for blood glucose level detection in the literature, ranging from radio frequencies to millimetre waves. Although some applications at terahertz and infrared range have also been investigated (e.g., [44,45]), the scope of this review is limited to RF/microwave and some millimetre-wave applications. Most of the work reported focusses on narrow-band applications, with a few reporting wide-band behaviour. Since microwave diagnostic and treatment applications are based on the dielectric property discrepancies between the anomalous and healthy tissues, the behaviour of dielectric properties that is dispersive with respect to frequency is one of the primary constraints for frequency of choice.

Another related factor in frequency selection is penetration depth: as conductivity increases with frequency for all tissues, the electromagnetic wave encounters greater loss at higher frequencies, which can be related directly to how much tissue the wave can pass through and still be detectable at the system's minimum threshold for detection. (A related parameter is the skin depth; we do not discuss this here, but the penetration depth is always greater than the skin depth.) For most implementations of sensors for glucose monitoring, a reflection mode is used; a few use a transmission mode (e.g., for systems placed on the ear lobe). The penetration depth is essentially a reflection-mode parameter; transmission-mode systems can be expected to have a maximum allowed sample thickness approximately twice that of the penetration depth (because the reflected wave passes through the tissues twice). Penetration depth decreases with frequency for all tissues. At low frequencies (e.g., below 100 MHz), the penetration depths for skin, fat and muscle would be more than thicknesses typically encountered; above 10 GHz, however, very little penetration into muscle can be expected, while penetration depths for skin and fat are of less than or equal to typical thicknesses [46]. We note that the limits on exposure, particularly the Specific Absorption Rate [SAR], place an upper bound on transmit power, which translates into a maximum penetration depth for a tissue of given loss.

As noted before, microwave frequencies have been employed for breast cancer imaging and treatment purposes due to the dielectric property discrepancy between the benign and malign tissues [47]. In microwave imaging, the employed frequency range is between 3 GHz and 7 GHz. The resolution of the microwave images increases at higher frequencies; however, penetration depth and wavelength decrease. To illustrate the penetration depth and wavelength in tissue, we plotted the behaviour two values with respect to frequency in muscle tissue. The muscle tissue dielectric properties have been utilized before in the literature to represent the lossy medium of the human body [40]. The relative permittivity and conductivity of muscle tissue is shown in Figure 4a; the change of wavelength and penetration depth in muscle tissue medium with respect to frequency is shown in Figure 4b. Similar to high water-content tissues, the relative permittivity of the muscle tissue decreases with the increase in frequency, while the conductivity of the muscle tissue increases. Both the dielectric property change and the increase in frequency affects the wavelength and penetration depth. From Figure 4b, it can be seen that both the wavelength and the penetration depth is less than 5 mm. This demonstrates that, above 10 GHz, the body tissues will be even more lossy and the propagating wave will quickly attenuate.

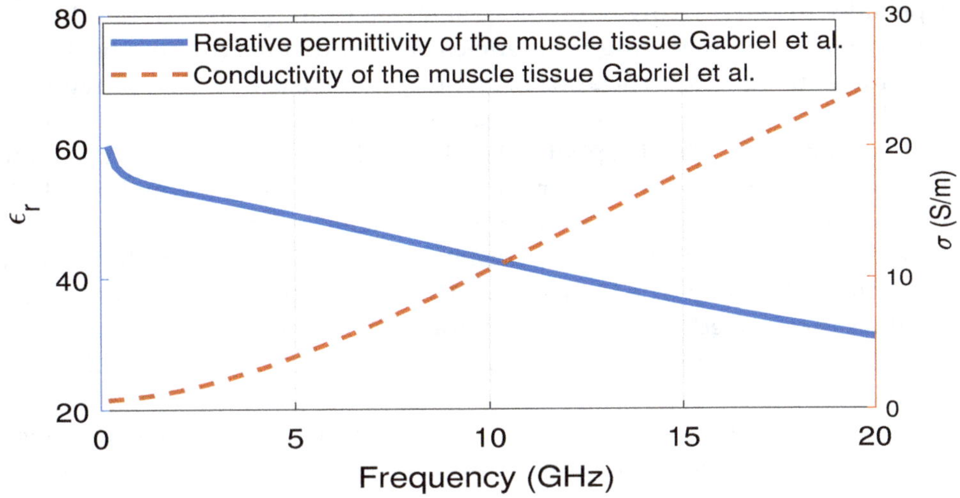

(a)

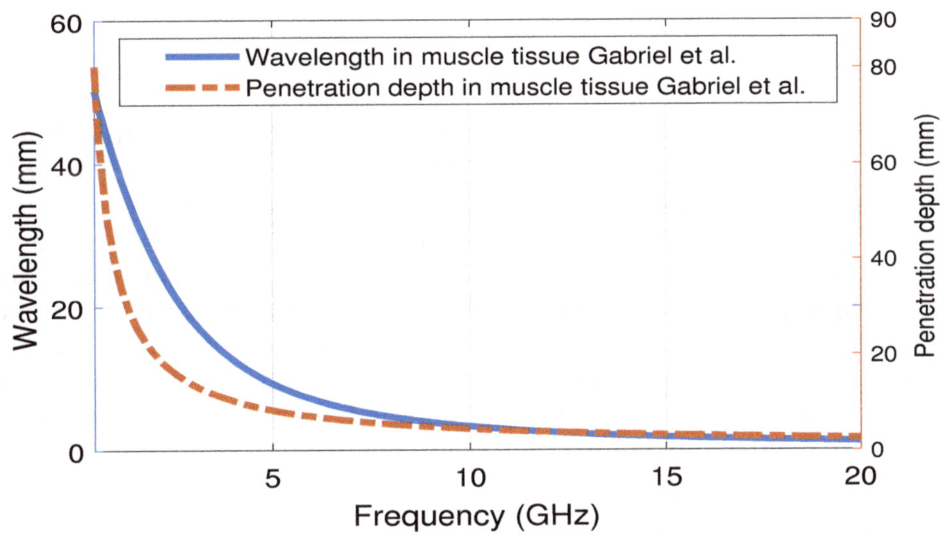

(b)

Figure 4. Muscle tissue dielectric properties and wave behaviour in muscle tissue medium: (**a**) relative permittivity and conductivity of muscle tissue between 200 MHz and 20 GHz; (**b**) wavelength and penetration depth in muscle medium.

One other criterion that can be considered while choosing the frequency of operation is looking into the utilization of the bands. For example, the US Federal Communications Commission's MedRadio spectrum allocation covers the 413–419 MHz, 426–432 MHz, 438–444 MHz, 451–457 MHz and 2360–2400 MHz ranges. These bands are specifically useful for implants and body-worn devices for off-body, on-body and in-body communications, since the signal is still quite strong for these bands. Other possible bands include the license-exempt 2.4–2.5 GHz and 5.725–5.875 GHz ISM bands. At 2.45 GHz, the wavelength and penetration depth in muscle tissue is around 22 mm for both quantities. At 5.8 GHz, the wavelength and penetration depth in muscle tissue is around 7.6 mm and 7.4 mm, respectively.

Lastly, it can be concluded from Section 2 that the glucose-dependent dielectric property change is very limited, especially in the microwave region, such that the glucose-dependent change does not display a significant variation between the frequencies. This indicates that the limited change in blood dielectric properties due to the glucose variations can only be measured by employing a highly sensitive technique. Broadband dielectric property measurement techniques, such as the open-ended coaxial probe, are known to suffer from accuracy and repeatability limitations, whereas narrow band measurement techniques are known to be more precise. Therefore, empirically we can conclude that a narrow-band technique will be more sensitive to glucose-dependent dielectric property changes. Ultimately, the sensitivity of a resonator also depends on the measurement technique and the performance of the employed technique at the operation frequency. The Q factor, which is indicative of the measurement sensitivity, of narrow-band resonators is expected to increase at higher frequencies (that is, higher order modes for a given resonator tend to have higher Q factors). Considering the constraints imposed by the lossy nature of the biological tissue media (higher loss and smaller penetration depth with increasing frequency) and the band availability, plus the fact that resonators tend to be some multiple of a half-wavelength in size (hence, physically larger at lower frequencies), a narrow-band resonator operating at a narrow band frequency between 4 GHz and 7 GHz can be a viable option. Of course, it is still possible to employ other frequencies, both higher and lower, as can been seen in the literature. We now review these choices, with a discussion following in Section 3.3.

3.2. *Frequencies Employed in the Literature*

Different frequencies have been employed in the literature to sense the glucose change. For example, in [48], a monopole antenna operating between 1–6 GHz was designed. The antenna response between 1.5–3 GHz was observed to shift during simulations and while testing it with blood mimicking phantoms. However, it is known that the response of wideband and ultra-wideband antennas are less sensitive to the dielectric property changes in a medium. For instance, Vivaldi antennas are frequently employed for microwave medical imaging applications to both provide a wideband signal and prevent the antenna detuning due to close proximity to human body. Additionally broadband dielectric property measurement methods known to suffer from low measurement accuracy. Considering that the realistic dielectric property change with respect to change in glucose levels is very limited, there is a need to employ more sensitive techniques.

As mentioned above (Section 2.3), an impedance spectroscopy approach was used in [38]; here, we describe the second set of measurements using the bio-impedance parameter directly, measured using a system from Biopac. Initially, measurements were performed on agar phantoms with aqueous solutions using varying quantities of glucose: 0 mmol/L, 50 mmol/L (900 mg/dL), 100 mmol/L (1800 mg/dL) and 200 mmol/L (3600 mg/dL); again, it must be stated that these are not realistic values, so questions regarding the sensitivity are not addressed. The bio-impedance of glucose solutions with solutions having different glucose concentrations were calculated at 10 Hz and supported the expectation that the change in bio-impedance decreased with increasing glucose concentration. An additional set of measurements were performed on a non-diabetic test subject, in conjunction with direct measurements with a commercial portable blood glucose meter (ACCU-CHEK Performa). Measurements were taken over the course of a 135-minute period, at five-minute intervals for the bio-impedance and thirty-minute intervals for the blood meter, during a type of oral glucose tolerance test. After some signal processing and curve-fitting, it was observed that there was an inverse correlation between the measured bio-impedance and the measured glucose level [38]. This work reported that the temperature, minimum and maximum blood volume and other components of blood (such as haemoglobin) might effect the bio-impedance calculations.

A spiral resonator operating between 628 and 677 MHz was introduced in [30]. This resonator was not tested with realistic glucose values and the response was explored to retrieve the relative permittivity of the tissues. The sensitivity of the resonator can not be judged. It should be noted that the wavelength and penetration depth is quite large at these frequencies. Therefore, the response of the structures operating close to MedRadio bands can be affected by other factors, such as the size of the tissue loaded to the resonator. When the final application is considered, this could emerge as a problem when setting a calibration standard.

Another resonator was presented in [26,43], operating close to 2.45 GHz when loaded with four- and five-layer tissue-mimicking materials (composed of dry skin, wet skin, fat, blood and muscle tissue). This resonator, which was not optimised for the wearable glucose monitor application, consisted of a microstrip patch resonator with two capacitively coupled feeding strips and had a Q-factor of around 4, making it relatively poor in terms of sensitivity. The penetration depth and wavelength at this frequency is still quite large (around 20 mm in muscle tissue); therefore, the calibration problem may still emerge at a smaller scale. One option to achieve matching for different loads is to utilize a impedance-matching circuit at these frequencies. However, this approach should be implemented so that glucose-dependent change in impedance will not be masked.

A serpentine-shaped capacitive structure operating between 3.0 GHz and 6.0 GHz was presented in [33,49]. The sensitivity of this structure was analysed for the best matching. Initially, the structure was designed to operate at 4.8 GHz; this frequency was chosen after analysing the penetration depth and reflections between different tissue boundaries. It is worth noting that most of the simulations were performed in commercial electromagnetic simulation programs; when the RF/microwave sensors are loaded with lossy materials (such as four-layered tissue-mimicking materials with frequency-dispersive dielectric properties), the simulations take longer to complete than simulations in air. Therefore, it is advised to run such simulations on workstations; even then, the cost of optimizing these sensors to operate at a certain frequency is high.

Two patch antennas operating at 2.45 GHz and 5.8 GHz were designed and tested with dextrose solutions in an attempt compare the performance of the antennas at these two frequencies [50]. The antennas are mounted at the bottom of two 3D printed cups. The cups were filled with dextrose solutions having concentrations ranging from 0 mg/dL to 5000 mg/dL. From 0 mg/dL to 1000 mg/dL, the amount of dextrose was increased by 200 mg/dL. When the behaviour of the patch antenna was analysed while changing the dextrose amount, it was observed the operation frequency did not change. However, the matching of the antennas changed with the increase in dextrose levels. Although the change was not linear, it was observed that the matching of the antenna operating at higher frequency was more sensitive to the dextrose change. The response of both antennas are given in Table 4. Since the antenna types were identical, the glucose-dependent change in antenna matching is attributed to the frequency of operation.

Table 4. Comparison of patch antennas operating at 2.45 GHz and 5.8 GHz tested with deionized water–dextrose solutions [50].

Dextrose Levels (mg/dL)	S_{11} Response (dB) at 2.45 GHz	S_{11} Response (dB) at 5.8 GHz
0	−14.87	−26.32
200	−14.82	−30.19
400	−15.4	−38.85
600	−14.45	−38.52

A resonator operating at 1.4 GHz was proposed in [51]. The sensor, which had a Q-factor of about 800 in air [51], was proposed to be placed on the abdomen region of the body, where its Q-factor was reduced to about 80 [51]. The sensor was tested with humans and the response compared with the commercial glucose sensors. Also, an in vitro interference test technique was proposed to test the sensor performance with glucose and other materials. The resonator response shifted 600 kHz when the glucose levels were increased from 0 mg/dL to 600 mg/dL. The in vitro performance of this resonator does not only depend on the frequency; the structure itself also has an important role. Therefore, in the abdomen region the tissue should not be considered homogeneous in the 1.4 GHz frequency range. Changes in other parameters are likely to affect the resonator response. In [51], the effect of other parameters was mitigated with a reference structure that was separated spatially from the tissue and main resonator, but otherwise identical to it. Hence, the change in resonant response (frequency and bandwidth) for the reference resonator can be used to track temperature via a calibration curve, thus allowing detection of permittivity changes with the main resonator caused by other factors. A clinical trial of this sensor involving 24 human subjects (eight non-diabetics, four Type-1 diabetics and 12 Type-2 diabetics) undergoing an oral tolerance test was reported [52] and assessed using the Clarke Error Grid and the mean absolute relative difference (MARD) parameter. Two versions of the sensor were used (12 subjects per sensor); some differences between sensors were possibly evident, based on MARD values of 11% and 14% for the respective test groups, although no detail is provided on the test subject groups to allow identification of other possible causes. An overall MARD value of 12.5% was calculated. Although the majority of test samples were in regions A and B of the Clarke Error Grid, there were some values in the upper C region (attributed to unexpected movement by the test subjects in [52]), demonstrating further work is necessary to enhance robustness. The comparison in time between the sensor and the reference glucose readings (taken using a YSI 2300 Glucose and Lactate Analyzer) was visually close in both papers [51,52]; curve-fitting models were developed in [51] that have presumably been used in [52] to produce estimated blood glucose levels (in mg/dL) directly.

Another microwave resonator operating at 6.53 GHz was proposed in [53]. When a container of de-ionized water–glucose solution, with a concentration of 0.75 mg/mL, was placed on the resonator, the resonance frequency shifted to 3.43 GHz. The glucose concentration was then increased to 1 mg/mL, then in 1 mg/mL increments to 5 mg/mL. The resonance frequency shifted to 3.53, 3.93, 4.23 and 5.03 GHz for glucose concentrations of 1 mg/mL, 2 mg/mL, 3 mg/mL, 4 mg/mL and 5 mg/mL, respectively. Although a very good resonance shift is observed, it should be noted that the sensitivity can not be merely attributed to frequency of operation. Both the resonator structure and the frequency of operation, thus, the Q factor, are all parameters that needs to be considered in this work. The readers should note the units used, which have a factor of 100 difference to those used in this work, such that the normal range of glucose concentration is stated as from 0.75 mg/mL to 2.16 mg/mL by the authors of [53]. The concentrations used are therefore similar to the values used in this review for quantitative comparisons.

A microstrip-line-based multi-band resonator, operating between 100 MHz and 500 MHz and 1.4 GHz to 1.8 GHz, was proposed in [54]. The resonator was tested using glucose solutions, with concentrations from 0 mg/dL to 5000 mg/dL. The resonance shift, as well as the matching of the resonator, was observed for both frequencies. It was concluded that the resonator displayed a better sensitivity to the glucose change at higher frequencies.

In [55], three versions of a resonator, operating at 1.92 GHz, 5.16 GHz and 7.16 GHz, was designed for measurement of glucose concentrations in microlitre volume solutions. A dielectric sensing cup with a microlitre volume was designed and integrated to these structures to hold the liquid. The Q factor of all three structures was investigated with solutions having different glucose concentrations. The Q factor changed by up to five units for glucose concentration ranging from 0% to 10%.

A spiral resonator was proposed in [56], operating at 7.65 GHz when placed in aqueous glucose solution and operating at 7.77 GHz when placed in a sample of pig blood. During the tests, the sample under test was put into a Petri dish with a diameter of 8 mm, which was placed in turn on the resonator (first, the aqueous solutions were tested, followed by the blood samples). Glucose concentrations for the aqueous solutions were from 0 mg/dL to 600 mg/dL; for the pig blood samples, concentrations from 100 mg/dL to 600 mg/dL were tested. The observed shift in operating frequency was negligible; thus, the authors reported the change in matching of the resonator. For the aqueous samples, with concentrations ranging from 0 mg/dL to 600 mg/dL; the S_{11} response decreased from −40 dB to −55 dB; for pig blood samples (concentrations ranging from 100 mg/dL to 600 mg/dL), the S_{11} response decreased from −18 dB to −25 dB. The change in the S_{11} response with respect to volume was also reported in this work. To the best of the authors' knowledge, the sample volume should be chosen in such way that the electromagnetic energy completely attenuates within the material under test (MUT) at the operating frequency, in order to explore the true performance of the structure during such experiments. The effective permittivity of the medium measured by the resonator will then only depend on the permittivity of the substrate and the permittivity of the MUT. Since the glucose-dependent dielectric property change is very limited, this is a paramount parameter to explore the full potential of a microwave sensor for blood glucose monitoring.

A metamaterial-based resonator operating at 2 GHz was proposed in [57]. In this work, the change in both amplitude and phase of S_{21} was tracked. The resonator was simulated with digital phantoms, with the relative permittivity of the digital phantoms changed based on the glucose-dependent dielectric property change equations described in [24]. To simulate the change in blood glucose levels between 0 mg/dL and 250 mg/dL, the relative permittivity of the digital blood-mimicking phantom was changed from 69.4 units to 47.5 units, respectively. When compared to the conclusions drawn in [26], where the change in relative permittivity was expected to be 1 unit for glucose levels from 0 mg/dL to 216 mg/dL, these changes in permittivity values are very large. Since no experimental validation was performed, the performance of the proposed structure can not be fully judged.

The millimetre-wave part of the spectrum, specifically around 60 GHz, is the operating band selected by a company called MediWise for their GlucoWise system [58,59]. This was chosen "*... as the wavelength is short enough for a relatively compact antenna sensor and the penetration depth is large enough for interrogation of thin human tissue regions with sufficient blood concentration*" (Saha et al., 2017 [59]). The developed sensors are intended to work either on the ear lobe or the fleshy part of the hand between thumb and first finger and are based on a pair of patch antennas (resonators) acting in transmission mode. Standard in vitro measurements were conducted using aqueous solutions of glucose and the authors stated the system "*can detect as low as 0.025 wt% of glucose in water*" [59]. Ten non-diabetic male subjects underwent an intravenous glucose tolerance test (IVGTT) while wearing the system. Results for two subjects showed reasonable correlation; poor results for the other test subjects were attributed to hand motion and "*... gradual sliding of the holder during the session, possibly due to fatigue or stress*" [59], emphasising the challenges introduced by external factors. The lag between direct blood measurements and indirect tissue measurements was also evident [59]. A more recent study involving an anaesthetised pig was reported [58], again using an IVGTT to introduce glucose 'spikes' to the blood stream. The sensor was compared with a "*spectrophotometric clinical blood chemistry analyzer (iLab 650 by Diamond Diagnostics) and a commercially available glucometer (Contour Next EZ by Bayer)*" [58]. The antennas were located at different positions on the ear of the pig and with varying separations, to investigate variability and the detuning effect. The spikes in glucose level were evident in the sensor response, with a lag of about thirteen minutes. This lag was attributed, in part, to the distance from the injection site and to the known lag between venous blood samples and interstitial fluid. It was also stated that "*although the area is convenient for the sensor placement, it is not particularly rich in blood and contains significant amounts of interstitial fluid*" [58].

3.3. Discussion

As seen from the literature reviewed above, there is no settled choice of frequency for non-invasive blood glucose monitoring using dielectric spectroscopy. Some systems use lower frequencies to gain tissue penetration, others use higher frequencies to avoid penetration and most do not specify the reason behind the frequency selection, or else are making it for pragmatic reasons related to design issues, such as device size (a lower frequency means a larger resonator), cost of electronic components (higher frequency components are generally more expensive than lower-frequency components), or wanting to operate in licence-exempt ISM bands. The question of measurement location is affected by and affects, the choice of frequency, via the penetration depth: a finger tip or ear lobe, for example, may require a smaller penetration depth, thus, supporting selection of a higher frequency (e.g., [58,59]). The electronic system must also be capable of sufficient accuracy and precision at the proposed frequency (have sufficient dynamic range and be low-noise).

While there are various arguments for using lower or higher frequencies, it should be mentioned that no system chooses the operating frequency based on the observed spectroscopic behaviour of the glucose molecule. Ideally, measurements would be performed at a frequency 'near' to a resonance in the spectroscopic response for glucose, as this would maximise the dielectric property change induced by a change in glucose concentration. We say 'near', as it is possible that the human tissues modify the response. Unfortunately, these molecular resonances are almost entirely in the terahertz (THz) part of the spectrum, between roughly 1 THz and the lower end of the infra-red part of the spectrum [10,60]. This is problematic for a number of reasons, including the extremely poor tissue penetration and current technological limitations for operating in this band. Although selective detection of glucose (and other similar molecules) has been successfully demonstrated using THz nano-antennas [60], with resonances between 0.5–2.5 THz, this approach has yet to be translated for work with human tissues, to the authors' knowledge. Given the poor penetration depth, it remains far from clear that a change in blood glucose concentration could be detected in this band. There would also need to be studies to determine how these resonances appear within tissue samples and whether the resonances of other molecules might obscure that of glucose.

4. Utilized Microwave Resonators and Antennas

In this section, we review the resonator geometries utilised in the literature, to try and identify any useful trends. We note that there are different terms used for the microwave sensor in the literature, namely 'antenna' and 'resonator'. Since most antennas are resonant elements, the distinction is somewhat vague (even artificial). Nevertheless, to avoid confusion from the respective camps, we have split the review along these lines, which perhaps arises from the respective backgrounds of the researchers: antennas researchers see the sensor as 'radiating' into the body tissues and its response being 'de-tuned' by those tissues; resonator designers, perhaps coming from filter design or material characterisation backgrounds, may think in terms of loaded and unloaded Q factors, field distribution across the sample under test and similar things. Essentially, these describe the same responses, but there can be some subtleties in the descriptions.

4.1. Antennas

Antennas employed for glucose-dependent dielectric property change include both wide and narrow-band antennas. A wideband monopole antenna operating between 1 GHz and 6 GHz was proposed in [48]. This antenna was simulated with a hand phantom and the S_{11} response of the antenna was tracked during the simulations. In addition to the drawbacks listed for employing a wideband method, a monopole antenna has an omnidirectional radiation pattern, suggesting that the S_{11} response of the antenna will be vulnerable to the changes in the vicinity of human body and the antenna. Considering that the glucose levels are only slightly changing the dielectric properties, the variations in S_{11} response due to glucose-dependent dielectric property change might be lost in uncontrolled environment.

Patch antennas, operating at 2.45 GHz and 5.8 GHz when loaded with deionized water and glucose solutions, are given in [50]. The antennas were printed on FR4 substrate and also covered with an FR4 superstrate to prevent the shorting of the antenna. When the end application is considered, a superstrate can be useful for managing the SAR within the allowed limits. As a side note: since non-invasive measurements are also envisioned for continuous use, the proposed materials should either be built with bio-compatible materials or should be covered with a bio-compatible material. During the experiments, it was observed that the matching of the antennas were changing with the change in glucose levels. The change was non-linear and the antenna operating at a higher frequency was more responsive to the change in glucose levels.

In [61], a patch antenna was proposed, operating at 5 GHz in air and around 2 GHz (depending on glucose concentration) when loaded with a phantom. The antenna was tested with two liquid phantoms, namely physiological solutions and pig blood, with glucose levels ranging from 0 mg/dL to 500 mg/dL. Simulations predicted a linear shift in resonant frequency of 5 MHz for the physiological solution; measurements did not display any correlation, which was attributed to possible differences in temperature and volume between test samples. Simulations using pig blood digital phantom predicted shifts of 200 MHz (comparing 125 mg/dL to 0 mg/dL) and 300 MHz (comparing 250 mg/dL to 125 mg/dL). When the antenna was tested with pig blood, smaller shifts were observed. A linear fit was performed; the resonant frequency increased by 43 MHz when increasing the concentration from 0 mg/dL to 125 mg/dL and from 125 mg/dL to 250 mg/dL and by 86 MHz when increasing glucose concentration from 250 mg/dL to 500 mg/dL. The number of sample points is relatively low, however and further experimental investigations seem advisable.

In [33], a serpentine-shaped antenna with passive coupling was proposed, designed to operate at 4.8 GHz in air. The antenna was envisioned to be placed on the finger tip in the end application. The proposed structure was simulated with a finger model and measured in vivo, with the S_{11} response tracked (with no monitoring of glucose). It was observed that the antenna had a very narrow bandwidth when operating in air; however, when the antenna was loaded with the finger (finger model), it was observed that the bandwidth increased (a result of the loss of the loading tissues) and it becomes impedance-matched (at the 10 dB return loss level) between 2.8 GHz and 5.5 GHz (or roughly 2.6–3.6 GHz for the simulation). This suggests that the proposed sensor essentially has a wideband behaviour. Since the human body is lossy, the permittivity and conductivity affects the characteristics of the antenna. To quantify the response of the antenna to the change in glucose levels, it was simulated with phantoms representing glucose solutions using de-ionized water. The glucose concentration changed from 0 mg/dL to 2000 mg/dL, resulting in a maximum shift in resonant frequency of 32 MHz. Simulations using a four-layer tissue model of the finger were also performed. The resonance peak shifted from 3.288 GHz to 3.292 GHz when the glucose levels were increased from 0 mg/dL to 2000 mg/dL, a shift of only 4 MHz, demonstrating again the sensitivity challenge.

One other aspect was discussed, namely the effect of the geometry on the electric field, by comparing the proposed serpentine geometry with the patch resonator from [43]. The serpentine resonator was seen to have a higher sensitivity to glucose variation, which is in accord with the idea that geometries with narrow-band responses give more sensitivity. Another way of understanding this is in the effect on the electric field, with the serpentine structure having both greater field intensity and greater field localisation in the central portion of the resonator, when compared with the patch structure. This illustrates another trade-off in the design process: compact geometries tend to achieve greater field intensities in smaller cross-sections, implying greater penetration depths and, potentially, improved sensitivity to changes in effective permittivity. The proviso is that smaller cross-sections also imply less averaging across the monitored volume, implying sensitivity to sensor location (and subject variability) could also increases. (SAR limits obviously still apply, as a constraint on the field intensity.) This study was recently extended in [62] to include the spiral resonator from [30,63] (see Section 4.2), with similar results. The spiral was deemed to be more sensitive than the patch structure and less sensitive than the serpentine structure (again in accord with the Q-factors), with the patch structure achieving greater field intensities. The greater uniformity of electric field for the spiral (compared to the patch) was seen as a contributing factor in the greater sensitivity, as well as in improving measurement uncertainties [62].

4.2. Resonators

An open-ended spiral resonator was presented in [63]. The resonator is basically a spiral-shaped microstrip transmission line and has two ports, with two straight microstrip lines capacitively coupled to the spiral line. The spiral shape was chosen to minimize contact orientation errors, due to the symmetry of the structure and to form a standing wave. The amplitude of the standing wave was tracked by measuring the amplitude of S_{21}. The resonator was modified to accommodate typical human thumbs and tested with human subjects. The tests were performed with healthy subjects using an informal oral glucose tolerance test, where the subjects were given a soda drink and the sensor response tracked over time, while the blood glucose levels were tracked with a commercial glucometer. A good agreement was reported in this study.

Following the reported study in [63], an open-ended spiral resonator with direct coupling was designed and tested with flour-and-water phantoms with varying permittivities in [30], as described in Section 2.2. The goal in this study was to retrieve the dielectric properties from the response of the resonator for a single frequency. This is performed by using polynomials that related the S_{11} response to the permittivity of the material placed on the resonator. The dielectric properties of the material were retrieved around 600 MHz.

A patch resonator operating in the 2.45 GHz ISM Band (when placed on a four-layered tissue-mimicking phantom) was designed and tested in [26]. The input impedance of the resonator was tracked at the operating frequency to quantify the blood glucose change. The blood layer of the four-layered phantom was changed, with the blood-mimicking materials having different concentrations of dextrose. It was concluded that the change in the real part of the input impedance was approximately 0.04% per unit change in glucose concentration of the blood-mimicking material.

Printed resonators operating at three different frequencies were proposed in [55], with dielectric microlitre cups to hold the liquid samples. The resonators were tested with deionized water and glucose solutions, with concentrations ranging from 0% to 10%. The response of the resonator to glucose concentration change was quantified by tracking the Q factor of the resonator. The maximum change in Q-factor (comparing 10% to 0%) was less than seven units, but the response was fairly linear and good agreement between simulation and measurement was observed. This reported study is not suitable for measuring the blood glucose levels continuously, however.

In [51], a ring resonator sensor was proposed. As noted before (Section 3.3), a reference resonator is used to calibrate the sensor for temperature changes in the sensing environment. An interference test system was proposed and the fabricated resonator tested with water solutions to quantify the change in sensor response, both with respect to glucose change and with respect to change of other vitamins and sugars present in the blood. It was concluded that the glucose levels caused greater changes in the resonant frequency and bandwidth of the resonator than other factors, such as ascorbic acid and maltose.

A resonator designed by combining a spiral inductor and interdigital capacitor was introduced in [64]. The resonator was printed on a GaAs substrate and operated at 5.8 GHz in air. The resonator was tested with glucose–water solutions by dropping the solution on the resonator. The experiments were also repeated with the blood plasma (denoted as human serum/human sera) with varying glucose levels. When the blood plasma was placed on the resonator, the resonant frequency shifted to 0.642 GHz; the resonant frequency then increased with the increase in the glucose levels. A sensitivity of 199 MHz per mg/mL change in glucose levels of the sample was reported.

In [53], a cross-coupled stepped-impedance resonator was designed and printed on a GaAs substrate. The resonator operated at 6.53 GHz in air: when loaded with the lossy material (that is, deionized-water and glucose solutions and blood plasma, denoted as human sera in the reported work) with varying glucose levels, the resonance frequency shifted to 3.4 GHz. The sample was dropped on the resonator and the relative permittivity of the samples retrieved from the resonator response. A change in the shunt capacitance of the resonator corresponds to an effective permittivity change and thus, the change in glucose levels. The S_{11} response of the resonator was tracked; the resonance peak shifted 978.7 MHz per mg/mL change in glucose levels of the sample.

4.3. Discussion

The majority of the work reported in the literature has used 'standard' geometries (e.g., ring resonators, patch resonators, strip/line resonators, spiral resonators). The geometries with greater Q-factors (more narrow-band responses) show greater sensitivities to glucose changes, as suggested throughout this paper. Resonators with spirals and interdigitated capacitors may have the greater sensitivities [33,62]. There seems to be an opportunity to further investigate the resonator geometries most suited for the glucose-monitoring application. There is also no real discussion of electrode geometries for systems using impedance spectroscopy for glucose monitoring in the engineering literature, although the body of literature for monitoring bio-electric signals (such as from the heart and muscles) may be of use. Some allusion to this issue is also made in patent documents and publications by Biovotion, with minimal or no detail or justification; Biovotion are discussed below in Section 5.1.

One aspect not widely considered or explained in any depth is the effect of resonator geometry on the field distribution around the resonator and into the tissues, the notable exceptions being [33,62]. (Again, some allusion to this issue is also made in patent documents and publications by Biovotion, with minimal or no detail or justification.) This also stands out as a research opportunity.

Although some of the sensors described have undergone some optimisation (e.g., for the intended body location, such as the finger [41,62,63]), much of the reported work has not considered this aspect. This is a gap in the literature, in the opinion of the authors, indicating a research opportunity. This is particularly true for sensors intended for wearable continuous glucose-monitoring systems. Here, there should be some consideration for the form factor of the final device. For wearable systems, there seem to be two main possibilities: a device strapped to the arm (e.g., a smart watch, or a specific device, as in [65,66]) or a 'smart plaster' for use on the torso, (upper) arm or (upper) leg. Such a smart plaster could offer greater surface area for accommodating larger resonator structures, but the issue of powering the sensor becomes more complicated.

5. Addressing the Selectivity Challenge

Thus far, we have described (in Section 2) the ability to detect changes in glucose level via dielectric spectroscopy and emphasised the challenge of sensitivity. Although there is possibly some scope for improvements in recipes for tissue-mimicking materials, we believe the sensitivity issue has been clearly demonstrated in the literature and that future research must have a greater focus on addressing the sensitivity and selectivity challenges. We further suggest that a multi-band approach seems preferable to single narrow or wide band sensors (Section 3). The justification for this is that narrow band resonators will give greater sensitivity to the observed small changes in effective permittivity than wide-band sensors, but insufficient selectivity against other factors affecting the relative effective permittivity. This limitation would be mitigated, in part, by multiple narrow-band resonances. The research (not to say, commercial) challenge then becomes the selection of the resonant frequencies and realisation of the resonator, which are affected partly by the form-factor and location of the wearable device on the body (Section 4). The use of multiple frequencies is unlikely to be sufficient, however, even with improved electromagnetic models for extracting the permittivity (e.g., compensating for small air-gaps). Additional sensors are almost certainly required to compensate for the 'external factors' and substantial (large-scale) studies required to understand the 'internal factors' (Section 2.4). In the following, we briefly review some existing approaches to multi-parameter sensing, before discussing how the remaining limitations may be overcome and then describing how this might work within an integrated diabetes management system, through comparison with studies conducted using commercial glucose monitors.

5.1. Multi-Parameter Sensing

The monitoring of various physiological signals is of broad interest, with applications in healthcare, sports (elite/professional and amateur), security and space [67,68]. Indeed, the growth of fitness trackers and smart watches attest to the growing trend to monitor personal activity in order to meet personal 'well-ness' goals. The value of monitoring such factors for use in glucose monitoring has also been recognised in the literature. For example, Choi et al. account for the effect of temperature via a dual-resonator approach [51,52], while the GlucoWise system "*includes two thermometers (one to measure the sample or skin temperature and one to monitor the ambient air temperature) and a solid-state three-axis accelerometer to detect movement*" (Saha et al., 2017) [59]. This system of additional sensors is not yet used to automatically correct the data, however, which would be required for realistic use.

One of the more developed systems in the literature is the 'Multi-Sensor' by Biovotion [65,66,69–73]. This has a long history, with predecessor companies being Pendragon and Solianis (some of the principals for Biovotion were involved in one or both of these predecessors) [10] and patent applications dating back to 2001. The elements of the Multi-Sensor are [65,66]

- dielectric property monitoring using resonators optimised for three frequency ranges:
  - 1–200 kHz, to 'monitor sudomotor activity' [65] (that is, sweat monitoring);
  - 0.1–100 MHz, to 'monitor the effect of glucose variations' (using three different resonators at the low, high and central parts of the band) [65];
  - 1 GHz and 2 GHz (separate electrodes), to 'monitor water migration' [65];
- two temperature sensors;
- one humidity sensor;
- an accelerometer (it is unclear how many axes);
- optical 'diffuse reflectance' sensors, to 'monitor hemodynamic changes' [65].

A sketch of the layout of the bottom of a printed circuit board used to form the various resonators is shown in Figure 5, based on drawing of a recent iteration of the Multi-Sensor from a patent document [74]. A number of different geometries have been used, including ring-type, line-type and inter-digitated capacitor 'electrodes' (this term is used to describe the Multi-Sensor resonators in the various publications and reflects the impedance spectroscopy perspective).

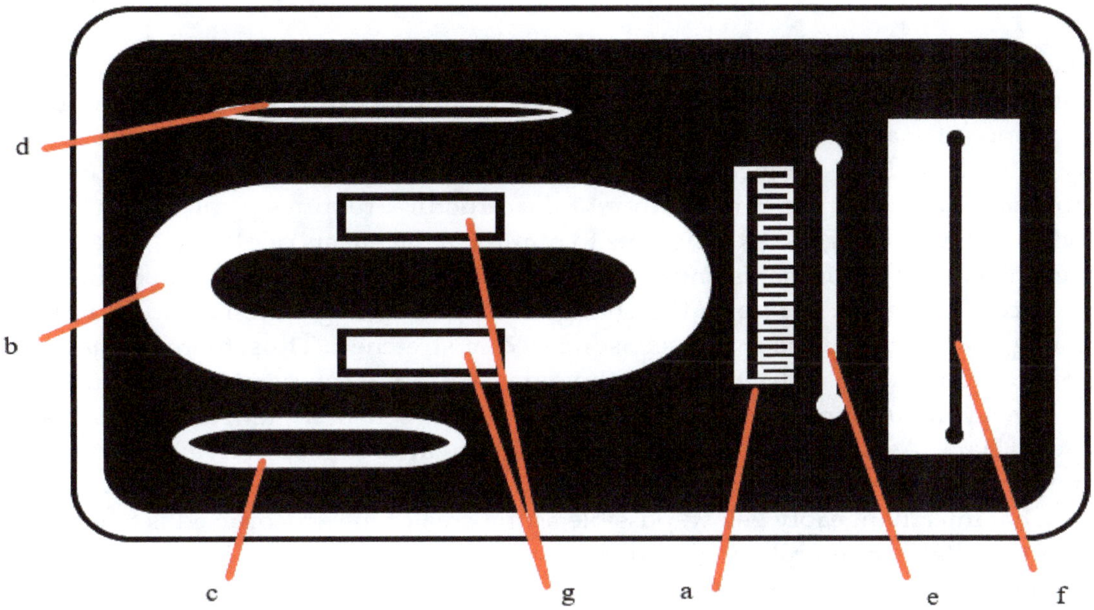

Figure 5. A sketch of the Biovotion Multi-Sensor arm-band, showing the various electromagnetic sensors (some of the sensors described in the text, including the humidity sensor and accelerometer, are within the housing and not visible in this image), based on a drawing from a recent patent document [74]: (a) inter-digital electrode operating in 1–20 kHz band as a sweat sensor; (b) 'short', (c) middle and (d) 'long' MHz-band electrodes; (e) 'short' and (f) 'long' GHz electrodes; (g) optical reflection sensors consisting of light sources and detectors. (Not to scale; geometries have been simplified) [65,74].

The Multi-Sensor is designed to be worn on the upper arm and has daily calibration requirements [65,66]. It is relatively bulky and not necessarily suited for continuous monitoring on some practical and aesthetic criteria, but it can be argued that the important task is to develop a fully functioning and reliable non-invasive monitoring device, with such considerations left as future refinements. In the most recent study, twenty Type-1 patients used the system for a total of 1072 study days in home and clinical settings. Training was required to ensure the patients could place the Multi-Sensor on the arm comfortably. One of the objectives of the study was to obtain a larger dataset, over a longer period, than currently available, to guide further refinements and this is an objective that should be considered by other researchers as well.

The results of the study were evaluated using the mean absolute relative deviation (MARD) and the Clarke Error Grid. As expected, there were subject/device-specific variations and a lower accuracy in uncontrolled (home) compared to controlled (clinical) settings. An overall MARD of 35.4 mg/dL was reported, which is still higher than the current state-of-the-art minimally invasive devices (using biosensors); furthermore, although 86.9% of points fell in the A and B zones of the Clarke Error Grid, 0.6% fell in the C zone, 12.1% in the D zone and 0.4% in the E zone. The algorithm used to modify the raw impedance spectroscopy data based on the other sensor inputs is not disclosed in detail, although the improvements in mean absolute deviation (MAD) are discussed. Previous papers suggest the use of principal component analysis and linear regression models (e.g., [73,75]), suggesting one possible source of error is an inadequate sample population. Thus, the potential to detect changes in glucose has again been clearly demonstrated, but not yet in a system that is clinically viable.

5.2. Case Study

In this case study illustrating the above issues, we present previously unpublished results from a small-scale study with human subjects conducted by the authors in 2014, investigating the effect of pressure on the response of a patch resonator placed on the wrist. As described above, the patch resonator was previously tested with tissue-mimicking phantoms to verify the proper functioning [26]. The ultimate test domain, to understand the true performance of the structure, requires measurements with human subjects, implying carefully designed experiments to minimize the effects of other changes in the body to the resonator response. One factor that is known to affect the resonator response from earlier observations is the applied force. This effect is due to the change in superstrate geometry and in return effective permittivity changes when the tissue is pressed, squeezed or stretched. Thus, there is a need to calibrate the response of the resonator in order to gather the data relating to the permittivity change due to the glucose levels. However, this approach requires both a multiple sensor system and a smart algorithm to detect the relevant data. As a necessary preliminary step towards this objective, this study conducted initial human experiments performed under controlled conditions. We will use the terms 'force' and 'pressure' somewhat interchangeably below, possible as the area of the sensor used is fixed.

A measurement platform monitoring both the applied force and the resonator response was built by embedding the patch resonator inside a wooden block and placing two commercial force sensors on the two ends of the resonator. Measurements were performed on one male and four female subjects. The subjects were asked to fast overnight; this was deemed necessary so that the blood glucose levels of the subjects were at the minimum level before the experiment. The effect of the applied force to the resonator response was measured for the different subjects while the blood glucose levels were at a minimum, to establish a baseline and understand the potential measurement uncertainties due to changes in pressure. For this preliminary study, however, the focus was on the development of a robust and reliable test procedure for use in clinical environments; hence, no direct blood glucose measurements were made at this stage.

The patch resonator presented in [26] was mounted on a wooden test bench with the dimensions of $140.5 \times 360 \times 18$ mm^3. The dielectric properties of the wooden bench were measured at the design frequency of 2.45 GHz, giving $\varepsilon_r = 1.8$ and $\tan(\delta) = 0.15$. Two force sensors were taped at both end of the resonator, leaving 2 mm space between the resonator and the force sensors. The force sensors were identical and the length, width and thicknesses of the sensors were 100 mm, 14 mm and 0.203 mm, respectively. Both of the force sensors used in this study were A201 type FlexiForce^{TM} commercial thin-film type sensors [76]. The transparent cover of the commercial sensors was polyester (Mylar) with dielectric properties of $\varepsilon_r = 3.2$ and $\tan(\delta) = 0.005$. The experimental configuration of the test bench is shown in Figure 6. The simulation configuration is identical to the experimental set-up. Note that the force sensors were considered as homogeneous Mylar materials during the simulations.

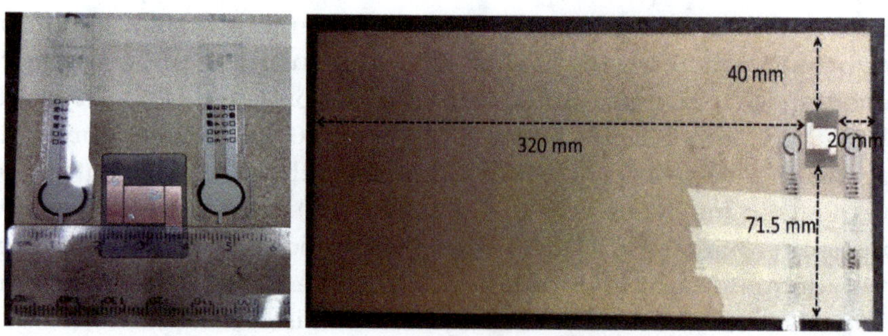

(a) (b)

Figure 6. Configuration of the test bench: (**a**) the resonator and force sensors; (**b**) wooden test bench.

The commercial force sensors can measure applied forces between 0 N and 440 N. The conditioning circuit, used for each force sensor, is shown in Figure 7. The conditioning circuits were built on a breadboard and output voltage of the force sensors were measured with multimeters. The variable resistances were fixed to 203 kΩ.

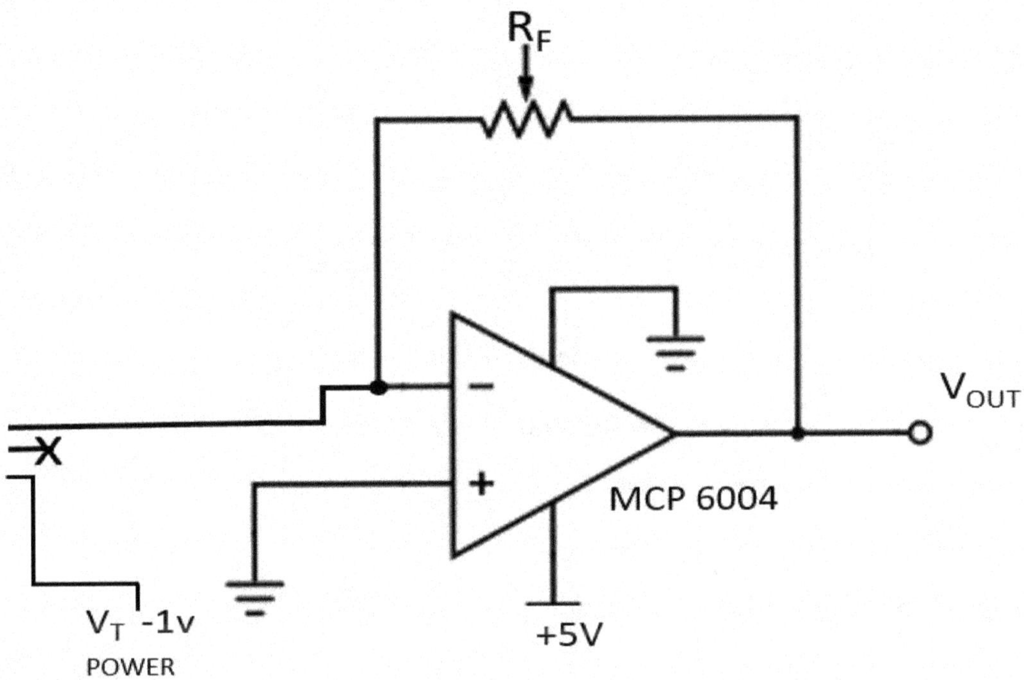

Figure 7. Conditioning circuit for thin-film force sensors [76].

The sensors were calibrated to express the applied force, as given by the output voltage, in terms of weight. Calibration was performed by placing a disk of known mass onto the sensing area of the force sensors to concentrate the weight only on the sensing area of the sensors; precise masses were then placed on top of the disk and the output voltages of the sensors measured with multimeters. The calibration graph for the sensor are shown in Figure 8a, where the plotted points are the median values of two sets of data taken from the first and second sensors. The coefficients for the power fitting function is a = 0.085 and b = 0.678. The R-square value is 0.965, quantifying the goodness of the fitting. Residual plots are given in Figure 8b.

Force measurements were performed with one male and four female healthy subjects. The Body Mass Index (BMI) of the each subject is given in Table 5. The age of the subjects were ranging from 25 to 40. The blood glucose levels of the subjects were expected to be constant and low (around 72 mg/dL, or 4–5 mmol/L), as the subjects were fasting overnight before the experiment. The subjects were asked to press the inner part of their right arms to the bench where the resonator and the sensors were mounted. The subjects' arms were also marked with arm bands, to ensure the same tissue block on each subject was measured and to ensure the placement of the arm matched with the previous measurements for each subject, maximising the repeatability.

Table 5. Body mass index (BMI) of the subjects.

Subject	BMI	Subject	BMI
$Female_1$	22.1	$Female_4$	21.9
$Female_2$	25.0	$Male_1$	22.1
$Female_3$	22.5		

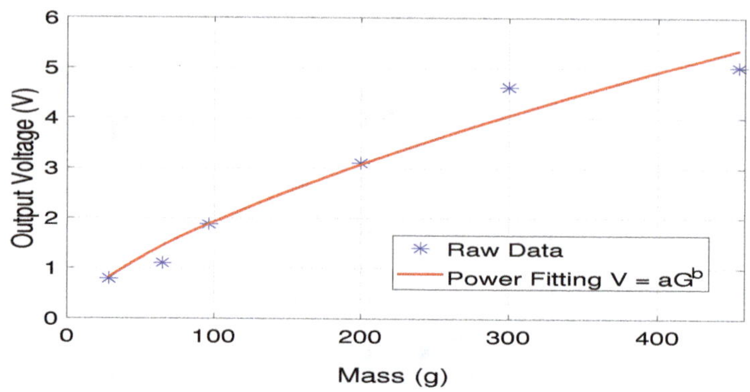

(a)

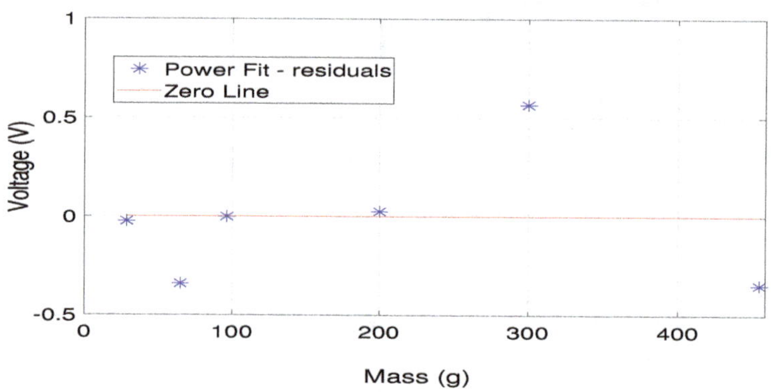

(b)

Figure 8. Calibration measurements: (**a**) the power fitting to the calibration values; (**b**) residuals of the power fitting.

During the force experiments, the subjects were asked to apply the same amount of force to both force sensors on either side the resonator. The experimenter recorded the resonator response when the same level of force was reached on both sensors (implying an equivalent force was applied evenly across the resonator). For each force level, the resonator response was recorded five times. The subjects applied four different levels of force as determined by the force sensor output voltages, from 0.5 V to 2 V in 0.5 V increments, with force determined from the calibration curve in Figure 8a when required (the results given below are expressed in terms of the directly measured sensor output voltages). The median of the collected response was taken for each force level for each subject, shown in Figure 9. In Figure 9, the red curve, expressed by $y = ax^b + c$ where $a = 0.12$, $b = -1.13$, $c = 2.49$, shows the median of all measurements.

The median fitting indicates that the superstrate permittivity increases with the increase in applied force. When the applied force is very low, for example at 0.5 V output, an air gap might be introduced between the tissue and the resonator, minimising the effect of the tissue superstrate on the resonator output (note that the resonance shift has a 5.3% decrease between 0.5 V and 1 V outputs). As the applied force increased, the magnitude of the resulting resonance shift decreases. The decrease in resonance is 1.7% and 0.8% for an increase in applied force from 1 V to 1.5 V and from 1.5 V to 2 V, respectively. This could be due to the tissue displacement: it is hypothesized that the fat tissue is displaced with the increase in applied force (also suggested recently in the literature [42,62]). This experiment was important to assess the effect of the applied force to the resonator. From the change observed in Figure 9, it is clear that the applied force has a significant effect on the resonator response; thus, it should be kept constant to differentiate the effect of the glucose change to the resonator response, ideally. In real-world scenarios, appropriate models should be utilised to remove the effect of pressure changes. Note that during the experiments subjects were not be able to apply greater forces consistently (the sensor output can reach up to 5 V).

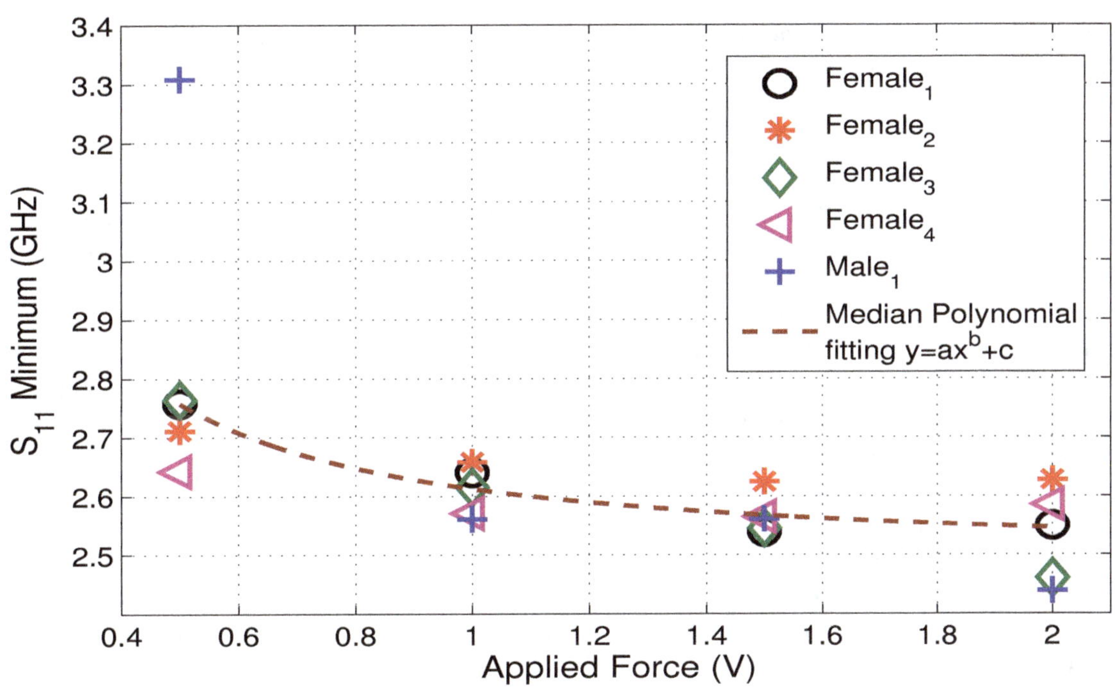

Figure 9. Change in sensor S_{11} response with the applied force voltage output.

After the force measurements were completed, the subjects were asked which force level was most comfortable. The subjects reported that the 1 V output was the most comfortable force level. The standard deviation from the mean (σ) on each applied force level among the five measurement was also calculated and are shown in Table 6; the 1 V applied force level shows least deviation. Although obviously only a small and unrepresentative sample, this type of information could be useful in the design stage for resonators and effective permittivity models, by looking for deviations from the target pressure and having models for changes in tissue properties (such as from compression) and air gaps.

Table 6. Standard deviation from the mean (σ) on each applied force level.

Force (V)	$Female_1$ σ (MHz)	$Female_2$ σ (MHz)	$Female_3$ σ (MHz)	$Female_4$ σ (MHz)	$Male_1$ σ (MHz)
0.5	25.954	9.5513	24.954	13.257	29.681
1	4.2943	4.6416	8.5015	1.1808	12.343
1.5	17.162	4.7459	25.373	12.159	10.428
2	6.7883	2.4348	2.7803	0.88977	19.459

5.3. Discussion

We have reached a point in this review where we believe we have demonstrated that the detection of glucose via dielectric spectroscopy requires highly sensitive systems that can account for a large number of external factors (such as temperature variability, the effect of pressure and the effect of sweat) to accurately determine the effective permittivity of glucose. This is independent of the frequency (or frequencies) used for the spectroscopic measurement, the optimum choice of which is far from clear. The fact that systems accounting for one or more of these external factors (e.g., [51,52,65,66]) still fall short of the required accuracy for acceptance by clinicians and regulatory bodies demonstrate that it is the biological factors—what we have called 'internal factors', plus issues of variation between subjects—that are the main hurdle (although we do not rule out the possibility for improvements in compensation of external factors, we do not believe these to be the primary limitation at this stage). Unfortunately, we do not believe that some clever design of wearable resonator operating at some 'special' frequency will overcome these limitations; hence, microwave engineers and other electromagnetic experts will not be able to address this challenge alone. We reiterate we are considering wearable microwave sensors for non-invasive monitoring; we are not considering implants, or whether THz sensors near the molecular resonance of glucose may be able to operate on the skin successfully. Even for these cases, of course, we would expect strong, multi-disciplinary teams to be necessary; it is possible, however, that the problems of sensitivity and selectivity would be less severe in these scenarios.

One possible research strategy to find answers to the above issues is as follows: in addition to continued improvements in capturing good permittivity data and isolating 'unexplained' variations from variations explained by other sensor outputs, more work is required to look at how the tissue permittivity varies with changes in other substances in tissues, both in vitro (including the use of phantoms) and in vivo. This will help build up a mass of knowledge that can be used to design better regression models, or even use in machine-learning and artificial intelligence techniques (e.g., fuzzy logic classifiers, neural networks and decision trees [8]), to build predictive systems. Real-time tracking is obviously important, but it is predictive capability that will save lives by warning of potential hypo- and hyperglycaemic events [10]—even if the action by (initial versions of) the system is to warn the user to confirm blood glucose level via a blood sample. Recent improvements in the use of technology in medical studies—such as the use of Apple's HealthKit, CareKit and ResearchKit (e.g., [77,78]) to capture data, the improvements in ambulatory monitoring devices in comfort and form-factor, the use of commercial wearables to provide activity and other data (although the accuracy of such systems has been questioned, they appear adequate, with the possible exception of low-intensity activities [79–81])—should all be leveraged to help achieve the required dataset. Commercially-available minimally invasive systems from the likes of Abbott, Dexcom and Medtronic now communicate with smart phones and to the cloud, allowing diabetics (as well others, such as spouses and healthcare professionals) to receive alerts for high and low glucose excursions, improving patient outcomes and peace-of-mind. A similar approach, potentially capturing other data, could be used to collect the necessary dataset across a wider sample population (e.g., [82–84]). Personalised models have been shown to have greater predictive power than global models (e.g., [73]), implying a period of calibration or learning by the system to realise the full potential. This would be in conjunction with traditional monitoring by blood samples and transition the system from the (acceptable but less accurate) global model to the personalised model.

6. Conclusions

In this review article, we have sought to convey both the potential and the challenges associated with measuring blood glucose levels non-invasively via microwave dielectric spectroscopy. We have shown (qualitatively, via the review of the literature and quantitatively, by applying realistic glucose levels to models from the literature) how changes in glucose levels produce only small changes in the dielectric properties, even under controlled conditions. This implies a highly sensitive sensor will be required to detect the small changes, which in turn implies low-noise electronics and a 'high-Q' (narrow-band) resonator to reduce the impact of noise and maintain the system dynamic range.

We have further discussed the issue of selectivity: the measured dielectric properties are the 'effective' properties of a medium equivalent to an average of the constituent tissues, each of which has biological process that affect the individual contributions. These 'internal factors' are temperature- and frequency-dependent and are coupled with 'external factors' that include such things as external temperature, activity level and even the fit of the clothes worn. A accurate method for retrieving the effective permittivity of the tissue(s) from the resonator response was briefly discussed (Section 2), but this is independent from relating the effective permittivity to the blood glucose level. We have described a number of 'multi-parameter' sensing strategies designed to mitigate or remove the effect of the 'external factors' and discussed the challenges of dealing with the 'internal factors'.

Given these challenges, it may seem that dielectric spectroscopy is unsuitable for the task at hand. Indeed, with the decision to suspend activities into a smart contact lens for glucose monitoring by Verily (part of Alphabet, owner of Google) [85], the dream of non-invasive monitoring may seem unachievable (although the early work by Noviosense, which also works with tears and notably uses an enzyme-based approach to achieve selectivity, offers some hope [9,86]). Rather than concede this, we have suggested avenues for further exploration that may enable true non-invasive, continuous monitoring of blood glucose levels to be achieved. In particular, we have suggested that a number of frequencies must be monitored and combined with data from other sensors in a suitable fashion.

Admittedly, there may be some scepticism [10] that adding additional sensors will overcome the fundamental issues of the low sensitivity of the effective dielectric to changes in blood glucose level and the sensitivity of the dielectric properties to other factors and this cannot be dismissed out-of-hand. On the other hand, it is certainly true that signal processing techniques can be used to 'clean up' a received message or radar return in order to extract low-amplitude variations in the presence of large-magnitude variations, given suitable measurements and models. Furthermore, there are now methods for identifying otherwise unrecognisable patterns in data that could help tease out the relationship between blood glucose level and effective permittivity, given a large enough dataset. As the availability of computational resources and machine-learning techniques is far greater now than even five years ago, as are new ways of collecting the data required from a suitably large sample population at a reasonable cost (e.g., using Apple's ResearchKit, coupled with smart watches that can collect other data, including heart rate and activity level). We suggest that there is still scope for progress, but believe that it will ultimately require even greater cross-disciplinary collaboration than seen to date. It has been suggested [10] that, for non-invasive continuous monitoring of blood glucose to be realised,

> "...a reasonable chance at success requires in-depth knowledge of all the following disciplines:

- The engineering disciplines related to [the] primary technology, e.g., optics, electronics, software, mechanical engineering, etc.
- Biochemistry, especially knowledge of the glucose molecule and its relation to the chosen field of technology.
- Physiology, especially the distribution of glucose in fluids and tissue.
- Metabolism, especially glucose sources and sinks.
- Diabetes, especially aspects of the disease that will affect [the primary] technology—the more understanding of endocrinology, the better.
- The history of non-invasive investigations, especially in [the primary] technology field—what didn't work and why.
- The regulatory requirements for a diagnostic device and the evolving structure of the market for existing devices." (Smith, 2018 [10])

We also suggest the engineering expertise required must include specialists in signal processing and computational intelligence, as well as microwave and electromagnetics specialists, medical professionals and patients. Attention should focus on the design of compact, highly sensitive resonators (preferably at multiple frequencies, although the selection of these frequencies remains an open research question), coupled with methods of removing the effect of the various external factors from the measured signal and then analysing the signal in the context of a sufficiently large dataset to extract reliable glucose data while accounting for subject-specific variations and the complex internal factors also affecting the effective permittivity.

Acknowledgments: The authors wish to thank M. Munoz Torrico for practical assistance in the measurements with the force sensors and to the test subjects who participated.

References

1. Diabetes: Key Facts—World Health Organization. Available online: http://www.who.int/news-room/fact-sheets/detail/diabetes (accessed on 15 October 2018).
2. Bruen, D.; Delaney, C.; Florea, L.; Diamond, D. Glucose Sensing for Diabetes Monitoring: Recent Developments. *Sensors* **2017**, *17*, 1866, doi:10.3390/s17081866. [CrossRef]
3. Comer, J. Semiquantitative specific test paper for glucose in urine. *Anal. Chem.* **1956**, *28*, 1748–1750. [CrossRef]
4. Yao, H.; Shum, A.J.; Cowan, M.; Lähdesmäki, I.; Parviz, B.A. A contact lens with embedded sensor for monitoring tear glucose level. *Biosens. Bioelectron.* **2011**, *26*, 3290–3296. [CrossRef]
5. Galassetti, P.R.; Novak, B.; Nemet, D.; Rose-Gottron, C.; Cooper, D.M.; Meinardi, S.; Newcomb, R.; Zaldivar, F.; Blake, D.R. Breath ethanol and acetone as indicators of serum glucose levels: an initial report. *Diabetes Technol. Ther.* **2005**, *7*, 115–123. [CrossRef] [PubMed]
6. Wang, C.; Sahay, P. Breath analysis using laser spectroscopic techniques: breath biomarkers, spectral fingerprints and detection limits. *Sensors* **2009**, *9*, 8230–8262. [CrossRef] [PubMed]
7. Wang, C.; Mbi, A.; Shepherd, M. A study on breath acetone in diabetic patients using a cavity ringdown breath analyzer: Exploring correlations of breath acetone with blood glucose and glycohemoglobin A1C. *IEEE Sens. J.* **2010**, *10*, 54–63. [CrossRef]
8. Todd, C.; Salvetti, P.; Naylor, K.; Albatat, M. Towards Non-Invasive Extraction and Determination of Blood Glucose Levels. *Bioengineering* **2017**, *4*, 82, doi:10.3390/bioengineering4040082. [CrossRef]

9. Waltz, E. Why Noviosense's In-Eye Glucose Monitor Might Work Better Than Alphabet's. Available online: https://spectrum.ieee.org/the-human-os/biomedical/devices/why-noviosenses-ineye-glucose-monitor-might-work-better-than-googles (accessed on 18 November 2018).
10. Smith, J. *The Pursuit of Noninvasive Glucose: "Hunting the Deceitful Turkey"*, 6th ed.; 2018. Self-published; Available online: https://www.researchgate.net/publication/327101583_The_Pursuit_of_Noninvasive_Glucose_Hunting_the_Deceitful_Turkey_Sixth_Edition (accessed on 18 November 2018).
11. ISO 15197:2013—In Vitro Diagnostic Test Systems—Requirements for Blood-Glucose Monitoring Systems for Self-Testing in Managing Diabetes Mellitus. Available online: https://www.iso.org/standard/54976.html (accessed on 19 November 2018).
12. Gao, Y.; Ghasr, M.T.; Nacy, M.; Zoughi, R. Towards Accurate and Wideband In Vivo Measurement of Skin Dielectric Properties. *IEEE Trans. Instrum. Meas.* **2018**, *PP*, 1–13.10.1109/TIM.2018.2849519. [CrossRef]
13. Güren, O.; Çayören, M.; Ergene, L.T.; Akduman, I. Surface impedance based microwave imaging method for breast cancer screening: Contrast-enhanced scenario. *Phys. Med. Biol.* **2014**, *59*, 5725–5739. [CrossRef]
14. Paglione, R.W. Coaxial Applicator for Microwave Hyperthermia. U.S. Patent 4,204,549, 27 May 1980.
15. Hall, P.S.; Hao, Y. *Antennas and Propagation for Body-Centric Wireless Networks*, 1st ed.; Artech House: Norwood, MA, USA, 2006; ISBN 1-58053-493-7.
16. Gabriel, C.; Gabriel, S.; Corthout, E. The dielectric properties of biological tissues: I. Literature survey. *Phys. Med. Biol.* **1996**, *41*, 2231–2249. [CrossRef]
17. Gabriel, S.; Lau, R.; Gabriel, C. The dielectric properties of biological tissues: II. Measurements in the frequency range 10 Hz to 20 GHz. *Phys. Med. Biol.* **1996**, *41*, 2251–2269. [CrossRef]
18. Gabriel, S.; Lau, R.; Gabriel, C. The dielectric properties of biological tissues: III. Parametric models for the dielectric spectrum of tissues. *Phys. Med. Biol.* **1996**, *41*, 2271–2293. [CrossRef] [PubMed]
19. Lazebnik, M.; Popovic, D.; McCartney, L.; Watkins, C.B.; Lindstrom, M.J.; Harter, J.; Sewall, S.; Ogilvie, T.; Magliocco, A.; Breslin, T.M.; et al. A large-scale study of the ultrawideband microwave dielectric properties of normal, benign and malignant breast tissues obtained from cancer surgeries. *Phys. Med. Biol.* **2007**, *52*, 6093–6115. [CrossRef] [PubMed]
20. Topsakal, E.; Karacolak, T.; Moreland, E.C. Glucose-dependent dielectric properties of blood plasma. In Proceedings of the IEEE 2011 XXXth URSI General Assembly and Scientific Symposium, Istanbul, Turkey, 13–20 August 2011; pp. 1–4.
21. Keysight Technologies. Agilent 85070E Dielectric Probe Kit 200 MHz to 50 GHz. Available online: http://literature.cdn.keysight.com/litweb/pdf/5989-0222EN.pdf (accessed on 18 November 2018).
22. Karacolak, T.; Moreland, E.C.; Topsakal, E. Cole—Cole model for glucose-dependent dielectric properties of blood plasma for continuous glucose monitoring. *Microw. Opt. Technol. Lett.* **2013**, *55*, 1160–1164. [CrossRef]
23. Cole, K.S.; Cole, R.H. Dispersion and absorption in dielectrics I. Alternating current characteristics. *J. Chem. Phys.* **1941**, *9*, 341–351. [CrossRef]
24. Venkataraman, J.; Freer, B. Feasibility of non-invasive blood glucose monitoring: In-vitro measurements and phantom models. In Proceedings of the 2011 IEEE International Symposium on Antennas and Propagation (APSURSI), Spokane, WA, USA, 3–8 July 2011; pp. 603–606.
25. Philis-Tsimikas, A.; Chang, A.; Miller, L. Precision, accuracy and user acceptance of the OneTouch SelectSimple blood glucose monitoring system. *J. Diabetes Sci. Technol.* **2011**, *5*, 1602–1609. [CrossRef]
26. Yilmaz, T.; Foster, R.; Hao, Y. Broadband tissue mimicking phantoms and a patch resonator for evaluating noninvasive monitoring of blood glucose levels. *IEEE Trans. Antennas Propag.* **2014**, *62*, 3064–3075. [CrossRef]
27. Lazebnik, M.; Madsen, E.L.; Frank, G.R.; Hagness, S.C. Tissue-mimicking phantom materials for narrowband and ultrawideband microwave applications. *Phys. Med. Biol.* **2005**, *50*, 4245–4258. [CrossRef]
28. Beam, K.; Venkataraman, J. Phantom models for in-vitro measurements of blood glucose. In Proceedings of the 2011 IEEE International Symposium on Antennas and Propagation (APSURSI), Spokane, WA, USA, 3–8 July 2011; pp. 1860–1862.
29. Gund, A.; Lindqvist, S. *Phantom Making and Modeling of Monopole Antennas in FD-TD for Breast Cancer Studies*; Department of Signals and Systems, Chalmers University of Technology: Göteborg, Sweden, 2005.

30. Yilmaz, T.; Foster, R.; Hao, Y. Towards accurate dielectric property retrieval of biological tissues for blood glucose monitoring. *IEEE Trans. Microw. Theory Tech.* **2014**, *62*, 3193–3204. [CrossRef]
31. Yilmaz, T.; Hao, Y. Electrical property characterization of blood glucose for on-body sensors. In Proceedings of the 5th European Conference on Antennas and Propagation (EUCAP), Rome, Italy, 11–15 April 2011; pp. 3659–3662.
32. Smulders, P.F.; Buysse, M.G.; Huang, M.D. Dielectric properties of glucose solutions in the 0.5–67 GHz range. *Microw. Opt. Technol. Lett.* **2013**, *55*, 1916–1917. [CrossRef]
33. Turgul, V.; Kale, I. Permittivity extraction of glucose solutions through artificial neural networks and non-invasive microwave glucose sensing. *Sens. Actuators A Phys.* **2018**, *277*, 65–72. [CrossRef]
34. Turgul, V.; Kale, I. On the accuracy of complex permittivity model of glucose/water solutions for non-invasive microwave blood glucose sensing. In Proceedings of the IEEE E-Health and Bioengineering Conference (EHB), Iasi, Romania, 19–21 November 2015; pp. 1–4.
35. Turgul, V.; Kale, I. Characterization of the complex permittivity of glucose/water solutions for noninvasive RF/Microwave blood glucose sensing. In Proceedings of the 2016 IEEE International Instrumentation and Measurement Technology Conference Proceedings (I2MTC), Taipei, Taiwan, 23–26 May 2016; pp. 1–5.
36. Medical Device Radiocommunications Service (MedRadio) | Federal Communications Commission. Available online: https://www.fcc.gov/medical-device-radiocommunications-service-medradio (accessed on 22 November 2018).
37. Wireless Medical Telemetry Service (WMTS) | Federal Communications Commission. Available online: https://www.fcc.gov/wireless/bureau-divisions/mobility-division/wireless-medical-telemetry-service-wmts (accessed on 22 November 2018).
38. Li, J.; Igbe, T.; Liu, Y.; Nie, Z.; Qin, W.; Wang, L.; Hao, Y. An Approach for Noninvasive Blood Glucose Monitoring Based on Bioimpedance Difference Considering Blood Volume Pulsation. *IEEE Access* **2018**, *6*, 51119–51129. [CrossRef]
39. Vander Vorst, A.; Rosen, A.; Kotsuka, Y. *RF/Microwave Interaction with Biological Tissues*; John Wiley & Sons, Inc.: Hoboken, NJ, USA, 2005.
40. Yilmaz, T. Wearable RF Sensors for Non-Invasive Detection of Blood-Glucose Levels. Ph.D. Thesis, Queen Mary, University of London, London, UK, 2013.
41. Turgul, V.; Kale, I. Influence of fingerprints and finger positioning on accuracy of RF blood glucose measurement from fingertips. *Electron. Lett.* **2017**, *53*, 218–220. [CrossRef]
42. Turgul, V.; Kale, I. Simulating the Effects of Skin Thickness and Fingerprints to Highlight Problems With Non-Invasive RF Blood Glucose Sensing from Fingertips. *IEEE Sens. J.* **2017**, *17*, 7553–7560. [CrossRef]
43. Yilmaz, T.; Foster, R.; Hao, Y. Patch resonator for non-invasive detection of dielectric property changes in biological tissues. In Proceedings of the IEEE Antennas and Propagation Society International Symposium (APSURSI), Chicago, IL, USA, 8–14 July 2012; pp. 1–2.
44. Jepsen, P.U.; Møller, U.; Merbold, H. Investigation of aqueous alcohol and sugar solutions with reflection terahertz time-domain spectroscopy. *Opt. Express* **2007**, *15*, 14717–14737. [CrossRef] [PubMed]
45. Tarr, R.V.; Steffes, P.G. Non-Invasive Blood Glucose Measurement System and Method Using Stimulated Raman Spectroscopy. US Patent 5,243,983, 14 September 1993.
46. Psychoudakis, D.; Chen, C.C.; Lee, G.Y.; Volakis, J.L. Epidermal Sensor Paradigm: Inner Layer Tissue Monitoring. In *Handbook of Biomedical Telemetry*; John Wiley & Sons, Inc.: Hoboken, NJ, USA, 2014; Chapter 18, pp. 525–548.
47. Yilmaz, T.; Kılıç, M.A.; Erdoğan, M.; Çayören, M.; Tunaoğlu, D.; Kurtoğlu, İ.; Yaslan, Y.; Çayören, H.; Arıkan, A.E.; Teksöz, S.; et al. Machine learning aided diagnosis of hepatic malignancies through in vivo dielectric measurements with microwaves. *Phys. Med. Biol.* **2016**, *61*, 5089–5102. [CrossRef] [PubMed]
48. Freer, B.; Venkataraman, J. Feasibility study for non-invasive blood glucose monitoring. In Proceedings of the 2010 IEEE Antennas and Propagation Society International Symposium (APSURSI), Toronto, ON, Canada, 11–17 July 2010; pp. 1–4.
49. Turgul, V.; Kale, I. A novel pressure sensing circuit for non-invasive RF/microwave blood glucose sensors. In Proceedings of the 2016 IEEE 16th Mediterranean Microwave Symposium (MMS), Abu Dhabi, UAE, 14–16 November 2016; pp. 1–4.

50. Yilmaz, T.; Ozturk, T.; Joof, S. A Comparative Study for Development of Microwave Glucose Sensors. In Proceedings of the 32nd URSI GASS, Montreal, QC, Canada, 19–26 August 2017; pp. 1–4.
51. Choi, H.; Naylon, J.; Luzio, S.; Beutler, J.; Birchall, J.; Martin, C.; Porch, A. Design and in vitro interference test of microwave noninvasive blood glucose monitoring sensor. *IEEE Trans. Microw. Theory Tech.* **2015**, *63*, 3016–3025. [CrossRef]
52. Choi, H.; Luzio, S.; Beutler, J.; Porch, A. Microwave noninvasive blood glucose monitoring sensor: Human clinical trial results. In Proceedings of the 2017 IEEE MTT-S International Microwave Symposium (IMS), Honololu, HI, USA, 4–9 June 2017; pp. 876–879.
53. Adhikari, K.K.; Kim, N.Y. Ultrahigh-sensitivity mediator-free biosensor based on a microfabricated microwave resonator for the detection of micromolar glucose concentrations. *IEEE Trans. Microw. Theory Tech.* **2016**, *64*, 319–327. [CrossRef]
54. Huang, S.Y.; Yoshida, Y.; Garcia, A.; Chia, X.; Mu, W.C.; Meng, Y.S.; Yu, W. Microstrip Line-based Glucose Sensor for Noninvasive Continuous Monitoring using the Main Field for Sensing and Multivariable Crosschecking. *IEEE Sens. J.* **2018**. [CrossRef]
55. Juan, C.G.; Bronchalo, E.; Potelon, B.; Quendo, C.; Ávila-Navarro, E.; Sabater-Navarro, J.M. Concentration Measurement of Microliter-Volume water–Glucose Solutions Using Q Factor of Microwave Sensors. *IEEE Trans. Instrum. Meas.* **2018**, 1–14. [CrossRef]
56. Melikyan, H.; Danielyan, E.; Kim, S.; Kim, J.; Babajanyan, A.; Lee, J.; Friedman, B.; Lee, K. Non-invasive in vitro sensing of d-glucose in pig blood. *Med. Eng. Phys.* **2012**, *34*, 299–304. [CrossRef] [PubMed]
57. Vrba, J.; Vrba, D. A Microwave Metamaterial Inspired Sensor for Non-Invasive Blood Glucose Monitoring. *Radioengineering* **2015**, *24*. [CrossRef]
58. Cano-Garcia, H.; Saha, S.; Sotiriou, I.; Kosmas, P.; Gouzouasis, I.; Kallos, E. Millimeter-Wave Sensing of Diabetes-Relevant Glucose Concentration Changes in Pigs. *J. Infrared Millim. Terahertz Waves* **2018**, *39*, 761–772, doi:10.1007/s10762-018-0502-6. [CrossRef]
59. Saha, S.; Cano-Garcia, H.; Sotiriou, I.; Lipscombe, O.; Gouzouasis, I.; Koutsoupidou, M.; Palikaras, G.; Mackenzie, R.; Reeve, T.; Kosmas, P.; et al. A Glucose Sensing System Based on Transmission Measurements at Millimetre Waves using Micro strip Patch Antennas. *Sci. Rep.* **2017**, *7*, 6855, doi:10.1038/s41598-017-06926-1. [CrossRef] [PubMed]
60. Lee, D.K.; Kang, J.H.; Lee, J.S.; Kim, H.S.; Kim, C.; Hun Kim, J.; Lee, T.; Son, J.H.; Park, Q.H.; Seo, M. Highly sensitive and selective sugar detection by terahertz nano-antennas. *Sci. Rep.* **2015**, *5*, 15459, doi:10.1038/srep15459. [CrossRef]
61. Vrba, J.; Karch, J.; Vrba, D. Phantoms for development of microwave sensors for noninvasive blood glucose monitoring. *Int. J. Antennas Propag.* **2015**, *2015*, 570870. [CrossRef]
62. Turgul, V.; Kale, I. Sensitivity of non-invasive RF/microwave glucose sensors and fundamental factors and challenges affecting measurement accuracy. In Proceedings of the 2018 IEEE International Instrumentation and Measurement Technology Conference (I2MTC), Houston, TX, USA, 14–17 May 2018; pp. 1–5.
63. Buford, R.J.; Green, E.C.; McClung, M.J. A microwave frequency sensor for non-invasive blood-glucose measurement. In Proceedings of the 2008 IEEE Sensors Applications Symposium (SAS), Atlanta, GA, USA, 12–14 February 2008; pp. 4–7.
64. Kim, N.Y.; Adhikari, K.K.; Dhakal, R.; Chuluunbaatar, Z.; Wang, C.; Kim, E.S. Rapid, sensitive and reusable detection of glucose by a robust radiofrequency integrated passive device biosensor chip. *Sci. Rep.* **2015**, *5*, 7807. [CrossRef]
65. Caduff, A.; Zanon, M.; Zakharov, P.; Mueller, M.; Talary, M.; Krebs, A.; Stahel, W.A.; Donath, M. First Experiences With a Wearable Multisensor in an Outpatient Glucose Monitoring Study, Part I: The Users' View. *J. Diabetes Sci. Technol.* **2018**, *12*, 562–568, doi:10.1177/1932296817750932. [CrossRef]
66. Zanon, M.; Mueller, M.; Zakharov, P.; Talary, M.S.; Donath, M.; Stahel, W.A.; Caduff, A. First Experiences With a Wearable Multisensor Device in a Noninvasive Continuous Glucose Monitoring Study at Home, Part II: The Investigators' View. *J. Diabetes Sci. Technol.* **2018**, *12*, 554–561, doi:10.1177/1932296817740591. [CrossRef]

67. Hao, Y.; Foster, R. Wireless body sensor networks for health-monitoring applications. *Physiol. Meas.* **2008**, *29*, R27–R56. [CrossRef]
68. Yilmaz, T.; Foster, R.; Hao, Y. Detecting Vital Signs with Wearable Wireless Sensors. *Sensors* **2010**, *10*, 10837–10862, doi:10.3390/s101210837. [CrossRef] [PubMed]
69. Caduff, A.; Hirt, E.; Feldman, Y.; Ali, Z.; Heinemann, L. First human experiments with a novel non-invasive, non-optical continuous glucose monitoring system. *Biosens. Bioelectron.* **2003**, *19*, 209–217, doi:10.1016/S0956-5663(03)00196-9. [CrossRef]
70. Pfützner, A.; Caduff, A.; Larbig, M.; Schrepfer, T.; Forst, T. Impact of posture and fixation technique on impedance spectroscopy used for continuous and noninvasive glucose monitoring. *Diabetes Technol. Ther.* **2004**, *6*, 435–441, doi:10.1089/1520915041705839. [CrossRef] [PubMed]
71. Caduff, A.; Dewarrat, F.; Talary, M.; Stalder, G.; Heinemann, L.; Feldman, Y. Non-invasive glucose monitoring in patients with diabetes: A novel system based on impedance spectroscopy. *Biosens. Bioelectron.* **2006**, *22*, 598–604, doi:10.1016/j.bios.2006.01.031. [CrossRef] [PubMed]
72. Caduff, A.; Talary, M.S.; Mueller, M.; Dewarrat, F.; Klisic, J.; Donath, M.; Heinemann, L.; Stahel, W.A. Non-invasive glucose monitoring in patients with Type 1 diabetes: A Multisensor system combining sensors for dielectric and optical characterisation of skin. *Biosens. Bioelectron.* **2009**, *24*, 2778–2784, doi:10.1016/j.bios.2009.02.001. [CrossRef] [PubMed]
73. Caduff, A.; Zanon, M.; Mueller, M.; Zakharov, P.; Feldman, Y.; De Feo, O.; Donath, M.; Stahel, W.A.; Talary, M.S. The Effect of a Global, Subject and Device-Specific Model on a Noninvasive Glucose Monitoring Multisensor System. *J. Diabetes Sci. Technol.* **2015**, *9*, 865–872, doi:10.1177/1932296815579459. [CrossRef]
74. Caduff, A.; Talary, M.S.; Müller, M.; De Feo, O. Wide Band Field Response Measurement for Glucose Determination. U.S. Patent Number 9,247,905 B2, 2 February 2016. United States Patent Document, Available from the United States Patent and Trademark Office. Available online: www.uspto.gov (accessed on 22 November 2018).
75. Mueller, M.; Talary, M.S.; Falco, L.; De Feo, O.; Stahel, W.A.; Caduff, A. Data Processing for Noninvasive Continuous Glucose Monitoring with a Multisensor Device. *J. Diabetes Sci. Technol.* **2011**, *5*, 694–702, doi:10.1177/193229681100500324. [CrossRef]
76. Thin-film Force Sensors. Available online: https://www.tekscan.com/force-sensors (accessed on 28 December 2018).
77. Williams, R.; Quattrocchi, E.; Watts, S.; Wang, S.; Berry, P.; Crouthamel, M. Patient Rheumatoid Arthritis Data from the Real World (PARADE) Study: Preliminary Results from an Apple Researchkit^{TM} Mobile App-Based Real World Study in the United States. *Arthritis Rheumatol.* **2017**, *69*, 223–224.
78. Chan, Y.F.Y.; Wang, P.; Rogers, L.; Tignor, N.; Zweig, M.; Hershman, S.G.; Genes, N.; Scott, E.R.; Krock, E.; Badgeley, M.; et al. The Asthma Mobile Health Study, a large-scale clinical observational study using ResearchKit. *Nat. Biotechnol.* **2017**, *35*, 354–362, doi:10.1038/nbt.3826. [CrossRef]
79. Cadmus-Bertram, L. Using Fitness Trackers in Clinical Research: What Nurse Practitioners Need to Know. *J. Nurse Pract.* **2017**, *13*, 34–40, doi:10.1016/j.nurpra.2016.10.012. [CrossRef]
80. Alinia, P.; Cain, C.; Fallahzadeh, R.; Shahrokni, A.; Cook, D.; Ghasemzadeh, H. How Accurate Is Your Activity Tracker? A Comparative Study of Step Counts in Low-Intensity Physical Activities. *JMIR mHealth uHealth* **2017**, *5*, e106, doi:10.2196/mhealth.6321. [CrossRef] [PubMed]
81. Xie, J.; Wen, D.; Liang, L.; Jia, Y.; Gao, L.; Lei, J. Evaluating the Validity of Current Mainstream Wearable Devices in Fitness Tracking Under Various Physical Activities: Comparative Study. *JMIR mHealth uHealth* **2018**, *6*, e94, doi:10.2196/mhealth.9754. [CrossRef] [PubMed]
82. Fioravanti, A.; Fico, G.; Patón, A.G.; Leuteritz, J.P.; Arredondo, A.G.; Waldmeyer, M.T.A. Health-Integrated System Paradigm: Diabetes Management. In *Handbook of Biomedical Telemetry*; John Wiley & Sons, Inc.: Hoboken, NJ, USA, 2014; Chapter 22, pp. 623–632.
83. Fico, G.; Fioravanti, A.; Arredondo, M.T.; Leuteritz, J.P.; Guillen, A.; Fernandez, D. A user centered design approach for patient interfaces to a diabetes IT platform. In Proceedings of the IEEE 2011 Annual International

Conference of the IEEE Engineering in Medicine and Biology Society, Boston, MA, USA, 30 August–3 September 2011; pp. 1169–1172.

84. Fioravanti, A.; Fico, G.; Arredondo, M.T.; Leuteritz, J. A mobile feedback system for integrated E-health platforms to improve self-care and compliance of diabetes mellitus patients. In Proceedings of the 2011 Annual International Conference of the IEEE Engineering in Medicine and Biology Society, Boston, MA, USA, 30 August–3 September 2011; pp. 3550–3553.
85. Otis, B. Verily Blog: Update on Our Smart Lens Program with Alcon. Available online: https://blog.verily.com/2018/11/update-on-our-smart-lens-program-with.html?m=1 (accessed on 18 November 2018).
86. Kownacka, A.E.; Vegelyte, D.; Joosse, M.; Anton, N.; Toebes, B.J.; Lauko, J.; Buzzacchera, I.; Lipinska, K.; Wilson, D.A.; Geelhoed-Duijvestijn, N.; et al. Clinical Evidence for Use of a Noninvasive Biosensor for Tear Glucose as an Alternative to Painful Finger-Prick for Diabetes Management Utilizing a Biopolymer Coating. *Biomacromolecules* **2018**, *19*, 4504–4511, doi:10.1021/acs.biomac.8b01429. [CrossRef] [PubMed]

9

Anthropomorphic Breast and Head Phantoms for Microwave Imaging

Nadine Joachimowicz [1,*], Bernard Duchêne [2], Christophe Conessa [1,†] and Olivier Meyer [1]

[1] Group of Electrical Engineering, Paris (GeePs: CNRS—CentraleSupélec—Université Paris-Sud—Sorbonne Université), 91190 Gif-sur-Yvette, France; christophe.conessa@unicaen.fr (C.C.); olivier.meyer@geeps.centralesupelec.fr (O.M.)

[2] Laboratoire des Signaux et Systèmes (L2S, UMR 8506: CNRS—CentraleSupélec—Université Paris-Sud), 91190 Gif-sur-Yvette, France; bernard.duchene@l2s.centralesupelec.fr

[*] Correspondence: nadine.joachimowicz@geeps.centralesupelec.fr

[†] Current address: Laboratoire Morphodynamique Continentale et Côtière (M2C, UMR6143: CNRS, Université Caen Normandie, Université Rouen Normandie), 14000 Caen, France.

Abstract: This paper deals with breast and head phantoms fabricated from 3D-printed structures and liquid mixtures whose complex permittivities are close to that of the biological tissues within a large frequency band. The goal is to enable an easy and safe manufacturing of stable-in-time detailed anthropomorphic phantoms dedicated to the test of microwave imaging systems to assess the performances of the latter in realistic configurations before a possible clinical application to breast cancer imaging or brain stroke monitoring. The structure of the breast phantom has already been used by several laboratories to test their measurement systems in the framework of the COST (European Cooperation in Science and Technology) Action TD1301-MiMed. As for the tissue mimicking liquid mixtures, they are based upon Triton X-100 and salted water. It has been proven that such mixtures can dielectrically mimic the various breast tissues. It is shown herein that they can also accurately mimic most of the head tissues and that, given a binary fluid mixture model, the respective concentrations of the various constituents needed to mimic a particular tissue can be predetermined by means of a standard minimization method.

Keywords: microwave imaging; breast cancer detection; brain stroke monitoring; dielectric characterization; UWB breast and head phantoms

---

1. Introduction

Due their non-ionizing nature and to the low cost and portability of the equipment, microwaves arouse a keen interest for biomedical applications. Furthermore, several studies have shown that, at these frequencies, the various human biological tissues show significant differences in their dielectric properties [1]. This is the reason why, at the present time, a lot of work is devoted to biomedical microwave imaging, more specifically for breast cancer detection and brain stroke monitoring. It can be noted that in these last two applications, the interest of microwave imaging lies in the dielectric contrast which may exist between normal healthy tissues and malignant [2] or stroke-affected [3] ones and, in turn, the magnitude of this contrast depends upon the nature of the disease, i.e., ischemic or hemorrhagic for the stroke and located in fat or in fibroconnective-glandular tissues for the breast tumor. For the latter case, contrasts as high as 10:1 are reported in Reference [2] between malignant and healthy adipose breast tissues; however, those that can be found between tumors and normal fibroconnective–glandular tissues are less than 10%, which renders the detection of such tumors with microwave imaging challenging.

Although microwave imaging is still an emerging technique that is not yet recognized as an alternative to magnetic resonance imaging (MRI) or X-ray computerized tomography (CT), several microwave imaging systems dedicated to breast tumor detection [4–8] (see Reference [9] for a comprehensive comparison of the various systems that concern this application) and brain stroke monitoring [10–13] are already at the clinical trial level.

However, before such a trial, the imaging systems need to be tested on reference anthropomorphic phantoms in order to assess and compare their performances in controlled realistic configurations. These reference phantoms should satisfy several requirements: Particularly, their structure must be close to that of the targeted human body part (breast or head), the dielectric properties of their constitutive materials must be close to that of the various biological tissues of the abovementioned part, and finally, their shape and dielectric properties must be stable over time in order that the phantom can be used as a benchmark.

One of the main difficulties encountered when looking for a tissue mimicking material (TMM) is the large dispersivity of soft tissue dielectric properties in the microwave frequency range. Thus, a lot of mixtures have been considered as TMMs [14], among which jelly mixtures based upon oil-in-gelatin dispersions [15–18] or upon water–agar or water–gelatin blends [19] and gel substances based upon water–polythene powder-TX-151 mixtures [20] are certainly among the most promising materials, as, in addition to accurately simulating the dispersive dielectric properties of the various human tissues in a large frequency range, they are relatively easy to produce and their mechanical properties allow the construction of anthropomorphic phantoms. Hence, the abovementioned mixtures fulfill the first two requirements outlined in the previous paragraph; however, they fail in satisfying the last one. Indeed, the dielectric and mechanical properties of phantoms based upon these TMMs are unstable over time. This is due either to evaporation or diffusion phenomena between layers of different gelatin concentrations [15] for the water–gelatin-based mixtures or to interaction with air if they are not very carefully shielded from the environment for the oil-in-gelatin dispersions [21,22]. Furthermore, with these materials, it is not always easy to avoid air bubbles getting trapped in the mixtures without specific equipments. If such bubbles are present, they would behave as small high-contrasted diffractors, which would greatly perturb the electromagnetic field within the phantom. Solid TMMs do not present these drawbacks; however, phantoms made of such materials [23] are not reconfigurable as solid TMMs are not adjustable in order to account for changes linked, for example, to the appearance of a tumor or of a stroke. By contrast, liquid mixtures allow us to avoid air bubbles and stability problems and they are adjustable, as they can easily be replaced.

Fluid TMMs based upon mixtures of Triton X-100 (TX-100, a non-ionic surfactant) and water have already been used to mimic the various breast tissues [24,25]; however, they cannot account for the high conductivity of many tissues at high frequencies. We have shown that adding salt to these mixtures allows us to get both permittivity and conductivity close to that of the various breast tissues over the 0.5–6 GHz range [22]. It is shown herein that, in fact, these mixtures are also good TMMs for head tissues. Furthermore, the respective concentrations of the various constituents needed to mimic a given tissue can be approximately deduced from a binary fluid mixture model involving TX-100 and salted water. In Reference [22], the dielectric properties of such mixtures were also shown to be stable over time periods as long as 1 year. Such a time stability is obtained by taking the precaution of extracting the TMMs from the phantom rigid structure required to contain and separate the TMMs that correspond to the different tissues, and to keep them away from light in sealed containers to avoid evaporation.

Concerning the phantom's rigid structure, recent progress in additive manufacturing now allows us to build up relatively easily reproducible 3D-printed complex structures from STL (stereolithography) files that describe their surfaces. For anthropomorphic structures, these STL files can be obtained from MRI or X-ray CT scans. Finally, one further advantage of 3D-printed phantoms is that the STL file can also be used to perform numerical simulations along with experimental validations. Before the design of the breast and head phantoms presented herein, other phantoms had already been built up in this way [25–28]; however, their structures were not suitable to be filled up with several fluid TMMs, as one is made of a unique cavity while the others are made of several parts which are intended to be used as temporary molds where gel-based breast or head parts are formed. The novelty, herein, was that the phantoms comprise several cavities intended to be filled up with different fluid TMMs. Since then, similar breast phantoms have been proposed [29–31].

2. The Phantoms

2.1. 3D-Printed Structures

Both breast and head phantoms are produced in the same way. Their structures are made of acrylonitrile butadiene styrene (ABS) and built up by additive manufacturing from STL files obtained by modifying original files available in the literature that describe anatomically realistic breast and head structures derived from MRI scans. Hence, the original file corresponding to the breast phantom comes from the University of Wisconsin–Madison [25], while that corresponding to the head phantom comes from the Athinoula A. Martinos Center for Biomedical Imaging at Massachusetts General Hospital [32]. These files have been modified by means of a computer-aided design software so as to separate three distinct cavities. This results from a trade-off between the preservation of highly dielectrically contrasted regions around the area of interest (i.e., the brain for the head phantom) and the minimization of the number of ABS internal walls that raise leakage and field perturbation issues. The phantoms are printed in several parts that are clipped and glued together and the seals are weatherproofed. Figure 1 displays sagittal sections of the breast and head phantoms produced from the original and modified STL files, while Figures 2 and 3 display exploded views that show the different parts of the latter, respectively.

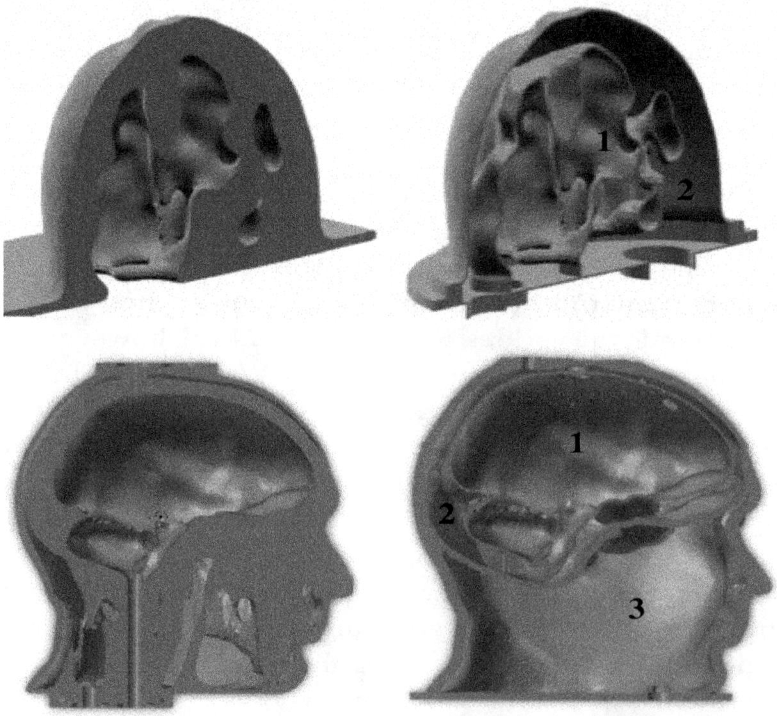

Figure 1. Sagittal sections of the breast (**up**) and head (**down**) phantoms derived from the original STL (stereolithography) files (**left**) and from the modified ones (**right**). The red numbers indicate the various cavities that contain the different TMMs corresponding to: (1) fibroglandular or heterogeneous mix tissues, (2) fatty tissues (**up-right**), and (1) brain, (2) cerebrospinal fluid, (3) miscellaneous tissues (**down-right**).

Concerning the breast structure, it is denoted as the GeePs-L2S (or Supelec) breast phantom. It has already been used as a reference phantom in the framework of Cost Action TD1301 MiMed (http://cost-action-td1301.org) and several publications report experimental results collected with this phantom by means of various microwave imaging systems [33–36].

In this phantom, cavities 2 and 1 (Figure 1—top right) correspond to a typical distribution of fatty and fibroglandular or heterogeneous mix tissues, respectively, while the third one (Figure 2c) can be placed at different locations in order to account for the presence of a tumor.

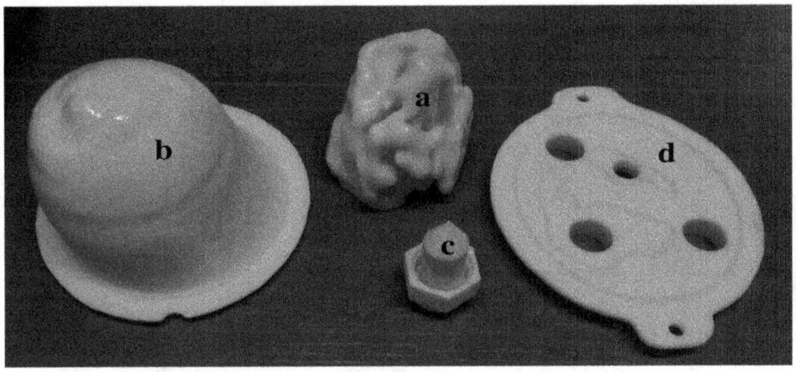

Figure 2. The different parts of the GeePs-L2S breast phantom: (**a**) The inner part contains the fibroglandular or heterogeneous mix tissue mimicking material (TMM); (**b**) the outer shell contains the fatty TMM; (**c**) the removable inclusion contains the tumor-like TMM; and (**d**) the support plate holds the different parts in place.

As for the head structure, it includes three fixed cavities. Cavities 1 and 2 (Figure 1—down right) are filled up from the top with brain and cerebrospinal fluid (CSF) TMMs, respectively, and cavity 3 can be filled from the bottom of the structure with mixtures whose dielectric properties can be adjusted in order to fit those of various tissues, such as bone, muscle, blood or a medium whose properties are an average of that of these tissues. Of course, the latter cavity must filled up before the former ones with the head upside down and the filling hole must be tightly closed before turning the phantom right side up. It can be noted that during this operation, it is difficult to avoid a little bit of air remaining in the cavity; however, once the phantom is right side up, this air will rise to the level of the nasal cavity where it is naturally present in a real human head.

Except for the outer shell of the head, which is relatively thick ($\approx$8 mm, i.e., the thickness of the skull) in order to get a good rigidity, for both phantoms, the thickness of the ABS structures is 1.5 mm. This results from a trade-off between wall stiffness, structure tightness, and low field perturbation. Indeed, at a frequency of 2.45 GHz, the values of the ABS dielectric parameters are $\epsilon_r = 3$ and $\sigma = 4 \times 10^{-3}$ S/m, which is far from the dielectric properties of the various biological tissues and, hence, leads us to opt for a thin structure in order to minimize the perturbation of the field inside the phantoms. However, this trade-off is not satisfactory. Indeed, on one hand, a 1.5-mm thickness is not sufficient to ensure a perfect waterproofing of the phantom, but leakages can be avoided by smoothing the structure by means of acetone vapor and by coating it with epoxy resin. On the other hand, despite their thinness, it has been experimentally [37] and numerically [38] shown that due to the high dielectric contrast with respect to the various biological tissues, the ABS walls perturb the field significantly. Concerning the breast structure, a solution proposed in Reference [29] consists of using conductive ABS whose dielectric parameters (i.e., $\epsilon_r \approx 10$ and $\sigma \approx 0.4$ S/m at 2.45 GHz, see [29]) are closer to that of adipose tissues ($\epsilon_r \approx 5$ and $\sigma \approx 0.1$ S/m, see Table 1) than the normal one. It can be noted that at 1 GHz, which should be the central frequency of the band considered for brain stroke monitoring, as will be seen later on, the parameters of conductive ABS are also very close to that of the bone ($\epsilon_r \approx 12$ and $\sigma \approx 0.2$ S/m, see Table 2 and Reference [29]); hence, this material is appropriate for the outer shell of the head that represents the skull and it could be used to print parts "b" and "c" (see Figure 3) of future versions of the head phantom. However, this material is not adequate for the inner walls of the phantom and a printable material whose parameters are close to that of the brain is still to be found. Finally, although this has not been done therein, the phantoms can be improved by plastering their external shell with flexible skin mimicking mixtures based upon graphite, carbon black, and silicone rubber [29,39] or urethane [40], that, in addition, could also solve the problems of leakage through the external wall.

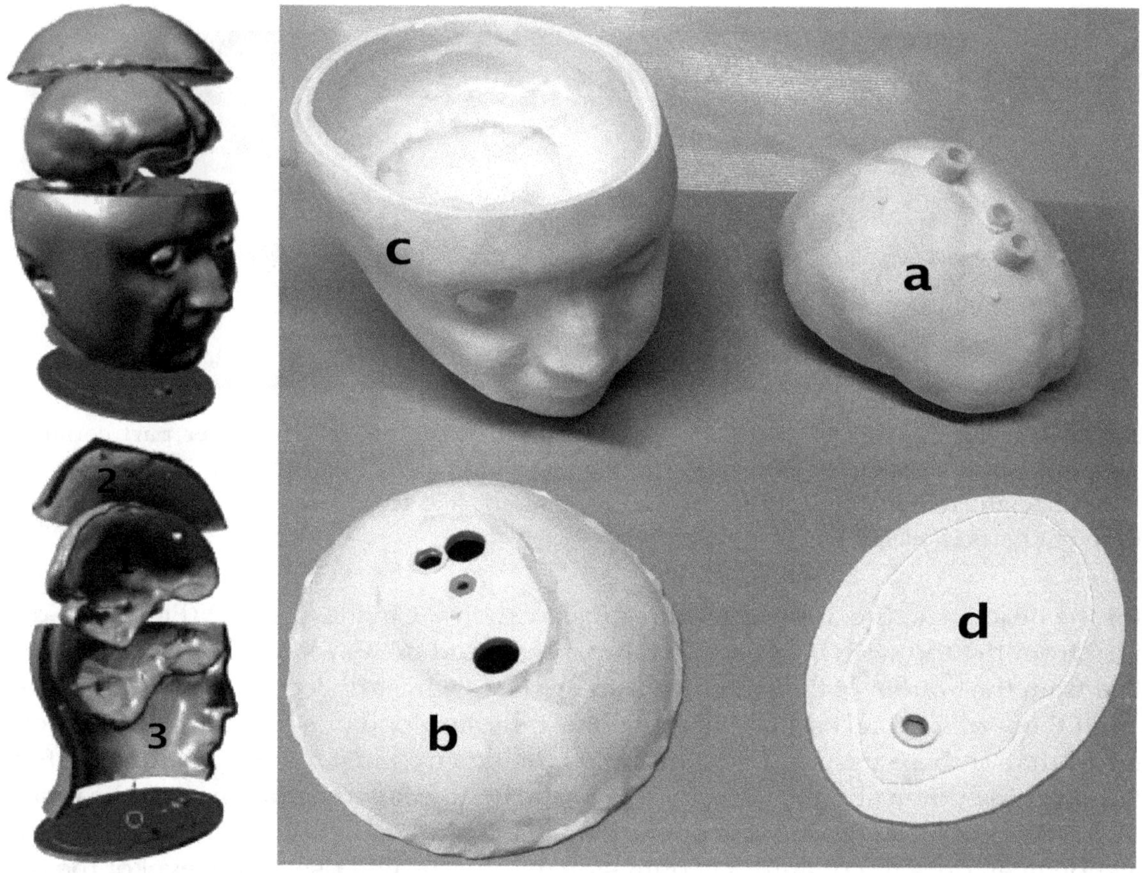

Figure 3. The different parts of the head phantom: (1) The inner tank (**a**) contains the brain TMM, (2) the upper cavity contains the cerebrospinal fluid (CSF) TMM, and (3) the lower one contains an average tissue medium mimicking mixture. The top and bottom of part (**c**) are clipped, respectively, to the part (**b**) and to the plate (**d**) by means of a tenon–mortise system that runs all around the joints, and the different parts are glued once in place, while the brain tank is held in place by several stops.

Table 1. Composition and properties of breast TMMs at 2.45 GHz and 37 °C (group: T = tumor, G1 = fibroglandular tissue, G2 = heterogeneous mix tissue, G3 = fatty tissue).

Group	Mixture Composition		Averaged Measurements		Debye Model	
	TX-100 (vol %)	NaCl (g/L)	ϵ_r	σ (S/m)	ϵ_r	σ (S/m)
T	18	4.0	56 ± 2	1.79 ± 0.06	53	1.8
G1	28	3.5	47 ± 1	1.61 ± 0.08	46	1.6
G2	41	0	37.8 ± 0.3	1.12 ± 0.05	37	1.1
G3	100	0	4.76 ± 0.04	0.18 ± 0.03	5	0.1

Table 2. Composition and properties of head TMMs at 1 GHz and 37 °C versus the values inferred from Cole–Cole models.

Tissue	Mixture Composition		Averaged Measurements		Cole-Cole	
	TX-100 (vol %)	NaCl (g/L)	ϵ_r	σ (S/m)	ϵ_r	σ (S/m)
Brain	38	5.2	44 ± 2	0.84 ± 0.03	42	0.7
CSF	6	13.7	70 ± 7	2.7 ± 0.2	68	2.5
Muscle	24	5.0	54 ± 2	0.97 ± 0.03	55	1.0
Bone	75	0.8	16.7 ± 0.8	0.30 ± 0.04	12	0.2
Blood	14	9.4	61 ± 3	1.72 ± 0.07	61	1.6

2.2. Tissue Mimicking Mixtures

As underlined above, in addition to being good TMMs for breast tissues, liquid mixtures made of TX-100 and salted water can mimic almost all the head tissues over a large frequency band with good precision. Furthermore, given a temperature and a frequency band, the concentrations of TX-100 and salt in the mixture needed to mimic a specific tissue can be approximately predetermined with a binary mixture model, such as the Böttcher's one [41] that yields ϵ_m, the complex permittivity of the TMM, as a function of (ϵ_1, V_1) and (ϵ_2, V_2), the permittivities and volume fractions of TX-100 and salted water, respectively. By accounting for the fact that $V_1 + V_2 = 1$, ϵ_m can be expressed without V_2:

$$\epsilon_m = \epsilon_2 + [3\ V_1\ \epsilon_m(\epsilon_1 - \epsilon_2)/(2\epsilon_m + \epsilon_1)]\,. \tag{1}$$

Elsewhere, Debye [42] and Cole–Cole [43,44] models have been developed for most of the human body tissues to describe the behavior of their complex permittivities ϵ_t as functions of the frequency. Particularly, in Reference [42], an accurate Debye model can be found to describe the permittivity of breast tissues with adipose tissue content in the range 85–100%, defined as group 3 in Reference [2], and it has been shown in Reference [22] that, in the 0.5–6 GHz frequency band, the complex permittivity of this tissue group is very close to that of TX-100, so that we have a model for ϵ_1:

$$\epsilon_1(\omega) = 3.14 + 1.6/(1 + j\,13.56 \times 10^{-12}\,\omega) + 0.036/(j\,\omega\epsilon_0), \tag{2}$$

where ω is the angular frequency, j is the imaginary unit, and ϵ_0 the dielectric permittivity of vacuum. It has been shown that the permittivity of TX-100 varies only very slightly with the temperature in the range 15–37 °C. Concerning the salted water, a parametric model can be found in Reference [45] that expresses ϵ_2 as a function of the frequency, the salinity, and the temperature.

Hence, the mixture component concentrations needed to mimic a specific tissue can be determined by fitting the mixture model ϵ_m to the permittivity of the tissue ϵ_t at several discrete frequencies f over the frequency range of interest, i.e., by minimizing the following cost functional:

$$J = \textstyle\sum_f w_f |\epsilon_m - \epsilon_t|_f^2\,, \tag{3}$$

where $w_f = 1/|\epsilon_t|_f^2$.

This can be done in an iterative way by means of a Gauss–Newton method [46]. The solution $\boldsymbol{x} = (V_1, S_m)^{\dagger}$ (where † indicates the transposition, V_1 the volume fraction of TX-100, and S_m the NaCl concentration of the mixture) at iteration step $k+1$ then reads:

$$\boldsymbol{x}^{k+1} = \boldsymbol{x}^k - \boldsymbol{H}^{-1}(\boldsymbol{x}^k)\boldsymbol{g}(\boldsymbol{x}^k). \tag{4}$$

In the above equation, $\boldsymbol{g}$ and $\boldsymbol{H}$ are the gradient and the approximate Hessian of J, respectively:

$$\begin{aligned} \boldsymbol{g} &= 2\sum_f w_f\, \Re e[(\epsilon_m - \epsilon_t)^*_f\, \boldsymbol{\epsilon}'_m]_f\,, \\ \boldsymbol{H} &= 2\sum_f w_f\, \Re e(\boldsymbol{\epsilon}'^*_m\, \boldsymbol{\epsilon}'^\dagger_m)_f\,, \end{aligned} \tag{5}$$

where $\boldsymbol{\epsilon}'_m = (\partial\epsilon_m/\partial V_1, \partial\epsilon_m/\partial S_m)^\dagger$ and * indicates the conjugate. By accounting for Equation (1), $\boldsymbol{\epsilon}'_m$ becomes:

$$\boldsymbol{\epsilon}'_m = \begin{pmatrix} 3\,\gamma\,(\epsilon_1 - \epsilon_2)\,/\,(4\delta) \\ [(\gamma\,(3V_2 - 1) + 4\epsilon_1)\,/\,(4\,V_2\,\delta)]\;\partial\epsilon_2/\partial S_2 \end{pmatrix}, \tag{6}$$

with:

$$\begin{aligned} \gamma &= \delta - \eta\,, \qquad \delta = (\eta^2 + 8\,\epsilon_1\,\epsilon_2)^{1/2} \\ \eta &= \epsilon_1 - 2\,\epsilon_2 - 3\,V_1\,(\epsilon_1 - \epsilon_2). \end{aligned}$$

The term $\partial\epsilon_2/\partial S_2$ can be straightforwardly deduced from the salted water parametric model. The above described iterative method converges very rapidly towards a stable solution that generally depends very little on the initial guess, which allows us to choose $\boldsymbol{x}^0$ in an empirical way. It can be noted that for a given mixture, due to the discrepancy between the dielectric parameter measured values and those given by Böttcher's model, the TX-100 and salt concentrations must be experimentally refined around the solution given by the latter in order to get closer to the expected permittivity values.

Table 1 recalls the results of Reference [47] concerning the breast TMMs at a temperature of 37 °C and a frequency of 2.45 GHz. It displays the TX-100 and salt concentrations obtained by fitting the Böttcher's and Debye models over the 0.5–6 GHz range and the measured and expected (given by the Debye model) dielectric properties of the various mixtures. The "measured" values are the means of measurements performed with three different apparatuses dedicated to the characterization of liquid dielectric material properties, several measurements being made with each system. The first one, denoted as S1 in the following, consists of a coaxial waveguide coupled to an Agilent E8364C (Keysight Technologies, Santa Rosa, CA, USA) vector network analyzer (VNA) on one side and, on the other side, to a circular cylindrical cell by means of a dielectric coaxial tight window; this cell is made of a 7-mm-diameter circular waveguide intended to be filled up with the liquid dielectric under test and is ended by a short circuit [48]. The other two systems consist of open-ended coaxial sensors: A Keysight 85070D high-temperature dielectric probe coupled to an HP 8753E VNA (Keysight Technologies, Santa Rosa, CA, USA) and a homemade one connected to a Rodhe & Schwarz ZVB8 VNA (Rodhe & Schwarz France, Meudon-la-forêt, France) and built up from a 3.6-mm-diameter, 15-cm-long, Teflon-filled copper rigid coaxial cable. The uncertainties that appear in Table 1 are the standard deviations of all the measurements performed by means of the three systems and, below 4.5 GHz, these deviations are generally less than 5% of the mean values, except for the conductivity of group G3, as the latter is very low.

The TX-100–salted water mixtures are very easy to produce; however, for TX-100 volume percentages in the range 40–50%, at low temperature and salt concentration, the mixture is rather viscous. It can be noted that very few TMMs are concerned by this problem (among those presented herein, only G2 of Table 1 falls into this category), but, for the latter, the mixture components are warmed separately, then mixed and vigorously stirred, left to rest at 45 °C for a few minutes until air bubbles vanish, and poured into the cavity while it is still warm.

Table 2 displays the results obtained in the same conditions for the head TMMs at 1 GHz. Note that the last two columns display the expected values given by the Cole–Cole models of References [43,44]. In this table, the brain is considered as a blend of white and grey matters (75% of white matter and 25% of grey matter) and "bone" refers to the cortical bone. Here again, the standard deviations are generally less than 5% of the mean values, except for CSF. This exception is linked to system S1, whose measurement results become less accurate as the permittivity increases, due to concomitant lowering of the cutoff frequency in the measuring cell.

Figure 4 displays the results obtained over the 0.5–6 GHz band. Measured, predicted (from Böttcher's model) and expected (from the Cole–Cole model) properties are in good agreement for almost all the tissues except, maybe, the measured values of conductivity for the brain and the bones that deviate a little bit from the expected values. It is worth noting that the variability of human tissue dielectric properties is very important. In the frequency band considered herein, it is evaluated in Reference [1] to be in the range $\pm\Delta\%$ (where $5 \leq \Delta \leq 10$) of the permittivity values given by the Cole–Cole models. Concerning the breast tissues considered in Table 1, the variability is even more important as each group spans tissues with a large heterogeneity in their adipose content (see [2]—Figures 9 and 10). This means that for almost all the TMMs considered herein except the bone mimicking one, the measured values fall within the uncertainty range of the Debye and Cole–Cole models, if the variability ranges of the tissue dielectric properties can be considered as the uncertainty ranges of the parametric models.

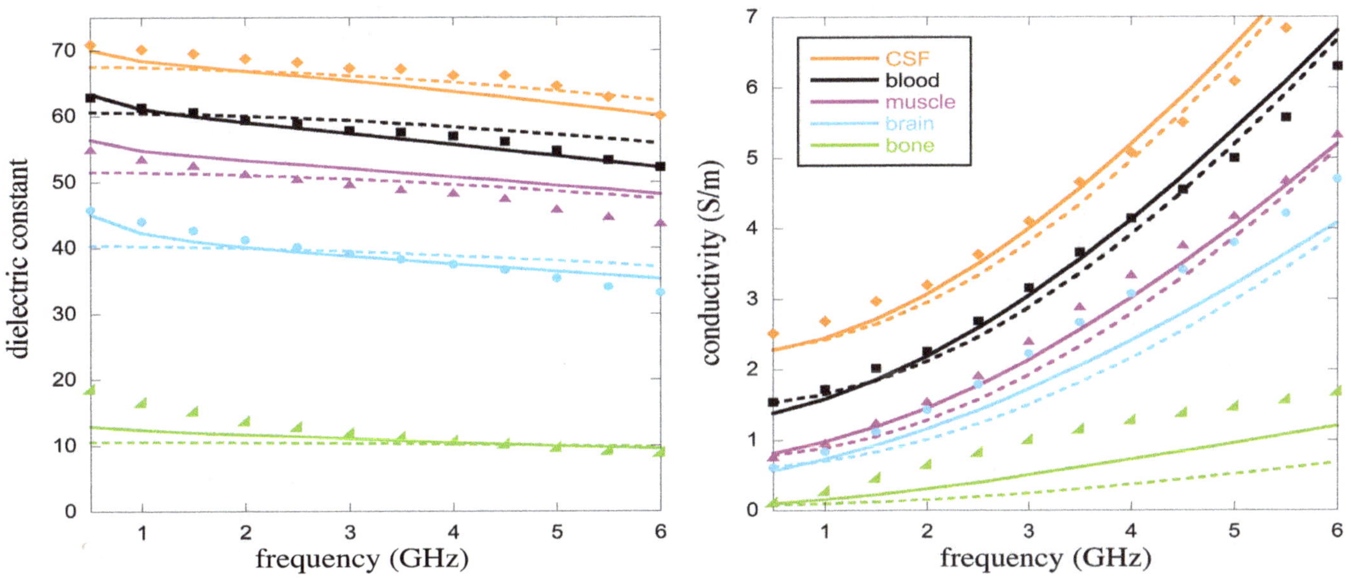

Figure 4. Means of the dielectric properties of various TMMs measured with three different set-ups (markers), compared to the results obtained by means of the tissue Cole–Cole models (full lines) and to those obtained with Böttcher's binary mixture law (dashed lines).

Furthermore, better fitting between predicted and expected properties of the various TMMs could be obtained with a narrower operating frequency range, and, although a lower resolution should be expected, the 0.6–1.5 GHz band would be more appropriate for brain stroke monitoring that requires an important penetration depth of the interrogating wave and where the range 1.5–4 GHz is a kind of "forbidden band" due to the strong attenuation of the waves within the head [3,49,50].

3. Conclusions

It has been shown herein that reference phantoms can be built up from 3D-printed structures and fluid TX-100–salted water mixtures. Such mixtures can mimic most of the breast and head tissues with a good precision concerning their dielectric properties over a large frequency range, and they are easily adjustable and reproducible. Furthermore, the respective proportions of the different mixture constituents needed to mimic a particular tissue can be approximately predetermined by means of a binary mixture model. Admittedly, these phantoms are very simplified compared to the real human breast or head and are less realistic than some other phantoms that can be found in the literature;

however, they have the advantage of being stable over time and easy to produce and, in addition, they preserve the areas of high dielectric contrast that are of interest to the applications considered herein, so that they can be considered as anthropomorphic. Note that they could be refined to be more realistic. Particularly for the head phantom, the lower part of the structure could be redesigned so as to delineate the buccal and nasal cavities, the eyeballs, and the muscles; however, this would need more ABS walls, which means field perturbation and leakage issues, for an improvement that should probably be minimal, as these parts are far from the area targeted by the brain stroke monitoring application. Furthermore, this would contradict the goal of this study that consists of the conception of simple phantoms that anyone involved in the field of microwave imaging could easily produce. The major drawback of these phantoms lies in the limited number of materials that can be used in additive manufacturing, which does not allow us to get rigid structures whose dielectric properties are close to that of some specific human tissues and particularly to that of the brain, but this drawback will certainly be overcome in the near future due to the rapid progress of 3D-printing technology that increasingly allows more and more materials to be processed.

Author Contributions: Study design and analysis, mixtures model, optimization, numerical and experimental validation, and manuscript preparation and revision, N.J. and B.D.; Design, development, and realization of phantom structures, N.J. and C.C.; Dielectric characterization, O.M. and C.C.

funding The part of this work that concerns the head phantom was partly supported by the Italian Ministry of University and Research under PRIN project "MiBraScan—Microwave Brain Scanner for Cerebrovascular Diseases Monitoring".

Acknowledgments: The authors would like to express their thanks to the University of Wisconsin–Madison and to the Athinoula A. Martinos Center for Biomedical Imaging for providing the original STL files of breast and head phantoms, respectively. This work has been developed under the framework of COST Action TD1301-MiMed. The authors would also like to thank V. Polledri and M. Police for carrying out measurements and 3D printings, respectively, and the anonymous reviewers for their constructive comments.

References

1. Gabriel, S.; Lau, R.; Gabriel, C. The dielectric properties of biological tissues: II. Measurements in the frequency range 10 Hz to 20 GHz. *Phys. Med. Biol.* **1996**, *41*, 2251–2270. [CrossRef] [PubMed]
2. Lazebnik, M.; Popovic, D.; McCartney, L.; Watkins, C.B.; Lindstrom, M.J.; Harter, J.; Sewall, S.; Ogilvie, T.; Magliocco, A.; Breslin, T.M.; et al. A large-scale study of the ultrawideband microwave dielectric properties of normal, benign and malignant breast tissues obtained from cancer surgeries. *Phys. Med. Biol.* **2007**, *52*, 6093–6115. [CrossRef] [PubMed]
3. Semenov, S.Y.; Corfield, D.R. Microwave tomography for brain imaging: Feasibility assessment for stroke detection. *Int. J. Antennas Propag.* **2008**. [CrossRef]
4. Meaney, P.M.; Fanning, M.W.; Li, D.; Poplack, S.P.; Paulsen, K.D. A clinical prototype for active microwave imaging of the breast. *IEEE Trans. Microw. Theory Tech.* **2000**, *48*, 1841–1853. [CrossRef]
5. Klemm, M.; Craddock, I.J.; Leendertz, J.A.; Preece, A.; Gibbins, D.R.; Shere, M.; Benjamin, R. Clinical trials of a UWB imaging radar for breast cancer. In Proceedings of the 4th European Conference on Antennas and Propagation (EuCAP), Barcelona, Spain, 12–16 April 2010.
6. Fear, E.C.; Bourqui, J.; Curtis, C.; Mew, D.; Docktor, B.; Romano, C. Microwave breast imaging with a monostatic radar-based system: A study of application to patients. *IEEE Trans. Microw. Theory Tech.* **2013**, *61*, 2119–2128. [CrossRef]
7. Porter, E.; Coates, M.; Popović, M. An early clinical study of time-domain microwave radar for breast health monitoring. *IEEE Trans. Biomed. Eng.* **2016**, *63*, 530–539. [CrossRef] [PubMed]
8. Fasoula, A.; Duchesne, L.; Gil Cano, J.D.; Lawrence, P.; Robin, G.; Bernard, J.-G. On-site validation of a microwave breast imaging system, before first patient study. *Diagnostics* **2018**, *8*, 53. [CrossRef] [PubMed]
9. O'Loughlin, D.; O'Halloran, M.J.; Moloney, B.M.; Glavin, M.; Jones, E.; Elahi, M.A. Microwave Breast Imaging: Clinical Advances and Remaining Challenges. *IEEE Trans. Biomed. Eng.* **2018**, *65*. [CrossRef]

10. Persson, M.; Fhager, A.; Trefná, H.D.; Yu, Y.; McKelvey, T.; Pegenius, G.; Karlsson, J.-E.; Elam, M. Microwave-based stroke diagnosis making global prehospital thrombolytic treatment possible. *IEEE Trans. Biomed. Eng.* **2014**, *61*, 2806–2817. [CrossRef] [PubMed]
11. Mobashsher, A.T.; Bialkowski, K.S.; Abbosh, A.M.; Crozier, S. Design and experimental evaluation of a non-invasive microwave head imaging system for intracranial haemorrhage detection. *PLoS ONE*, **2016**, *11*, e0152351. [CrossRef] [PubMed]
12. Hopfer, M.; Planas, R.; Hamidipour, A.; Henriksson, T.; Semenov, S. Electromagnetic tomography for detection, differentiation, and monitoring of brain stroke: A virtual data and human head phantom study. *IEEE Antennas Propag. Mag.* **2017**, *59*, 86–97. [CrossRef]
13. Scapaticci, R.; Tobon Vasquez, J.A.; Bellizzi, G.; Vipiana, F.; Crocco, L. Design and numerical characterization of a low-complexity microwave device for brain stroke monitoring. *IEEE Trans. Antennas Propag.* **2018**. [CrossRef]
14. Mobashsher, A.T.; Abbosh, A.M. Artificial human phantoms: Human proxy in testing microwave apparatus that have electromagnetic interaction with the human body. *IEEE Microw. Mag.* **2015**, *16*, 42–62. [CrossRef]
15. Lazebnik, M.; Madsen, E.L.; Frank, G.R.; Hagness, S.C. Tissue-mimicking phantom materials for narrowband and ultrawideband microwave applications. *Phys. Med. Biol.* **2005**, *50*, 4245–4258. [CrossRef] [PubMed]
16. Mashal, A.; Gao, F.; Hagness, S.C. Heterogeneous anthropomorphic phantoms with realistic dielectric properties for microwave breast imaging experiments. *Microw. Opt. Technol. Lett.* **2011**, *53*, 1896–1902. [CrossRef] [PubMed]
17. Abu Bakar, A.; Abbosh, A.; Bialkowski, M. Fabrication and characterization of a heterogeneous breast phantom for testing an ultrawideband microwave imaging system. In Proceedings of the IEEE Asia-Pacific Microwave Conference (APMC), Melbourne, Australia, 5–8 December 2011; pp. 1414–1417.
18. Hahn, C.; Noghanian, S. Heterogeneous breast phantom development for microwave imaging using regression models. *Int. J. Biomed. Imaging* **2012**, 6. [CrossRef] [PubMed]
19. Mohammed, B.J.; Abbosh, A.M. Realistic head phantom to test microwave systems for brain imaging. *Microw. Opt. Technol. Lett.* **2014**, *56*, 979–9824. [CrossRef]
20. Klemm, M.; Leendertz, J.A.; Gibbins, D.; Craddock, I.J.; Preece, A.; Benjamin, R. Microwave radar-based breast cancer detection: Imaging in inhomogeneous breast phantoms. *IEEE Antennas Wirel. Propag. Lett.* **2009**, *8*, 1349–1352. [CrossRef]
21. Porter, E.; Fakhoury, J.; Oprisor, R.; Coates, M.; Popović, M. Improved tissue phantoms for experimental validation of microwave breast cancer detection. In Proceedings of the 4th European Conference on Antennas and Propagation (EuCAP), Barcelona, Spain, 12–16 April 2010; pp. 1–5.
22. Joachimowicz, N.; Conessa, C.; Henriksson, T.; Duchêne, B. Breast phantoms for microwave imaging. *IEEE Antennas Wirel. Propag. Lett.* **2014**, *13*, 1333–1336. [CrossRef]
23. McDermott, B.; Porter, E.; Santorelli, A.; Divilly, B.; Morris, L.; Jones, M.; McGinley, B.; O'Halloran, M. Anatomically and Dielectrically Realistic Microwave Head Phantom with Circulation and Reconfigurable Lesions. *Prog. Electromagn. Res.* **2017**, *78*, 47–60. [CrossRef]
24. Romeo, S.; Di Donato, L.; Bucci, O.M.; Catapano, I.; Crocco, L.; Scarfì, M.R.; Massa, R. Dielectric characterization study of liquid-based materials for mimicking breast tissues. *Microw. Opt. Tech. Lett.* **2011**, *53*, 1276–1280. [CrossRef]
25. Burfeindt, M.J.; Colgan, T.J.; Mays, R.O.; Shea, J.D.; Behdad, N.; Van Veen, B.D.; Hagness, S.C. MRI-derived 3-D-printed breast phantom for microwave breast imaging validation. *IEEE Antennas Wirel. Propag. Lett.* **2012**, *11*, 1610–1613. [CrossRef] [PubMed]
26. Nguyen, P.T.; Abbosh, A.M.; Crozier, S. Thermo-dielectric breast phantom for experimental studies of microwave hyperthermia. *IEEE Antennas Wirel. Propag. Lett.* **2016**, *15*, 476–479. [CrossRef]
27. O'Halloran, M.; Lohfeld, S.; Ruvio, G.; Browne, J.; Krewer, F.; Ribeiro, C.O.; Inacio Pita, V.C.; Conceicao, R.C.; Jones, E.; Glavin, M. Development of anatomically and dielectrically accurate breast phantoms for microwave imaging applications. In *Radar Sensor Technology XVIII*; International Society for Optics and Photonics: Bellingham, WA, USA, 2014; p. 90770Y. [CrossRef]
28. Mobashsher, A.T.; Abbosh, A.M. Three-dimensional human head phantom with realistic electrical properties and anatomy. *IEEE Antennas Wirel. Propag. Lett.* **2014**, *13*, 1401–1404. [CrossRef]

29. Faenger, B.; Ley, S.; Helbig, M.; Sachs, J.; Hilger, I. Breast phantom with a conductive skin layer and conductive 3D-printed anatomical structures for microwave imaging. In Proceedings of the 11th European Conference on Antennas and Propagation (EuCAP), Paris, France, 19–24 March 2017; pp. 1065–1068. [CrossRef]
30. Rodriguez Herrera, D.; Reimer, T.; Solis Nepote, M.; Pistorius, S. Manufacture and testing of anthropomorphic 3D-printed breast phantoms using a microwave radar algorithm optimized for propagation speed. In Proceedings of the 11th European Conference on Antennas and Propagation (EuCAP), Paris, France, 19–24 March 2017; pp. 3480–3484. [CrossRef]
31. Fasoula, A.; Bernard, J.; Robin, G.; Duchesne, L. Elaborated breast phantoms and experimental benchmarking of a microwave breast imaging system before first clinical study. In Proceedings of the 12th European Conference on Antennas and Propagation (EuCAP), London, UK, 9–13 April 2018.
32. Graedel, N.N.; Polimeni, J.R.; Guerin, B.; Gagoski, B.; Wald, L.L. An anatomically realistic temperature phantom for radiofrequency heating measurements. *Magn. Reson. Med.* **2015**, *73*, 442–450. [CrossRef] [PubMed]
33. Rydholm, T.; Fhager, A.; Persson, M.; Meaney, P.M. A first evaluation of the realistic Supelec-breast phantom. *IEEE J. Electromagn. RF Microw. Med. Biol.* **2017**, *1*, 59–65. [CrossRef]
34. Koutsoupidou, M.; Karanasiou, I.S.; Kakoyiannis, C.G.; Groumpas, E.; Conessa, C.; Joachimowicz, N.; Duchêne, B. Evaluation of a tumor detection microwave system with a realistic breast phantom. *Microw. Opt. Technol. Lett.* **2017**, *59*, 6–10. [CrossRef]
35. Tobon Vasquez, J.A.; Vipiana, F.; Casu, M.R.; Vacca, M.; Sarwar, I.; Scapaticci, R.; Joachimowicz, N.; Duchêne, B. Experimental assessment of qualitative microwave imaging using a 3-D realistic breast phantom. In Proceedings of the 11th European Conference on Antennas and Propagation (EuCAP), Paris, France, 19–24 March 2017; pp. 2728–2731. [CrossRef]
36. Casu, M.R.; Vacca, M.; Tobon Vasquez, J.A.; Pulimeno, A.; Sarwar, I.; Solimene, R.; Vipiana, F. A COTS-based microwave imaging system for breast-cancer detection. *IEEE Trans. Biomed. Circuits Syst.* **2017**, *11*, 804–814. [CrossRef] [PubMed]
37. Rydholm, T.; Fhager, A.; Persson, M.; Geimer, S.; Meaney, P. Effects of the plastic of the realistic GeePS-L2S breast phantom. *Diagnostics* **2018**, *8*, 61. [CrossRef] [PubMed]
38. Joachimowicz, N.; Duchêne, B.; Tobon Vasquez, J.A.; Turvani, G.; Dassano, G.; Casu, M.R.; Vipiana, F.; Duchêne, B.; Scapaticci, R.; Crocco, L. Head phantoms for a microwave imaging system dedicated to cerebrovascular disease monitoring. In Proceedings of the IEEE International Conference on Antenna Measurements and Applications (IEEE CAMA), Västerås, Sweden, 3–6 September 2018.
39. Garrett, J.; Fear, E. Stable and flexible materials to mimic the dielectric properties of human soft tissues. *IEEE Antennas Wirel. Propag. Lett.* **2014**, *13*, 599–602. [CrossRef]
40. Garrett, J.; Fear, E. A new breast phantom with a durable skin layer for microwave breast imaging. *IEEE Trans. Antennas Propag.* **2015**, *63*, 1693–1700. [CrossRef]
41. Govinda Raju, G. Dielectric constant of binary mixtures of liquids. In Proceedings of the Conference on Electrical Insulation and Dielectric Phenomena, Ottawa, ON, Canada, 16–20 October 1988; pp. 357–363. [CrossRef]
42. Lazebnik, M.; Okoniewski, M.; Booske, J.H.; Hagness, S.C. Highly accurate Debye models for normal and malignant breast tissue dielectric properties at microwave frequencies. *IEEE Microw. Wirel. Comp. Lett.* **2007**, *17*, 822–824. [CrossRef]
43. Gabriel, S.; Lau, R.; Gabriel, C. The dielectric properties of biological tissues: III. Parametric models for the dielectric spectrum of tissues. *Phys. Med. Biol.* **1996**, *41*, 2271–2293. [CrossRef] [PubMed]
44. Andreuccetti, D.; Fossi, R.; Petrucci, C. Calculation of the Dielectric Properties of Body Tissues in the Frequency Range 10 Hz–100 GHz. Available online: http://niremf.ifac.cnr.it/tissprop/htmlclie/htmlclie.php (accessed on 17 December 2018).
45. Stogryn, A. Equations for calculating the dielectric constant of saline water. *IEEE Trans. Microw. Theory Tech.* **1971**, *19*, 733–736. [CrossRef]
46. Walter, E. *Numerical Methods and Optimization: A Consumer Guide*; Springer: Cham, Switzerland, 2014; ISBN 978-3-319-07670-6.

47. Joachimowicz, N.; Duchêne, B.; Conessa, C.; Meyer, O. Easy-to-produce adjustable realistic breast phantoms for microwave imaging. In Proceedings of the 10th European Conference on Antennas and Propagation (EuCAP), Davos, Switzerland, 10–15 April 2016; pp. 2892–2895. [CrossRef]
48. Belhadj-Tahar, N.E.; Fourrier-Lamer, A. Broad-band analysis of a coaxial discontinuity used for dielectric measurements. *IEEE Trans. Microw. Theory Tech.* **1986**, *34*, 346–350. [CrossRef]
49. Scapaticci, R.; Di Donato, L.; Catapano, I.; Crocco, L. A Feasibility Study on Microwave Imaging for Brain Stroke Monitoring. *Prog. Electromagn. Res. B* **2012**, *40*, 305–324. [CrossRef]
50. Bjelogrlic, M.; Volery, M.; Fuchs, B.; Thiran, J.P.; Mosig, J.R.; Mattes, M. Stratified spherical model for microwave imaging of the brain: Analysis and experimental validation of transmitted power. *Microw. Opt. Technol. Lett.* **2018**, *60*, 1042–1048. [CrossRef]

10

Monitoring Thermal Ablation via Microwave Tomography: An Ex Vivo Experimental Assessment

Rosa Scapaticci [1,*], Vanni Lopresto [2], Rosanna Pinto [2], Marta Cavagnaro [3] and Lorenzo Crocco [1]

1 National Research Council of Italy—Institute for the Electromagnetic Sensing of the Environment, 80124 Napoli, Italy; crocco.l@irea.cnr.it
2 Italian National Agency for New Technologies, Energy and Sustainable Economic Development, Division of Health Protection Technologies, Casaccia Research Center, 00123 Rome, Italy; vanni.lopresto@enea.it (V.L.); rosanna.pinto@enea.it (R.P.)
3 Department of Information Engineering, Electronics and Telecommunications, Sapienza University of Rome, 00184 Rome, Italy; marta.cavagnaro@uniroma1.it
* Correspondence: scapaticci.r@irea.cnr.it

Abstract: Thermal ablation treatments are gaining a lot of attention in the clinics thanks to their reduced invasiveness and their capability of treating non-surgical patients. The effectiveness of these treatments and their impact in the hospital's routine would significantly increase if paired with a monitoring technique able to control the evolution of the treated area in real-time. This is particularly relevant in microwave thermal ablation, wherein the capability of treating larger tumors in a shorter time needs proper monitoring. Current diagnostic imaging techniques do not provide effective solutions to this issue for a number of reasons, including economical sustainability and safety. Hence, the development of alternative modalities is of interest. Microwave tomography, which aims at imaging the electromagnetic properties of a target under test, has been recently proposed for this scope, given the significant temperature-dependent changes of the dielectric properties of human tissues induced by thermal ablation. In this paper, the outcomes of the first *ex vivo* experimental study, performed to assess the expected potentialities of microwave tomography, are presented. The paper describes the validation study dealing with the imaging of the changes occurring in thermal ablation treatments. The experimental test was carried out on two *ex vivo* bovine liver samples and the reported results show the capability of microwave tomography of imaging the transition between ablated and untreated tissue. Moreover, the discussion section provides some guidelines to follow in order to improve the achievable performances.

Keywords: microwave imaging; thermal ablation; microwave ablation; image-guided; monitoring; dielectric properties

---

1. Introduction

Thermal ablation is a therapeutic procedure used to destroy unhealthy tissue by way of a very high and localized temperature increase. In thermal ablation, the target temperature is close to 60 °C in the zone of ablation, which for tumor treatment should include the pathologic lesion plus a 5–10 mm safety margin of healthy tissue [1,2]. At this temperature, an almost instantaneous cell death by way of coagulative necrosis is achieved [1].

The increase in temperature can be obtained using different energy sources, such as radiofrequency currents, ultrasounds, lasers [3]. Among the others, microwave thermal ablation (MTA), in which the energy source is an electromagnetic field in the Industrial, Scientific and Medical (ISM) frequency band (typically at 915 MHz or 2.45 GHz), is gaining an increasing attention in the clinical practice [4,5], owing to its capability of treating larger tumors in a shorter time with respect to other ablation modalities [2].

As a matter of fact, MTA is increasingly used to treat different types of solid tumors, as those of the liver, kidney, lung, etc. [6–10].

The MTA clinical set-up is typically made by a minimally invasive interstitial applicator (i.e., a microwave ablation antenna), whose diameter is in the order of a few mm, a microwave power generator, and a cooling system used to keep the antenna's shaft at safe temperatures. The clinical procedure foresees the introduction of the antenna into the patient's body, percutaneously or following natural paths, and the onset of the microwave generator with a power value and for a time duration depending on the dimension of the tumor to be treated (typically, 60–100 W for about 5−10 min) [4,5]. Commercial systems give coagulative performances of the devices based on experiments performed either *ex vivo* or in vivo on animals [11,12]. Clinicians use these data to define the clinical protocol, i.e., the power value and time of irradiation to be used in a defined pathological situation. Moreover, software tools have been recently developed to help defining the best insertion path for the antenna [13].

Before the treatment, to help targeting the applicator in the center of the tumor to be treated, clinicians use image-guidance techniques such as ultrasounds (US), computerized tomography (CT), or magnetic resonance imaging (MRI). During the treatment, temperature is monitored by temperature sensors (usually thermocouples), whose positions are carefully chosen to assure safe temperatures in critical organs close to the tumor to be treated [14–24]. Techniques which could be used to monitor the evolution of the thermally ablated area during the treatment include US, CT, and MRI. However, all these techniques show drawbacks, which prevent their integration into MTA systems. In particular, US would be the most natural choice for MTA real-time monitoring, due to its widespread availability, low cost, and real-time imaging up to sub-millimeter resolutions [17]. However, US can be scarcely effective for the real-time monitoring of MTA procedures, because it is blinded by a hyper-echogenic cloud caused by water vaporization in the heated tissue, which conceals the applicator and the tumor [1,18].

With reference to CT, studies investigated the best sequences to be used for real-time thermometry of radiofrequency thermal ablation [19–21]. The contra-indications of CT are mainly related to the exposure of the patient and the clinician to the ionizing radiation of CT, with a dose that depends on the duration of the MTA procedure and on the number of performed scans. Moreover, CT scanners do not have real-time capabilities, and perform fixed imaging in the axial plane, which leads to difficulties in treatments to be performed under the diaphragm or in other areas where oblique imaging planes are desirable [17].

MRI is potentially the most accurate and safe technique to perform real-time thermometry during the procedure [14,23], since temperature can be obtained from T1 relaxation time or proton resonance frequency (PRF) shift [24]. However, MRI use is limited by technical difficulties related to (unavoidable) motion artefacts, electromagnetic compatibility issues with the microwave antenna, and, last but not least, the high cost of the MRI equipment, which entails a significant impact in terms of economical sustainability for health systems [18].

Accordingly, the lack of a reliable, low-cost, real-time imaging system represents a weak point of thermal ablation procedures, especially those using microwave power, thus impairing their widespread use in the clinics [16]. For this reason, research is pushing towards the development of a non-invasive real-time monitoring system, both trying to improve existing techniques and looking for brand new solutions.

Microwave tomography (MWT) has been recently proposed as an alternative imaging modality for non-invasive real-time monitoring of thermal ablation procedures [25–27]. MWT images the variation of the electromagnetic properties with respect to an unperturbed situation, by recording (and properly processing) the electromagnetic field backscattered by the region of interest when probed by a known incident wave. Given the experimentally observed evidence that tissues undergo dramatic changes during ablation treatments [28–30], MWT is in principle viable for thermal ablation monitoring. Moreover, MWT involves low-cost and portable equipment as it exploits standard components—such as microwave (MW) antennas, MW generators, amplifiers—whose size and cost have considerably reduced in the last years thanks to the progress in the field of telecommunications. Finally, MWT is completely harmless, being based on the use of low-power non-ionizing radiations.

The basic principle of MWT thermal ablation monitoring is to probe the treated region with an array of antennas, external to the patient body, and record the evolution of the back-scattered field during the treatment. The variations of the recorded data between different time instants are then processed by means of a suitable inverse scattering algorithm, whose output is an image of the changes occurring in the electromagnetic properties of the scenario under test. In particular, to enable real-time operations, linearized inversion models can be exploited, based on the circumstance than only localized variations occur during the treatment and that the main (or first) clinical goal is to detect the boundary between treated and untreated tissue.

The potential of MWT monitored thermal ablation has been so far investigated in silico. In particular, Scapaticci et al. [27] showed the possibility of imaging the evolution of thermal ablation within a sample of liver tissue, whereas [31] simulated the monitoring of an interstitial heating procedure of a brain tumor. In this paper, the first experimental proof-of-concept of thermal ablation monitoring via MWT is reported. In particular, the results from two MTA procedures carried out on *ex vivo* liver tissue are described and discussed. The tomographic approach is the same as the one assessed in the previous in silico study [27], properly adapted to the measurement configuration adopted in the experiments. In particular, the changes occurring in the samples before and after microwave ablation are imaged, with the aim of appraising the boundary between treated and untreated tissue.

The paper is structured as follows. In the next section, the adopted material and methods are described. In particular, the experimental set-up developed for the validation is described along with the protocol adopted for thermal ablation. Then, the MWT algorithm is recalled and particularized to the adopted configuration. The results are presented in the subsequent section, preceded by the visual analysis of the ablated specimens, which provides the information necessary to assess the imaging outcomes. Discussion and conclusions follow.

2. Materials and Methods

2.1. Experimental Set-Up

The conceptual scheme of the experimental setup developed for the present proof-of-concept experiments is depicted in Figure 1. The setup consisted of two main parts: the 'therapeutic' one, on the right side of the picture, which was in charge of performing MTA, and the 'monitoring' part, on the left side, which gathered the data required for the MWT processing.

The MTA subsystem was based on a commercial ablation apparatus (HS AMICA, HS Hospital Service S.p.A., Rome, Italy), consisting of a programmable microwave power generator (available power: 100 W continuous wave (CW), frequency: 2.45 GHz), connected through a coaxial cable to a 14-gauge cooled-shaft percutaneous applicator. The MTA applicator was a coaxial dipole antenna. The antenna was equipped with a mini-choke to confine the energy emission in the zone to be treated [32]. The applicator was cooled by means of water pumped by a peristaltic pump (at a constant velocity of 40 mL/min), circulating into the shaft up to the mini-choke section.

The MW power, fed to and reflected from the applicator, was monitored by a two-channel digital power meter (Agilent E4419B, Agilent Technologies Inc., Santa Clara, CA, USA) and a Type-N dual-coaxial reflectometer coupler (Narda 3022, Narda Microwave Corp., Hauppauge, NY, USA).

MTA was performed on specimens of *ex vivo* bovine liver taken from a slaughter house. A box of polymethyl-methacrylate (PMMA)—a material typically with negligible losses and low dielectric constant (e.g., about 2.9) [33], i.e., almost transparent to MW fields—with internal dimensions of $120 \times 100 \times 100$ mm^3, was used to hold the tissue specimens (size $120 \times 100 \times 80$ mm^3) and to allow an accurate and repeatable insertion of the MTA applicator (Figure 2). Specifically, the MTA applicator was introduced in the specimen through a hole located at the center of the front-side wall of the box, along the x-axis (see Figure 2), so that the distal tip of the applicator was inserted into the tissue specimen at a depth of about 7 cm, and the feed was approximately located in correspondence of the barycenter of the tissue specimen (Figure 2).

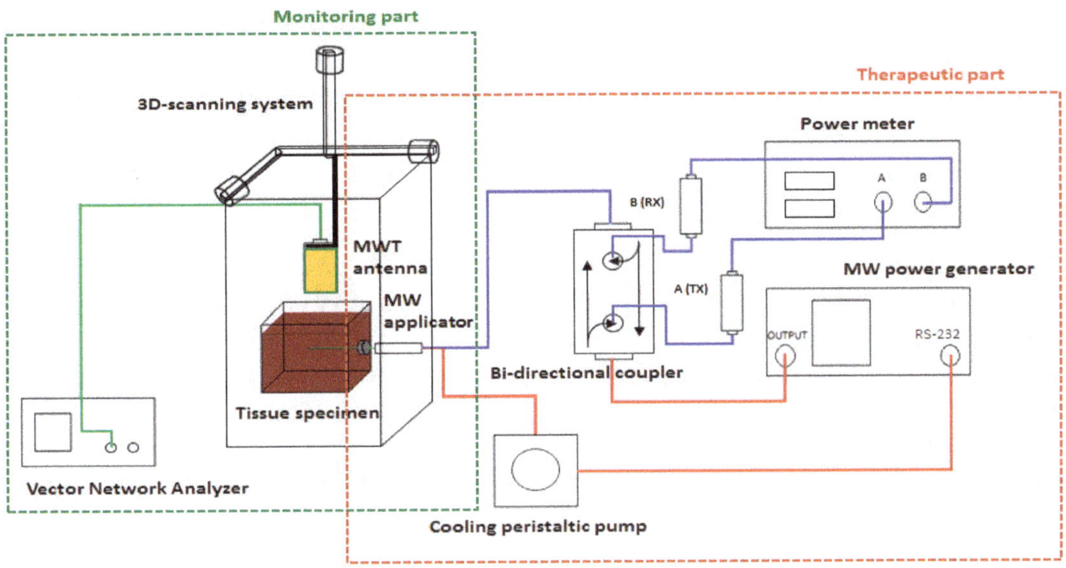

Figure 1. The experimental setup developed for the proof of concept. Tx and Rx denote part of the transmitted signal (Tx) and part of the reflected one (Rx) collected by the directional coupler to measure the actual power fed to the MTA antenna. The green line represents the connection between the vector network analyzed (VNA) and the MWT antenna. The red lines represent the connection of the MW power generator with the bidirectional coupler and with the peristaltic pump, and of the peristaltic pump with the MW applicator. The blue lines represent the connections of the power meter with the bidirectional coupler, and of the bidirectional coupler with the MW applicator. The black arrows refer to conventional symbols used for bidirectional coupler, which identify the directions of propagation of the direct power (forward) and of the reflected power (backward).

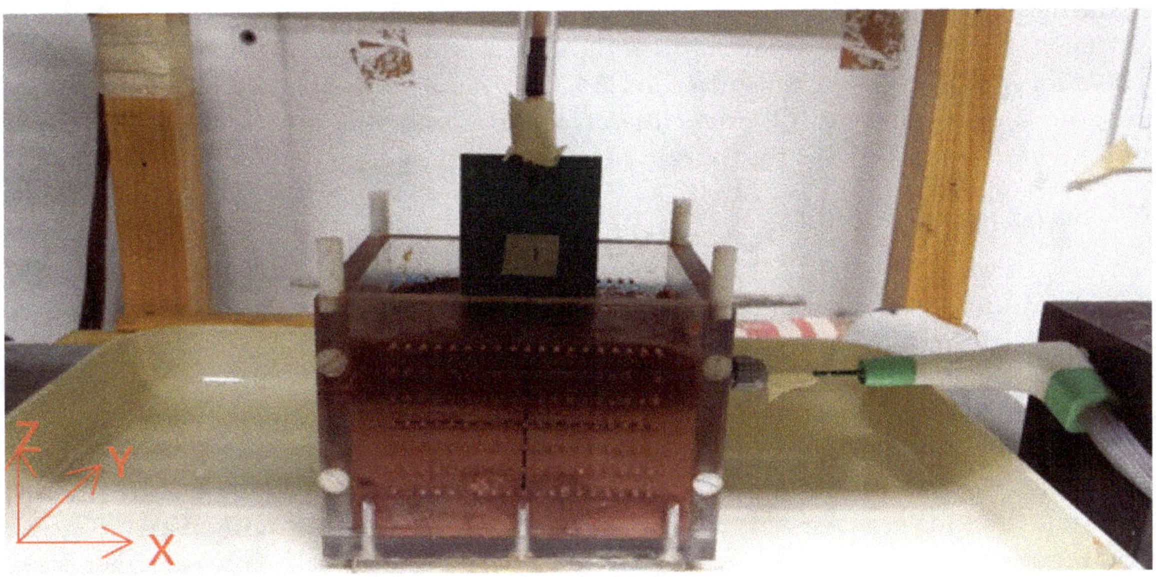

Figure 2. Plastic box containing an *ex vivo* tissue specimen of bovine liver. The MWT antenna is visible on the top of the specimen connected to the arm of the scanning system. The MTA applicator is visible on the right of the specimen, partially inserted into it. The reference system is shown on the bottom left in red color.

The MWT subsystem consisted of a microwave antenna connected to a vector network analyzer (VNA, Keysight E5071C ENA, 9 kHz–4.5 GHz, Keysight Technologies, Santa Clara, CA, USA) measuring the reflection coefficient (S_{11}, magnitude and phase). A multi-monostatic acquisition was performed moving the antenna along a rectilinear path (oriented along the y-axis) above the specimen surface (Figure 2), by means of a remotely controlled three-dimensional (3D) scanning system with 0.1-mm spatial resolution (ITALMETRON, Rome, Italy). The scanning system was controlled by a purposely developed routine in Labview^{TM}.

2.2. MTA Experiments

The MTA experiments were performed on two different *ex vivo* tissue specimens of bovine liver. In both cases, an average net power of about 60 W at 2.45 GHz (CW) for a time of 8 min was delivered to the applicator. The ablation protocol (power and time) was chosen in such a way to achieve an ablated zone completely included in the specimen, with a margin of untreated tissue between the boundary of the ablation and the surface of the specimen [34].

In order to assess the outcomes of the imaging procedure, the algorithm's results were compared to the actual scenario. To obtain a description of such a 'ground truth' a visual inspection of the zone of ablation was performed. To this end, at the end of the MTA procedure, the specimen was sectioned. In particular, the specimen was cut in the xy plane (see Figure 2), at a depth corresponding to the height at which the applicator was inserted. In the xy plane, the zone of ablation achieved with the considered cooled-shaft applicator typically consists in an ellipsoidal-shaped thermally coagulated area of ablated-but-not-carbonized tissue encompassing an arrow-shaped central region of carbonized tissue [29]. In the transversal plane—i.e., the plane orthogonal to the shaft of the applicator (yz in Figure 2)—the thermal lesion has typically a circular shape with a rim of white coagulated tissue surrounding the central carbonized area [29].

The characteristic dimensions of the ablated zone, defined in terms of maximum extension in the longitudinal (i.e., parallel to the shaft of the applicator, x-axis in Figure 2) and transverse (y-axis in Figure 2) directions, were measured with a ruler (accuracy ± 0.5 mm). Likewise, the maximum extension of the central carbonized region was measured in the longitudinal and transverse directions. Moreover, the height of the specimen in the antero-posterior direction (z-axis in Figure 2) was measured prior and after completion of the ablation procedure, to assess possible deformation of the specimen linked to ablation-induced tissue modifications [34,35]. The distance between the upper boundary of the ablated zone and the surface of the specimen was measured post-ablation to assess the extension in the antero-posterior direction of the margin of untreated tissue.

2.3. MWT Measurements

For each MTA experiment, MWT measurements (S_{11}, magnitude and phase) were performed in two different conditions, i.e., pre-ablation (untreated tissue) and right after completion of the MTA procedure. The resulting differential scattering parameters provide the data required for the MWT processing, since the changes in the dielectric properties of the specimen due to the ablation are expected to be reflected by the variations of the scattering coefficients [28].

MWT measurements were carried out in the 1–4 GHz frequency band (201 frequency points) at 13 evenly spaced positions along the y-axis, in correspondence of the applicator's feed ($x = 0$). In particular, the antenna was moved from $y = -30$ mm to $y = +30$ mm with a spatial step of 5 mm, as shown in Figure 3 (red dots in the figure). It is to be noted that both the measurements performed before and those performed after ablation were conducted with the applicator inserted into the specimen, but turned off.

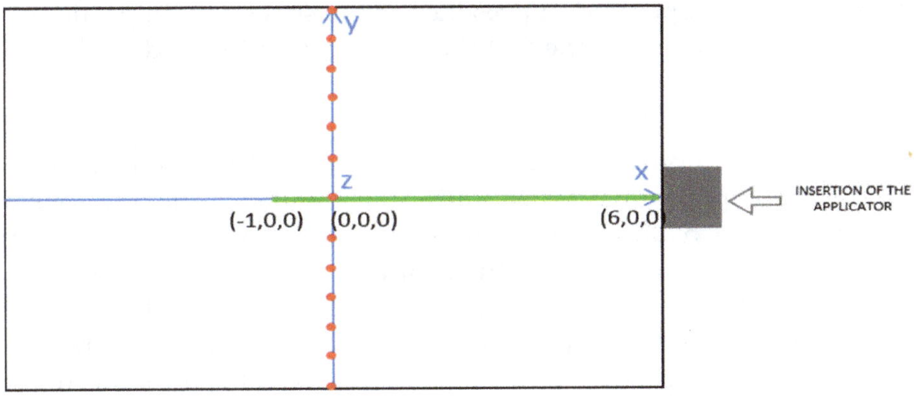

Figure 3. Positioning of the MTA applicator in the tissue specimen (green line) and MWT measurement points (red dots). View on a coronal plane at a height of about 40 mm from the applicator. Distances are expressed in cm. The blue lines denote the coordinate axes, while grey square and white arrow indicate the applicator and its insertion direction, respectively.

For each experiment, MWT measurements were carried out for two heights of the antenna. In particular, measurements were taken with the antenna in contact with the surface of the specimen, that is at $z = 30$ mm, putting the origin ($z = 0$) in correspondence to the shaft of the applicator, and with the antenna at a height $z = 40$ mm. For this latter case, considering the transverse dimension of the tissue specimen (height of about 8 cm) and the insertion position of the applicator (at the height of about 5 cm from the bottom of the specimen) and by neglecting not predictable ablation-induced tissue deformation [34,35], this corresponds to an average distance of about 10 mm between the distal edge of the MWT antenna and the surface of the tissue specimen.

In order to make fully independent experiments, the two MTA procedures were monitored employing two different ultra-wide band antennas. The first antenna (Figure 4a) consisted in a coplanar antipodal configuration with a 'half-heart' geometry (dimension 50 × 85 mm^2) printed on a Rogers substrate (RO4003, relative permittivity $\varepsilon_r = 3.38$) [36]. The second antenna (Figure 4b) is a coplanar Vivaldi configuration (dimension 54 × 68 mm^2) printed on a Taconic substrate (RF-35, $\varepsilon_r = 3.50$) [37].

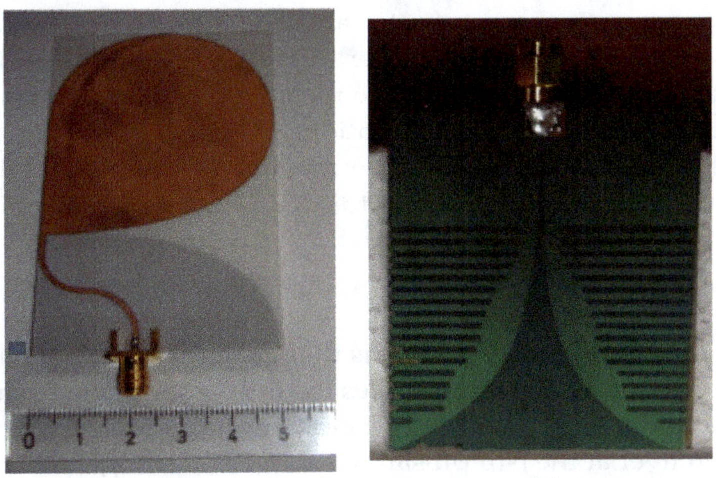

(a) (b)

Figure 4. MWT antennas: (**a**) half-heart shape; (**b**) Vivaldi shape.

It is worth noting that the two antennas were not specifically designed for the purpose of this experiment. Nevertheless, see Appendix A, they showed an acceptable behavior throughout the measurement bandwidth, when operated in presence of the specimen, in particular when they were not in contact with it (as expected, given the fact they were not optimized).

2.4. Imaging Algorithm and Assessment Criterion

To form the image of the monitored ablation scenario, a differential microwave tomography approach based on the Born approximation was adopted, similar to the one considered in previous studies [28,29]. Such an approach allows to image (in a qualitative fashion) the variations occurring in the scenario under test, which was indeed the scope of this initial experimental study. Notably, the approach uses the truncated singular value decomposition (TSVD) algorithm [38], which allows real-time results, since its computationally intensive part can be run off-line before data acquisition. In the following, the TSVD inversion algorithm, as particularized for the experimental configuration, is recalled, whereas the formulation details are given in Appendix B.

The experimental data were acquired along a rectilinear domain, hence, the available information was not adequate for imaging a 3D region. Accordingly, a 2D domain corresponding to the cross section of the specimen along the yz plane, i.e., orthogonal the applicator shaft, in correspondence of the line of scan, was taken as region of interest Ω. Such a domain was then discretized into $P = N_y \times N_z$ square pixels of 0.5 mm resolution. In particular, $N_y = 201$, and $N_z = 79$ when the antenna is at $z = 30$ mm and $N_z = 99$ when the antenna is at $z = 40$ mm.

In the TSVD scheme, the unknown vector is directly retrieved by applying the inversion formula to the data vector $\Delta\mathbf{S}$:

$$\Delta\boldsymbol{\chi} = \mathbf{K}_R^{+}\Delta\mathbf{S} \tag{1}$$

where $\Delta\boldsymbol{\chi}$ denotes the $P \times 1$ column vector of the unknowns (the 2D matrix encoding the contrast is rearranged into a 1D vector for the sake of implementation of the TSVD algorithm), whose generic element encodes the differential contrast value, assumed non-dispersive, in the relevant pixel, defined as

$$\Delta\chi_j = \frac{\Delta\varepsilon_j}{\varepsilon_L}, \qquad j = 1, \ldots, P \tag{2}$$

where $\Delta\varepsilon_j$ is the variation of the complex permittivity in the j-th pixel due to the ablation profile and ε_L is the complex permittivity of liver, assumed to be homogenous and with the properties of liver tissue at 2.45 GHz, as taken from the literature [28].

$\Delta\mathbf{S}$ is the $[N_f \times N_m] \times 1$ column vector of the (complex) differential data, given by the difference between the scattering parameter measured after ablation and the scattering parameter measured before ablation with $N_f = 201$ being the number of frequency points and $N_m = 13$ the number of antenna positions. The differences between the measured S-parameters are directly fed into the inversion algorithm, without any scaling or calibration.

$\boldsymbol{K}_R^{+}$ is the regularized pseudo inverse of the kernel matrix $\mathbf{K}$, which, in the adopted model, is an $M \times P$ matrix, whose rows are ordered according to $\Delta\mathbf{S}$ and whose generic entry K_{mp} is given by

$$K_{mp} = -\frac{j}{2}\pi k_f \rho J_1\left(k_f \rho\right) H_0^2\left(k_f |r_q - r_p|\right) H_0^2\left(k_f |r_q - r_p|\right) \tag{3}$$

where $f = 1, \ldots N_f$; $q = 1, \ldots N_m$; $p = 1, \ldots, P$; ρ is the radius of a circle having the same area of the pixel, J_1 is the first order Bessel function, H_0^2 denotes the 0-th order second kind Hankel function, r_q is the q-th position of the antenna and r_p denotes the position of the p-th pixel, $k_f = \omega_f \sqrt{\varepsilon_L \mu_o}$ is the (complex) wavenumber in liver at the f-th pulsation ω_f, μ_o is the magnetic permeability in vacuum.

To obtain $\boldsymbol{K}_T^{+}$, let us introduce the singular value decomposition (SVD) of $\mathbf{K}$, defined as

$$\mathbf{K} = \mathbf{U}\,\boldsymbol{\Sigma}\,\mathbf{V}^T \tag{4}$$

where $\mathbf{U}$ is the $M \times M$ matrix whose columns are the left singular vectors (which span the space of differential data), $\mathbf{V}$ is the $P \times P$ matrix whose columns are the right singular vectors (which span the space of visible contrast functions) and $\mathbf{\Sigma}$ is the $M \times P$ matrix of the singular values, whose elements are all zeros but for those lying on the diagonal of the $M \times M$ submatrix (being in our case $M < P$). These scalars, say $s_1, \ldots, s_M$ are ordered in decreasing fashion and accumulate to zero, that is $s_1 > s_2 \ldots, s_{M-1} > s_M$, with $s_n \to 0$, $n \to \infty$.

Due to the unavoidable presence of noise on data, the direct inversion of $\mathbf{K}$ is unstable, since the exponentially fast growth of $1/s_n$ for increasing values of n results in an uncontrolled amplification of noise. To overcome this drawback, the regularized pseudo inverse $\boldsymbol{K}_{\boldsymbol{R}}^{+}$ is introduced by truncating the singular value decomposition (SVD) to the first R values, with $R < M$, thus obtaining

$$\boldsymbol{K}_{\boldsymbol{R}}^{+} = \mathbf{V}_{\boldsymbol{R}}\, \mathbf{\Sigma}_{\boldsymbol{R}}^{-1} \mathbf{U}_{\boldsymbol{R}}^{T} \tag{5}$$

where $\mathbf{U}_{\boldsymbol{R}}^{T}$ is the $M \times R$ matrix whose columns are the first R left singular vectors, $\mathbf{V}_{\boldsymbol{R}}$ is the $P \times R$ matrix whose columns are the first R right singular vectors and $\mathbf{\Sigma}_{\boldsymbol{R}}^{-1}$ is the $R \times R$ diagonal matrix, whose elements are the inverse of the first R singular values, $1/s_i$ $i = 1, \ldots, R$.

Note that the SVD (4) is computed off-line (and only once), so that the solution (1) is achieved in real-time with a standard laptop, since it only involves (a few) matrix vector operations.

2.4.1. Choice of the Regularization Parameter R

The truncation index R is the regularization parameter of the TSVD algorithm, and represents a degree of freedom in its implementation. In particular, a threshold as large as possible is in principle desirable to improve the accuracy. On the other hand, as mentioned before, this may induce an error amplification effect. As such, the threshold R is chosen as a trade-off between accuracy and stability.

For the considered measurement configuration, R also affects the maximum depth of visible targets. Such a circumstance can be appreciated from the spatial coverage of $\boldsymbol{K}_{\boldsymbol{R}}^{+}$, defined as the squared amplitude of the elements of matrix $\mathbf{V}_{\boldsymbol{R}}$ summed along the columns and rearranged on the $N_y \times N_z$ grid. Figure 5 shows the spatial coverage of $\boldsymbol{K}_{\boldsymbol{R}}^{+}$ for different values of R in the yz plane at x = 0 (see Figure 2 for the reference system). In the adopted colormap, the black regions represent those portions of the imaging domain that are expected to be poorly retrieved. As can be observed, the larger the threshold, the larger the portion of the domain which is 'covered' by the imaging algorithm. In particular, it can be noted that $R = 20$ only allows imaging the shallow part of the specimen. Considering that the applicator is positioned in the origin of the reference system and that an ablation zone in the order of a few centimeters is typically dealt with, the threshold was set to $R = 48$, as this value allows imaging a sufficiently deep portion of the specimen, while keeping the number of unknown lower than $R = 60$, which is helpful to ensure a stable result in the unavoidable presence of noise.

2.4.2. Assessment Criterion

To assess the obtained imaging results, the ex-post visual inspection of the ablated specimen was exploited to build reference images to be compared with the one obtained from the processing of the experimental (differential) data. In particular, the observed size of the treated region, together with the expected values of the dielectric properties of ablated tissue [36] were used to build a 2D reference differential contrast $\Delta\chi_{ref}$. Then, the ideal imaging result is given by the projection onto the first R = 48 right singular functions, computed as

$$\Delta\chi_{id} = \mathbf{V}_{\boldsymbol{R}} \mathbf{V}_{\boldsymbol{R}}^{T} \Delta\chi_{ref}. \tag{6}$$

Equation (6) provides the ideal output of the adopted imaging procedure in the considered conditions.

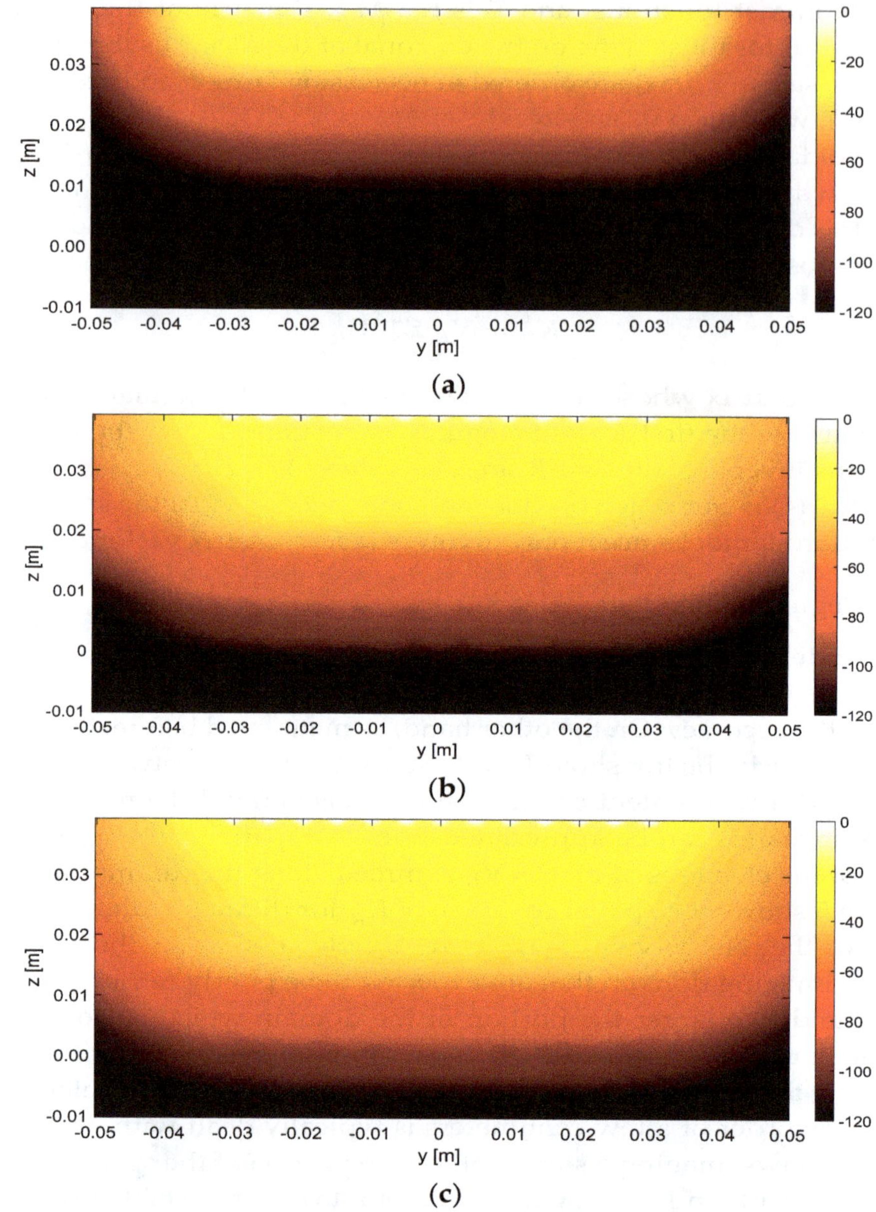

Figure 5. Spatial coverage of the operator K_R^+ for R equal to (**a**) 20; (**b**) 48; and (**c**) 60. In the study, $R = 48$ was set. Refer to Figure 2 for the reference system.

3. Results

3.1. Ex Vivo Post-Ablation Analysis

At the end of the MTA procedure, the specimens were sectioned along the *xy* plane, displaying the coagulative necrosis for visual inspection, and the characteristic dimensions of the zone of ablation were measured.

Figure 6 shows the sectioned specimens from the two experiments with the relevant measurement superimposed. In particular, L_A (mm) and D_A (mm) represent the maximum extension of the ablated zone in the longitudinal (i.e., the length) and transverse (i.e., the diameter) directions, respectively. Likewise, L_C (mm) and D_C (mm) represent the maximum extension of the central carbonized zone in the longitudinal and transverse directions, respectively. H (mm) represents the distance between the upper boundary of the ablated zone and the surface of the tissue specimen measured post-ablation, which is the upper margin of untreated tissue in the transverse direction.

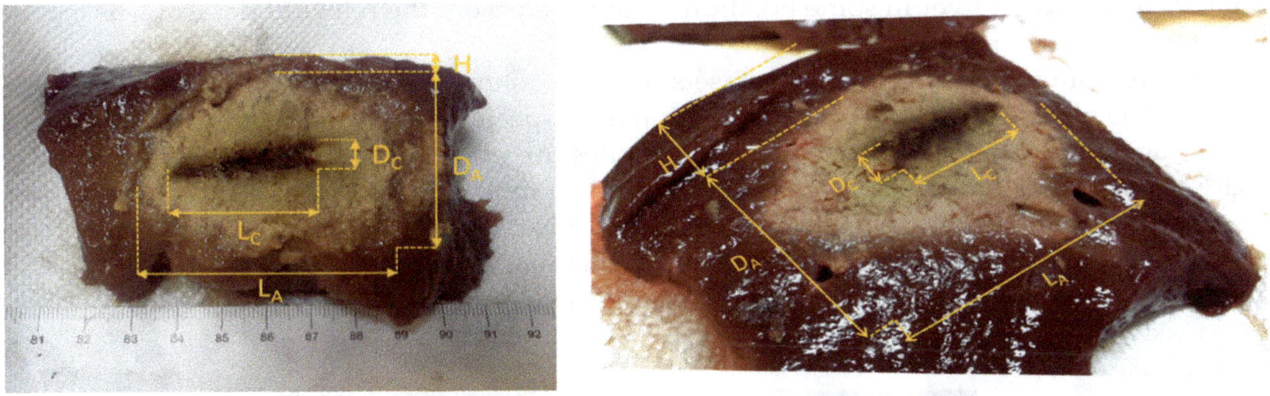

(a) (b)

Figure 6. Characteristic dimensions of the zone of ablation in a coronal plane as appraised from the visual inspection. (**a**) Vivaldi experiment. (**b**) Half-heart experiment. The yellow dotted lines denote the position of interfaces of interest, while the two-way arrows identified distances.

As it was shown in previous works [35], ablation-induced tissue deformation is highly heterogeneous and eventually not predictable, resulting in both tissue shrinkage and expansion, owing to interactions between the contracting thermally-coagulated tissue and the untreated tissue encompassing the zone of ablation, as well as to expansion of water steam diffusing from the inner zone of ablation. As discussed in the following, this aspect represents a non-trivial issue in the assessment pursued in this work.

In Table 1, the characteristic dimensions of the zone of ablation are summarized, along with the net power (mean value ± standard deviation, W) supplied to the applicator during the MTA procedure. From the reported data, it is apparent that in both MTA experiments tissue specimens showed ablation-induced deformation in the transverse direction ($D_A/2 + H - 30$, being 30 mm the distance pre-ablation between the applicator and the surface of the specimen). Specifically, in the experiment with the Vivaldi antenna the specimen was characterized by a contraction of about 7 mm, whereas in the half-heart antenna case, the specimen exhibited an expansion of about 5 mm. Such an outcome cannot be easily foreseen or modeled. As an ex-post observation, it can be noted that, as summarized in Table 1, the experiment with the half-heart antenna lead to a larger transverse ablation diameter (D_A) with respect to the one in the experiment with the Vivaldi antenna, i.e., 44 mm vs. 38 mm. Therefore, it can be argued that the more superficial ablation achieved in the experiment with the half-heart antenna may have facilitated the upwards propagation of vapor gases, thus causing tissue transverse expansion. However, such an outcome cannot be generalized, since the ultimate result of an ablation procedure (and then of ablation-induced tissue deformation) relies on heat propagation, which is also affected by tissue morphology around the applicator (e.g., presence of small blood vessels or local non-homogeneities).

Table 1. Characteristic dimensions of the ablation zone achieved in the MTA experiments

MWT Antenna	Power (W)	L_A (mm)	D_A (mm)	L_C (mm)	D_C (mm)	H (mm)	Remarks
Vivaldi	54.8 ± 0.8	56	38	36	8	4	transverse contraction ~7 mm
Half-heart	57.8 ± 1.2	54	44	31	8	13	transverse expansion ~5 mm

3.2. *Microwave Tomography Results*

The expansion of the liver sample observed in the post-ablation visual inspection in the case of half-hearth experiment confirmed a difficulty occurred when performing the MWT measurements with the antenna in contact with the liver. As a matter of fact, due to the swelling, the antenna was somehow 'immersed' in liver in some positions. For this reason, the relevant dataset was excluded from the tomographic processing.

For the remaining three available datasets, Figure 7 shows the ideal contrast functions $\Delta\chi_{ref}$ according to the visual analysis of the post-ablation liver specimens described in the previous section. In these images, the variations between the two states are evidenced: the green areas identify the ablated tissue, whereas the yellow areas correspond to modifications of the specimen caused by shrinkage in the Vivaldi experiment and swelling in half-heart case. Of course, given the heterogeneous and not predictable nature of tissue ablation and deformation, these images cannot provide an accurate model of the ground truth, nevertheless, they retain the features which are mostly relevant for the imaging task.

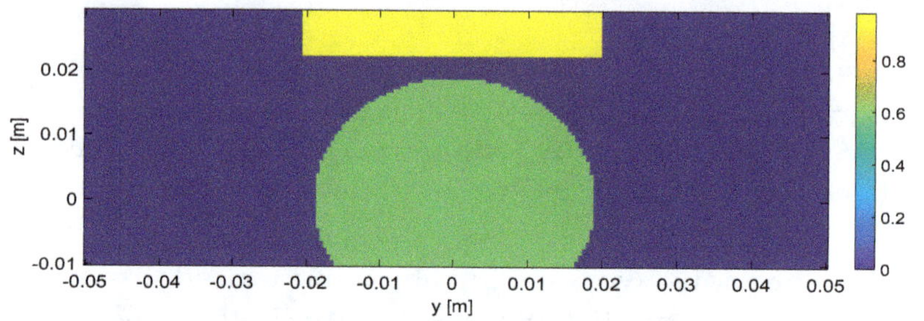

(a)

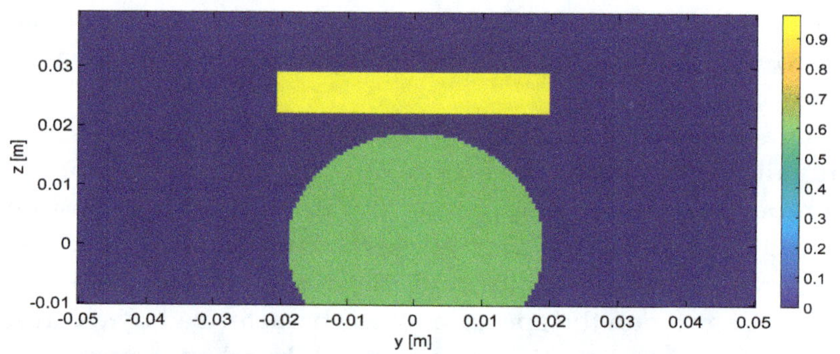

(b)

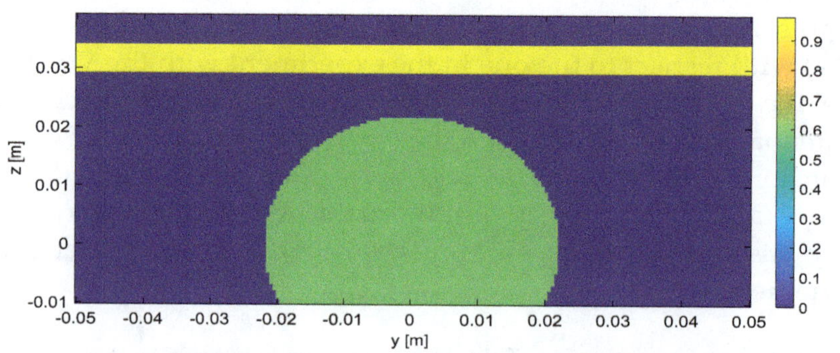

(c)

Figure 7. Ideal differential contrast for the analyzed cases. Each figure represents the yz cross-section of the ground truth as deduced from visual inspection. The green areas are ablated tissue, the yellow areas are specimen surface modifications. The MTA applicator is located at (0 m, 0 m). The MWT antenna moves along the top border of each figure. (**a**) Vivaldi experiment with antenna in contact; (**b**) Vivaldi experiment with antenna at 10 mm from the specimen; (**c**) Half-heart experiment with antenna at 10 mm from the specimen. The bar chart of each sub-figure are in the same scale and they denote the absolute value of the differential contrast for the three analyzed cases.

In Figure 8, the imaging results for the processed datasets are reported in terms of the normalized amplitudes of the estimated differential contrast, i.e., $|\Delta\chi|$ for the tomographic images and $|\Delta\chi_{id}|$ for the ideal reconstructions. As a matter of fact, while the algorithm actually provides an estimate of the (complex) differential contrast $\Delta\chi$, the very limited amount of available data and the aspect limited nature of the measurement configuration, which prevents a complete estimate of the unknown function, do not allow retrieving the actual quantitative values. For this reason, the images are given in terms of the retrieved differential contrast amplitude, as this provides a qualitative estimate of the main variations occurring in the imaged zone. As said, such information corresponds to the first clinically relevant goal to achieve.

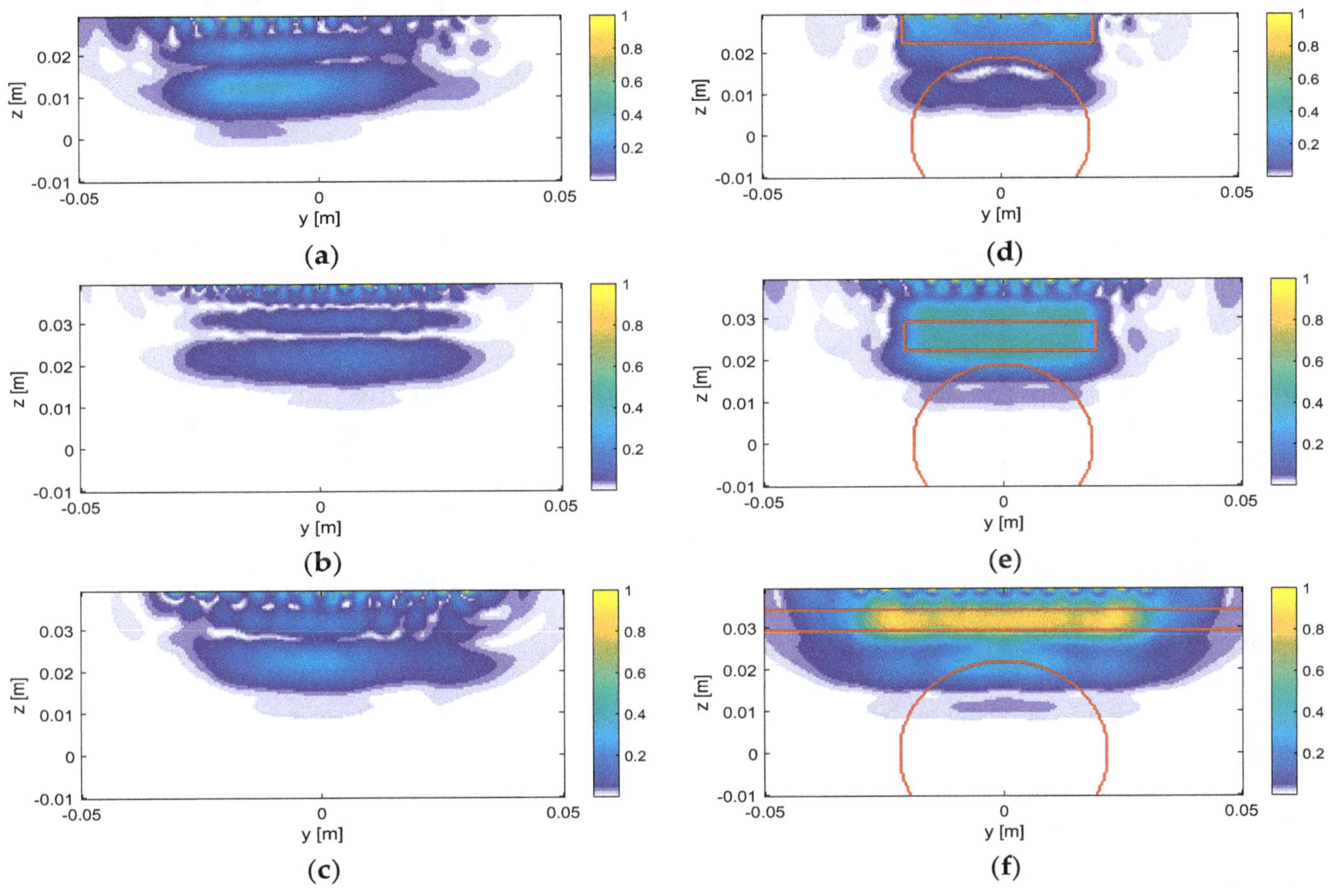

Figure 8. Comparison between tomographic results and ideal reconstructions. Each figure reports the plot of a cross-section in the *yz* plane of the retrieved contrast (normalized modulus). In the images, the main features (in terms of qualitative variations) of the differential contrast appear. Left side, tomographic images: (**a**) Vivaldi experiment with antenna in contact with liver sample; (**b**) Vivaldi experiment with antenna at 1 cm from sample; (**c**) Half-heart experiment with antenna at 1 cm height. Right side, (**d**–**f**) ideal reconstructions. Red contours denote the contour of the ideal differential contrast, as identified in Figure 7. All mps are normalized to their maximum. As such, colorbars range from 0 to 1. 0 values represent areas where no variation occurrs, while 1 values denote areas where the maximum variation is observed.

In the figure, the left column shows the tomographic image obtained from processing the experimental data, whereas the right column reports the ideal reconstructions, obtained by applying Equation (6) to the differential contrast of the relevant reference scenario shown in Figure 7. On the images on the right of the figure, the contour of the ablated area and the surface modifications are superimposed to facilitate interpretation. To allow better appraisal of the results, taking into account the differential nature of the imaging approach, the adopted color bar forces the false colors to white in the areas where the amplitude of the differential contrast is estimated as zero. It is worth noting that obtaining these images requires less than 1 s on a standard desktop pc.

4. Discussion

The comparison between the tomographic images and the ideal images allowed both to interpret the results as well as to appraise their quality and the open issues that emerged from the present study.

The ablated specimens underwent significant surface changes during the thermal treatment. In a differential imaging framework, such modifications are retrieved by the algorithm and appear as 'targets' in the images. As such, the obtained images will not just report the contrast variations due to the ablation of the tissue, but also the variations related to the post-ablation specimen deformation. Such a circumstance is confirmed by the observation of the ideal images in the right column of Figure 8, wherein the deformation is clearly visible. In the tomographic results, such features are also visible and are correctly positioned.

As far as the transition between treated and untreated tissue is concerned, in the Vivaldi experiment, the separation between the surface of the sample and the ablated tissue (i.e., the margin of untreated tissue in the z direction) is lower than 0.5 cm, due ablation-induced shrinkage of the specimen. Such a distance is in the order or even below the expected spatial resolution of MWT at the adopted frequency band ($\delta = \frac{C}{2B}$, with c being the velocity of propagation in the liver and B the bandwidth of the signal), which—for the case at hand—is about 8 mm. Accordingly, the experimental conditions did not allow to appreciate the separation between untreated (and shrunk) tissue and treated tissue. This is confirmed by the observation of the ideal images, wherein indeed the position of the treated-to-ablated tissue boundary cannot be discriminated. Nevertheless, despite this limitation, the tomographic images obtained from the experimental data are consistent with the ideal ones.

For the half-heart case, the swelling of the specimen had an opposite effect, so that no overlap is expected and the transition from treated to untreated tissue is expected to be properly imaged, as confirmed by the ideal images. This is fully confirmed by the experimental result, wherein both the effect of the swelling and the treated-to-untreated boundary are correctly imaged. Besides, a good agreement with the ideal results is obtained.

Accordingly, a first experimental evidence of the capability of MWT of detecting the transition between treated and untreated tissue was achieved, using a procedure which can be easily implemented in real time. This is indeed one of the main clinical goals to pursue, to propose a new technique for real-time monitoring the evolution of thermal ablation treatment.

5. Conclusions

In this paper, the outcomes of the first experimental proof-of-concept of thermal ablation monitoring via MWT were presented. The study aimed at assessing the feasibility of MWT as a real-time monitoring tool for thermal ablation treatments. To this end, a laboratory set-up was designed to set an *ex vivo* experiment in which the changes in the electromagnetic properties of two bovine liver specimens where imaged by means of MWT measurement and processing. Overall, the results confirmed the anticipated potential of MWT, but a number of interesting issues aroused, which deserve further investigation in future research work.

The main drawback occurred due to the modification of the specimen volume during ablation. Although this effect was to some extent expected in *ex vivo* experiments, whether it actually occurs in vivo or in clinical situations is not clear. In fact, the liver-air system herein dealt with is a much simpler scenario from a thermodynamic point of view than the actual scenario, wherein the treated region is surrounded by the parenchyma or other biological tissue. To partially cope with this issue, and also move to a more complex *ex vivo* scenario, future experiments will deal with a three-layer structure, in which a matching medium (whose properties have to be properly chosen) is positioned between the antennas and the liver specimen. This layer may both mimic the tissue surrounding the liver and provide a surrounding medium which may absorb the tissue deformation. In addition to this, the use of a matching medium can improve the performance of the antennas, which in turn can reduce uncertainty on data and therefore allow inspecting more in depth. To this end, the design of ad hoc antennas is of course a crucial aspect, since the antennas used in this study provide sub-optimal, yet acceptable, performances in the measurement frequency band.

The presented experiments aimed at pursuing the initial goal of observing and assessing the two extreme cases of non-ablated and ablated tissue. Their positive outcome stimulates a campaign of experiments that will address the monitoring of an ongoing treatment, by performing measurements at intermediate ablation stages also. In this respect, the need of coping with measurements taken during the operation of the thermal applicator represents an interesting issue to investigate, not only to understand the effect of the MW heating signal onto the measured data (possible interference), but also to examine the possible cooperative role of the applicator as well as the possibility of devising interleaved treatment/measurement protocols in which the thermal ablation and the monitoring are performed alternatively.

Finally, performing a number of linear scans along parallel rectilinear paths can be foreseen as way to gather a sufficient amount of data in order to build more accurate, possibly 3D maps of the monitored scenario. In this respect, the use of an array of antennas could be envisaged in order to keep the measurement time as low as possible, by resorting to electronic rather than mechanical scanning.

Author Contributions: The paper is the result of a collaborative effort amongst the authors. More specifically, Study Design & Methodology: L.C., M.C. and V.L., Experiments: V.L. and R.P.; Formal analysis, Software & Validation: R.S., Writing—original draft, R.S., M.C.; Writing—review & editing, R.S., V.L., R.P., M.C. and L.C., Supervision L.C.

Acknowledgments: The authors would like to thank Ibrahim Akduman and his colleagues at Istanbul Technical University for proving the Vivaldi antennas used in one of the experiments. The authors acknowledge the R&D Unit of HS Hospital Service S.p.A., Rome, Italy, for providing the applicators and the MW power generator used in the research.

Appendix A

In this appendix, the measured scattering parameters (S_{11}) for the two antennas adopted in the experiment are reported.

Figure A1 shows the scattering parameter measured with the antenna located in correspondence of the applicator axis ($y = 0$) in contact with the liver tissue or placed at 1 cm distance from the surface of the liver. In particular, Figure A1a reports the data for the half-heart antenna, while Figure A1b shows the data related to the Vivaldi antenna.

As can be seen, despite the antennas were not designed for this particular application, the value of the S_{11} parameter (on average) in the considered frequency band is below -5 dB which is quite acceptable. In addition, a better performance is observed for the half-hearth antenna trough out the whole band.

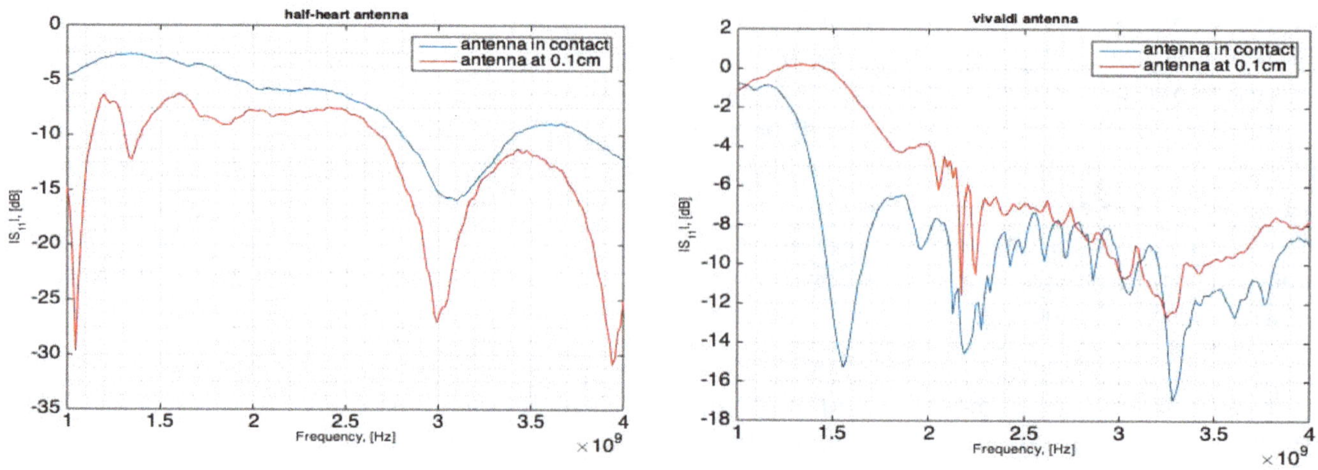

(a) (b)

Figure A1. Amplitude of the S_{11} scattering parameters as measured for the antenna in the central position (in correspondence of the applicator): (**a**) Half-heart antenna. (**b**) Vivaldi antenna.

Appendix B

This appendix provides the formulation of the inverse scattering method adopted to process the data gathered in the experimental study.

The input data is given by the difference between scattering parameters collected by each antenna before and after ablation. Hence, for each of the 201 frequency points in the measured bandwidth and for each of the 13 antenna positions, a differential scattering parameter, say S, is obtained.

For a given position r_x of the MWT antenna and for each pulsation ω in the measurement bandwidth, the differential scattering parameter can be expressed as

$$\Delta S = S_{11}^{a} - S_{11}^{0} = K[\Delta\chi] \tag{A1}$$

where S_{11}^{a} is the scattering parameter measured after ablation and S_{11}^{0} is the scattering parameter measured before ablation, respectively.

$\Delta\chi$ is the differential contrast, which encodes the changes occurring in the electromagnetic properties of the specimen due to the ablation. Such a function is defined as

$$\Delta\chi(r,\omega) = \frac{\varepsilon_a(r,\omega)}{\varepsilon_L(r,\omega)} - 1 \tag{A2}$$

where $r = (x,y)$ denotes the generic position in the imaged region Ω, ε_a is the complex permittivity profile in Ω after the ablation and ε_L is the complex permittivity profile in the liver specimen before ablation, which is assumed as homogeneous, with the same properties as liver tissue at 2.45 GHz. K is the short notation for the integral operator encoding the imaging kernel, whose explicit expression is given by

$$K[\Delta\chi] = \int_{\Omega} G(k, r_x, r) G\left(k_f, r, r_x\right) \Delta\chi(r,\omega) dr \tag{A3}$$

where r_x is the position of the antenna, $k = \omega\sqrt{\varepsilon_L \mu_o}$ is the (complex) wavenumber in liver at the working frequency and G is the Green's function for the unperturbed scenario, that is the solution of the Helmholtz equation

$$\nabla^2 G(r, r_x) - k^2 G(r, r_x) = -j\omega\mu_o\, \delta(r - r_x), \tag{A4}$$

with $G(r, r_x) = G(r_x, r)$ by virtue of reciprocity. The Born approximation is adopted to cast (A4), since the Green function both models the radiation of the induced current to the receiving antenna, $G(r_x, r)$, as well as the field induced by the antenna in the region of interest, $G(r, r_x)$.

In our approach, the Green function is simply modeled as the Green function pertaining to an unbounded homogeneous medium having the properties of liver, which reads

$$G(r, r_x) = H_0^2(k|r - r_x|), \tag{A5}$$

with H_0^2 denoting the 0th order second kind Hankel function. Of course, more sophisticated modeling could be adopted by using for instance a numerical model of the actual antennas placed on the specimen-filled box, but a simpler model is intrinsically more robust against uncertainties arising in the actual scenario (e.g., actual shape of the sample, actual radiation pattern of antenna in presence of the specimen).

The above model provides the basis for the equation to be inverted. In particular, by discretizing Ω into $N_x \times N_y$ square pixels and gathering all the differential data into a $[N_f \times N_m] \times 1$ column vector $\Delta\mathbf{S}$, with N_f being the number of frequency points and N_m the number of antenna positions, the discretized data-to-unknown relationship that has to be inverted is given by

$$\Delta\mathbf{S} = \mathbf{K}\,\Delta\chi \tag{A6}$$

References

1. Goldberg, S.N.; Gazelle, G.S.; Mueller, P.R. Thermal ablation therapy for focal malignancy: A unified approach to underlying principles, techniques, and diagnostic imaging guidance. *Am. J. Roentgenol.* **2000**, *174*, 323–331. [CrossRef] [PubMed]
2. Ahmed, M.; Brace, C.L.; Lee, F.T., Jr.; Goldberg, S.N. Principles of and advances in percutaneous ablation. *Radiology* **2011**, *258*, 351–369. [CrossRef] [PubMed]
3. Skinner, M.G.; Lizukay, M.N.; Koliosz, M.C.; Sherary, M.D. A theoretical comparison of energy sources—Microwave, ultrasound and laser—For interstitial thermal therapy. *Phys. Med. Biol.* **1998**, *43*, 3535–3547. [CrossRef]
4. Meloni, M.F.; Galimberti, S.; Dietrich, C.F.; Lazzaroni, S.; Goldberg, S.N.; Abate, A.; Sironi, S.; Andreano, A. Microwave ablation of hepatic tumors with a third generation system: Locoregional efficacy in a prospective cohort study with intermediate term follow-up. *Z Gastroenterol.* **2016**, *54*, 541–547. [CrossRef] [PubMed]
5. Ierardi, A.M.; Mangano, A.; Floridi, C.; Dionigi, G.; Biondi, A.; Duka, E.; Lucchina, N.; Lianos, G.D.; Carrafiello, G. A new system of microwave ablation at 2450 MHz: Preliminary experience. *Updates Surg.* **2015**, *67*, 39–45. [CrossRef] [PubMed]
6. Haemmerich, D.; Laeseke, P.F. Thermal tumour ablation: Devices, clinical applications and future directions. *Int. J. Hyperth.* **2005**, *21*, 755–760. [CrossRef] [PubMed]
7. Livraghi, T.; Meloni, F.; Solbiati, L.; Zanus, G. Complications of microwave ablation for liver tumors: Results of a multicenter study. *Cardiovasc. Intervent. Radiol.* **2012**, *35*, 868–874. [CrossRef] [PubMed]
8. Li, M.; Yu, X.; Liang, P.; Liu, F.; Dong, B.; Zhou, P. Percutaneous microwave ablation for liver cancer adjacent to the diaphragm. *Int. J. Hyperth.* **2012**, *28*, 218–226. [CrossRef] [PubMed]
9. Callstrom, M.R.; Charboneau, J.W. Technologies for ablation of hepatocellular carcinoma. *Gastroenterology* **2008**, *134*, 1831–1835. [CrossRef] [PubMed]
10. Jones, C.; Badger, S.A.; Ellis, G. The role of microwave ablation in the management of hepatic colorectal metastases. *Surgeon* **2011**, *9*, 33–37. [CrossRef]
11. Hoffmann, R.; Rempp, H.; Erhard, L.; Blumenstock, G.; Pereira, P.L.; Claussen, C.D.; Clasen, S. Comparison of four microwave ablation devices: An experimental study in ex vivo bovine liver. *Radiology* **2013**, *268*, 89–97. [CrossRef] [PubMed]
12. Brace, C.L.; Laeseke, P.F.; Sampson, L.A.; Frey, T.M.; van der Weide, D.W.; Lee, F.T., Jr. Microwave ablation with a single small-gauge triaxial antenna: In vivo porcine liver model. *Radiology* **2007**, *242*, 435–440. [CrossRef] [PubMed]
13. Emprint™ Ablation System with Thermosphere™ Technology. Available online: http://www.medtronic.com/covidien/en-us/products/ablation-systems/emprint-ablation-system.html (accessed on 4 December 2018).
14. Ahmed, M.; Solbiati, L.; Brace, C.L.; Breen, D.J.; Callstrom, M.R.; Charboneau, J.W.; Chen, M.H.; Choi, B.I.; De Baère, T.; Dodd, G.D., III; et al. Image-guided tumor ablation: Standardization of terminology and reporting criteria—A 10-year update. *J. Vasc. Interv. Radiol.* **2014**, *25*, 1691–1705. [CrossRef] [PubMed]

15. Saccomandi, P.; Schena, E.; Silvestri, S. Techniques for temperature monitoring during laser-induced thermotherapy: An overview. *Int. J. Hyperth.* **2013**, *29*, 609–619. [CrossRef] [PubMed]
16. Lopresto, V.; Pinto, R.; Farina, L.; Cavagnaro, M. Treatment planning in microwave thermal ablation: Clinical gaps and recent research advances. *Int. J. Hyperth.* **2017**, *33*, 83–100. [CrossRef]
17. Garrean, S.; Hering, J.; Saied, A.; Hoopes, P.J.; Helton, W.S.; Ryan, T.P.; Espat, N.J. Ultrasound monitoring of a novel microwave ablation (MWA) device in porcine liver: Lessons learned and phenomena observed on ablative effects near major intrahepatic vessels. *J. Gastrointest. Surg.* **2009**, *13*, 334–340. [CrossRef]
18. Han, Z.-Y.; Liang, P.; Yu, X.-L.; Cheng, Z.-G.; Liu, F.-Y.; Yu, J. A clinical study of thermal monitoring techniques of ultrasound-guided microwave ablation for hepatocellular carcinoma in high-risk locations. *Sci. Rep.* **2017**, *7*, 41246.
19. Cazzato, R.L.; Buy, X.; Alberti, N.; Fonck, M.; Grasso, R.F.; Palussière, J. Flat-panel cone-beam CT-guided radiofrequency ablation of very small (1.5 cm) liver tumors: Technical note on a preliminary experience. *Cardiovasc. Intervent. Radiol.* **2015**, *38*, 206–212. [CrossRef]
20. Pandeya, G.D.; Greuter, M.J.; de Jong, K.P.; Schmidt, B.; Flohr, T.; Oudkerk, M. Feasibility of noninvasive temperature assessment during radiofrequency liver ablation on computed tomography. *J. Comput. Assist. Tomogr.* **2011**, *35*, 356–360. [CrossRef]
21. Bruners, P.; Pandeya, G.D.; Levit, E.; Roesch, E.; Penzkofer, T.; Isfort, P.; Schmidt, B.; Greuter, M.J.; Oudkerk, M.; Schmitz-Rode, T.; et al. CT-based temperature monitoring during hepatic RF ablation: Feasibility in an animal model. *Int. J. Hyperth.* **2012**, *28*, 55–61. [CrossRef]
22. Fani, F.; Schena, E.; Saccomandi, P.; Silvestri, S. CT-based thermometry: An overview. *Int. J. Hyperth.* **2014**, *30*, 219–227. [CrossRef] [PubMed]
23. Clasen, S.; Pereira, P.L. Magnetic resonance guidance for radiofrequency ablation of liver tumors. *J. Magn. Reson. Imaging* **2008**, *27*, 421–433. [CrossRef]
24. McDannold, N. Quantitative MRI-based temperature mapping based on the proton resonant frequency shift: Review of validation studies. *Int. J. Hyperth.* **2005**, *21*, 533–546. [CrossRef] [PubMed]
25. Bucci, O.M.; Cavagnaro, M.; Crocco, L.; Lopresto, V.; Scapaticci, R. Microwave ablation monitoring via microwave tomography: A numerical feasibility assessment. In Proceedings of the 2016 10th European Conference on Antennas and Propagation (EuCAP), Davos, Switzerland, 10–15 April 2016; pp. 1–5.
26. Bellizzi, G.G.; Crocco, L.; Cavagnaro, M.; Farina, L.; Lopresto, V.; Scapaticci, R. A full-wave numerical assessment of microwave tomography for monitoring cancer ablation. In Proceedings of the 2017 11th European Conference on Antennas and Propagation (EUCAP), Paris, France, 19–24 March 2017; pp. 3722–3725.
27. Scapaticci, R.; Bellizzi, G.G.; Cavagnaro, M.; Lopresto, V.; Crocco, L. Exploiting Microwave Imaging Methods for Real-Time Monitoring of Thermal Ablation. *Int. J. Ant. Propag.* **2017**, *2017*, 5231065. [CrossRef]
28. Lopresto, V.; Pinto, R.; Lovisolo, G.A.; Cavagnaro, M. Changes in the dielectric properties of ex vivo bovine liver during microwave thermal ablation at 2.45 GHz. *Phys. Med. Biol.* **2012**, *57*, 2309–2327. [CrossRef] [PubMed]
29. Lopresto, V.; Pinto, R.; Cavagnaro, M. Experimental characterisation of the thermal lesion induced by microwave ablation. *Int. J. Hyperth.* **2014**, *30*, 110–118. [CrossRef] [PubMed]
30. Cavagnaro, M.; Pinto, R.; Lopresto, V. Numerical models to evaluate the temperature increase induced by ex vivo microwave thermal ablation. *Phys. Med. Biol.* **2015**, *60*, 3287–3311. [CrossRef] [PubMed]
31. Chen, G.; Stang, J.; Haynes, M.; Leuthardt, E.; Moghaddam, M. Real-Time Three-Dimensional Microwave Monitoring of Interstitial Thermal Therapy. *IEEE Trans. Biomed. Eng.* **2018**, *65*, 528–538. [CrossRef]
32. Cavagnaro, M.; Amabile, C.; Bernardi, P.; Pisa, S.; Tosoratti, N. A minimally invasive antenna for microwave ablation therapies: Design, performances, and experimental assessment. *IEEE Trans. Biomed. Eng.* **2011**, *58*, 949–959. [CrossRef] [PubMed]
33. Bur, J.A. Dielectric properties of polymers at microwave frequencies: A review. *Polymer* **1985**, *26*, 963–977. [CrossRef]
34. Amabile, C.; Farina, L.; Lopresto, V.; Pinto, R.; Cassarino, S.; Tosoratti, N.; Goldberg, S.N.; Cavagnaro, M. Tissue shrinkage in microwave ablation of liver: An ex vivo predictive model. *Int. J. Hyperth.* **2017**, *33*, 101–109. [CrossRef] [PubMed]

35. Lopresto, V.; Strigari, L.; Farina, L.; Minosse, S.; Pinto, R.; D'Alessio, D.; Cassano, B.; Cavagnaro, M. CT-based investigation of the contraction of ex vivo tissue undergoing microwave thermal ablation. *Phys. Med. Biol.* **2018**, *63*, 055019. [CrossRef]
36. Pittella, E.; Bernardi, P.; Cavagnaro, M.; Pisa, S.; Piuzzi, E. Design of UWB antennas to monitor cardiac activity. *ACES J.* **2011**, *26*, 267–274.
37. Abbak, M.; Akıncı, M.N.; Çayören, M.; Akduman, İ. Experimental Microwave Imaging with a Novel Corrugated Vivaldi Antenna. *IEEE Trans. Antennas Propag.* **2017**, *65*, 3302–3307. [CrossRef]
38. Bertero, M.; Boccacci, P. *Introduction to Inverse Problems in Imaging*; Institute of Physics: Bristol, UK, 1998.

11

On-Site Validation of a Microwave Breast Imaging System, before First Patient Study

Angie Fasoula *, Luc Duchesne, Julio Daniel Gil Cano, Peter Lawrence, Guillaume Robin and Jean-Gael Bernard

MVG Industries, 91140 Villebon sur Yvette, France; luc.duchesne@mvg-world.com (L.D.); julio_daniel.gil_cano@mvg-world.com (J.D.G.C.); peter.lawrence@mvg-world.com (P.L.); guillaume.robin@mvg-world.com (G.R.); jean-gael.bernard@mvg-world.com (J.-G.B.)

* Correspondence: angie.fasoula@mvg-world.com

Abstract: This paper presents the Wavelia microwave breast imaging system that has been recently installed at the Galway University Hospital, Ireland, for a first-in-human pilot clinical test. Microwave breast imaging has been extensively investigated over the last two decades as an alternative imaging modality that could potentially bring complementary information to state-of-the-art modalities such as X-ray mammography. Following an overview of the main working principles of this technology, the Wavelia imaging system architecture is presented, as are the radar signal processing algorithms that are used in forming the microwave images in which small tumors could be detectable for disease diagnosis. The methodology and specific quality metrics that have been developed to properly evaluate and validate the performance of the imaging system using complex breast phantoms that are scanned at controlled measurement conditions are also presented in the paper. Indicative results from the application of this methodology to the on-site validation of the imaging system after its installation at the hospital for pilot clinical testing are thoroughly presented and discussed. Given that the imaging system is still at the prototype level of development, a rigorous quality assessment and system validation at nominal operating conditions is very important in order to ensure high-quality clinical data collection.

Keywords: breast cancer diagnosis; microwave imaging; medical radar; on-site validation; breast phantoms

---

1. Introduction

Microwave imaging for medical applications has been of interest for many years. The microwave images are maps of the electrical property distributions in the body. The electrical properties of various tissues may be related to their physiological state; notably, there has been some evidence of changes in the properties of cancerous tissues when compared to normal tissues. Cancer detection with microwave imaging is based on this contrast in electrical properties. Microwave imaging, as an alternative imaging modality to X-ray mammography for breast cancer detection, has interested many researchers during the last 20 years [1–5].

Among them, at least four research teams have performed clinical testing of their experimental prototypes [6–11], demonstrating numerous positive results and a potential added value of the microwave technology toward a better specificity and/or sensitivity in breast cancer diagnosis when combined with the state-of-the-art modalities. The potential for regular follow-up of the patient during breast cancer treatment has also been envisaged using the microwave technology [8]. The interested reader is directed to a series of review papers that have been recently published [12–14]; these papers provide an extensive overview of the microwave breast imaging system prototypes that have been clinically tested, the principal technical features and differences among them, as well as the most important results reported so far.

One of the most appealing features of the microwave technology is the use of non-ionization radiation; thus, it is very safe for the patient and could open up the possibility for scheduling regular three-dimensional (3D) scans of the breast, as often as required, for optimal diagnostic and/or follow-up of rapidly evolving pathologies. In conjunction with the design of appropriate radar signal processing algorithms, automated tumor detection can be naturally integrated with the microwave image formation process, providing clinicians with useful tools for computer-aided diagnosis (CAD). Several CAD systems for breast cancer have been proposed during the last decade [15–17], especially on X-ray mammography systems. Although they are not yet part of the routine clinical practice, they have proved useful in aiding clinicians to diagnose breast cancers in cases where simple visual inspection is ambiguous. The Wavelia microwave breast imaging system, as presented in this paper, is being developed for such an intended future use.

The Wavelia system is a low-power electromagnetic wave breast imaging device for cancer screening purposes. The device consists of two subsystems, both performing a non-invasive examination: the microwave breast imaging subsystem, and the optical breast contour detection subsystem. The device has been recently installed at the Clinical Research Facility of Galway University Hospital (CRFG) in Ireland, for a first-in-human pilot clinical test. In this paper, the methodology and indicative results from the on-site validation of the device, using anthropomorphic breast phantoms, are presented. The developed methodology is meant to be applied after each installation of the device in hospital, in order for the device functioning to be carefully verified and validated, before any patient recruitment is authorized.

The paper is structured as follows. All of the materials and methods used for the on-site validation of the imaging system are presented in Section 2 of the paper. In Section 2.1, a description of the Wavelia imaging system is provided. In Section 2.2, the fundamental working principles of the microwave breast imaging technology are summarized. In Section 2.3, the anthropomorphic breast phantoms which have been used for the design and testing of the Wavelia imaging system are presented. In Section 2.4, the main steps of the microwave breast imaging algorithm are outlined. In Section 2.5, an introduction to the optical scanner which is integrated in the Wavelia system is included; indicative results as used for the on-site validation of the optical scanner, are also shown in this subsection. In Section 2.6, the on-site validation test procedure used for the site acceptance of the Wavelia microwave breast imaging system is detailed. In Section 3, indicative validation test imaging results are shown. The presented results are grouped into two parts: in Section 3.1, images formed at a single vertical position of the sensor network are presented, whereas in Section 3.2, images formed using data collected at multiple vertical scan positions of the sensor network are shown. In Section 4, a summary of quality assessment (QA) results from the on-site validation of the system is included, followed by a short discussion on the potential sources of mismodeling of the breast with the available phantoms, which may inevitably lead to adjustments of the system when working with clinical data.

2. Materials and Methods

2.1. The Wavelia Microwave Breast Imaging System Prototype

Wavelia is a prototype medical device that employs low-power electromagnetic waves for the detection of breast cancer. A photo of the device, as installed in the CRFG examination room, in Galway, Ireland for first-in-human pilot clinical testing, is shown in Figure 1.

As mentioned in the introduction, the device consists of the microwave breast imaging subsystem and the optical breast contour detection subsystem. The microwave breast imaging subsystem is an active device that illuminates the breast with non-ionizing low-power electromagnetic waves in the microwave frequency spectrum, which penetrate the breast under examination. The subsystem collects the scattered electromagnetic waves and recovers pertinent information about the breast tissue consistency based on the dielectric contrast of these tissues. The optical breast contour detection subsystem serves to provide the total volume and boundary contour of the breast, as a priori information for the microwave breast imaging subsystem.

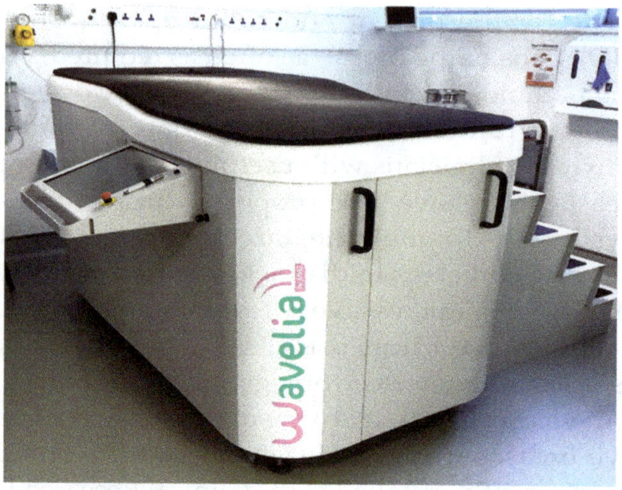

Figure 1. The Wavelia breast imaging system, which was recently installed in Galway University Hospital, for a first-in-human clinical test.

During the examination, the patient will be lying in a prone position on the examination table. A dedicated circular opening on the examination table will permit the immersion of the breast in a specific liquid, which will serve as a coupling (transition) medium between the imaging system and the breast. The coupling liquid has been appropriately manufactured such that it has electromagnetic properties favoring the penetration of the electromagnetic wave in the breast.

The intended performance of the device is to unambiguously detect the presence of breast malignant lesions and estimate their 3D location within a given level of accuracy. While the ultimate goal is the diagnosis of breast cancer at an early stage of development, in the course of the pilot first-in-human trial, the achievable performance of the device will only be verified against benchmark cases of prediagnosed palpable cancers. To this extent, co-registration of the imaging results with available images from reference modalities (X-ray mammogram and/or ultrasound scans) will be performed. Thus, a "ground truth" will be available to assess the performance of the prototype device under test.

In Figure 2, a top view of the Wavelia microwave breast imaging subsystem examination table, as well as a zoomed view on the transition liquid in which the breast is immersed during the scan, are shown.

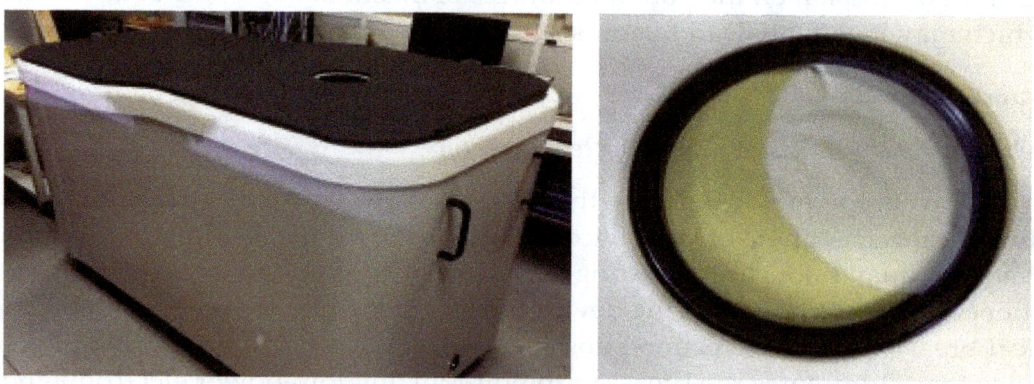

(a) (b)

Figure 2. Wavelia microwave breast imaging system: (**a**) Top view of the examination table; (**b**) Zoomed view on the transition liquid in which the breast is immersed during the scan.

2.2. *Microwave Breast Imaging at Prone Position: The Principle*

The microwave imaging scan is performed using a network of 18 wideband Vivaldi-type antennas in a horizontal circular configuration. The sensors are located outside a container that hosts the coupling liquid. The sensors are piloted to perform a vertical motion such that the full breast volume is appropriately illuminated during the scan. The scan takes approximately 10 min for a breast of medium size, as the breast phantom used for the on-site validation of the system.

A schematic description of the prone examination setup is shown in Figure 3.

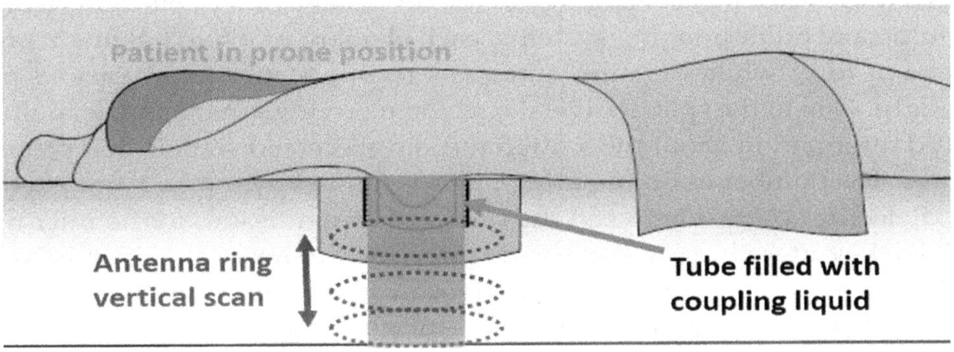

Figure 3. Microwave breast imaging examination: the principle.

The technology is very safe. The emitted microwave power level inside the breast is limited physically by the capacity of the radiofrequency components, such that the maximum radiated level inside the breast is always lower than 50 mW. Calculations have been performed for the localized specific absorption rate (SAR) in the breast. The maximum localized SAR in the breast complies with the International Commission on Non-Ionizing Radiation Protection (ICNIRP) recommendations and the European Union (EU) Directive 1999/519/CE on the limitation of exposure of the public to electromagnetic fields (compliance with a safety factor of four). The Radio-Frequency (RF) front end is based on vector network analyzer architecture. The resulting emission/reception RF chain has a dynamic range of 75 dB.

From the perspective of microwave imaging, the anatomy of the breast can be simplified to the following [14]:

- An adipose layer directly below the skin. This layer consists of vesicular cells filled with fat, which are aggregated into lobules and separated by Cooper's ligaments;
- The mammary glands: the innermost tissue of the breast consists of about 15–20 sections, termed lobes, with many smaller sections of mammary glands, which are arranged in a circular fashion. These lobes and ducts are also surrounded by Cooper's ligaments, which have the function of maintaining the inner structure of the breast and supporting the tissue attached to the chest wall;
- Posterior to the breast is the major pectoral muscle, as well as ribs two to six.

Breast tumors typically originate in the glandular tissue. The increased volume of water within the cancerous tissue is responsible for the strong electromagnetic scattering associated with microwave imaging. The increase of sodium and water, particularly inbound water within the tumor cells, leads to the greater conductivity and permittivity of the tumorous tissues [18,19].

Several studies have examined the dielectric properties of normal and cancerous breast tissue. Indicatively, in 1992, Campbell and Land measured in vitro the complex permittivity of female breast tissue at 3.2 GHz [20]. They reported a significant dielectric contrast between normal (fatty tissue and all other healthy breast tissues) and tumor tissue. They also suggested that due to the similarity in the dielectric properties of malignant and benign tumors, it might not be possible to distinguish between the two based on dielectric properties alone.

Some additional characteristics that are inherent to benign and malignant tumors have the potential to be helpful for tumor classification using microwave imaging, such as the tumor shape and surface texture [21–23]. Malignant tumors usually present the following characteristics: irregular and asymmetric shapes, blurred boundaries (lack of sharpness), rough and complex surfaces with spicules or microlobules, non-uniform permittivity, distortion in the structure of the breast, and irregular tissue density (due to masses and calcifications). Conversely, benign tumors tend to have the following characteristics: spherical, oval, or at least present well-circumscribed contours, compactness, and a smooth surface.

In the Wavelia microwave breast imaging device, multistatic radar detection technology [24,25] is employed. In multistatic radar imaging systems, each element of a fixed-element array illuminates the imaging scene in turn, while the other antennas record scattering at various angles from the transmitter boresight. Due to the spatial diversity of the receiving antennas, the multistatic approach acquires enhanced information about the scatterers, using received signals that propagate outwards via different routes. The number of illuminating paths is limited by the array geometry.

Due to the dielectric contrast between the different breast tissues at the microwave frequency range [19,20,26], back-scattered radar signals are physically generated. The received radar echoes are appropriately processed in order to detect and localize any significant scatterers (tumors) in the breast. An increased level of coherence of reflections originating from a given location results in the high intensity of the radar image at the given location in the breast, thus suggesting the presence of a significant scatterer.

Prior to radar imaging of the interior of the breast, pre-processing of the backscattered signals is performed to remove artifacts in order to accentuate the useful radar echoes of weak power level. The strong artifacts mainly consist of direct coupling between the antennas, skin reflections, and antenna reverberation. Following artifact removal, an effective radar-imaging algorithm is employed to unambiguously detect the presence of tumors and accurately localize them, while simultaneously suppressing clutter due to the normal heterogeneity of breast tissue.

Apart from using reflected microwave energy to reconstruct images of the breast, the radar target signatures may contain additional information on the shape, size, and other features of the tumor. This information could potentially be exploited for discrimination between benign and malignant lesions.

2.3. The Breast Phantoms

During the design phase, but also for the on-site validation, the imaging device has been deployed with phantoms, which simulate the real breast. These phantoms have been manufactured considering:

- Realistic breast shapes extracted from a publicly available database of real MRI breast images [27];
- The state-of-art knowledge in terms of dielectric properties of the breast normal and malignant tissues in the frequency range of interest [26,28–30];
- Realistic asymmetric tumor shapes and sizes [22,23,31];

The manufactured breast phantoms have been presented in further detail in [32,33], by A. Fasoula et al.

The breast phantom repository, as published by the University of Wisconsin [27], has been used to define MRI-based realistic breast geometries. Based on this, rigid plastic molds have been 3D-printed for the breast outer surface, as well as for the segmented fibroglandular tissue in the breast MRI image, after the minimum required simplification, such that the geometry is printable in a limited number of compartments. For the imaging tests, both molds are filled with liquids mimicking the adipose and fibroglandular tissue [34]. Either liquid is poured in the corresponding mold compartment; the compartment walls are sufficiently thin to avoid significant impact on electromagnetic wave propagation.

Solid mixtures of graphite, carbon black, and urethane are used to manufacture the skin and tumor phantoms. The formula published in [35] by J.Garrett et al. has been slightly adjusted to achieve solid mixtures with appropriate dielectric properties mimicking the corresponding types of tissues.

In Figure 4, the geometry of one of the breasts of class ACR3 (heterogeneously dense) that has been selected from the database for the on-site validation of the imaging system, as well as the corresponding 3D printed molds, are depicted. The selected adipose tissue-mimicking liquid has a mean dielectric constant $\varepsilon_r = 5$, while the fibroglandular tissue-mimicking liquid has a mean dielectric constant $\varepsilon_r = 36$.

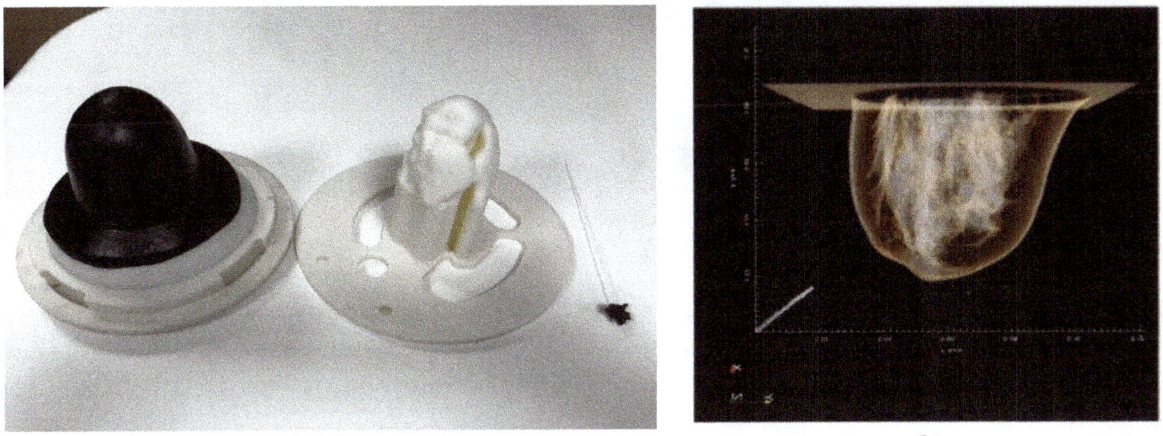

(a) (b)

Figure 4. The breast molds: (**a**) Bottom view of the outer breast surface mold (on the left), covered with the black 2-mm thick skin phantom, and the outer fibroglandular tissue mold; (**b**) Original geometry of the breast, segmented from an MRI breast image.

As depicted in Figure 4, a 2-mm thick skin layer with mean dielectric constant $\varepsilon_r = 38$ is attached to the breast outer surface mold. The selected material, apart from its adequate mean dielectric properties, also has a dispersive profile of complex permittivity well-fitting to the skin dielectric properties, as reported in the relevant literature [28].

A tumor is simulated by use of a microlobulated solid having a diameter of 14 mm and a mean dielectric constant $\varepsilon_r = 52$ within the frequency band of interest. The shape of the tumor phantom is based on a Gaussian random sphere (GRS) model of the breast lesions [21–23]. Aside from its adequate mean dielectric properties, the selected material used for this phantom has a dispersive profile of complex permittivity that fits well with the one of malignant breast tissue, as reported in the literature [29].

A photo of the tumor phantom used during the validation tests of the microwave breast imaging device is shown in Figure 5.

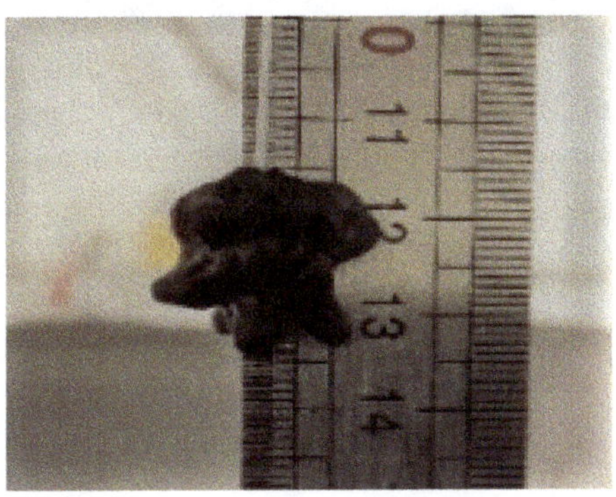

Figure 5. The tumor phantom: microlobulated shape, average radius of 14 mm, dielectric properties matching the measured dielectric properties of excised malignant tissue.

Two snapshots from the preparation of the experimental setup, before a typical validation test of the device, are shown in Figure 6.

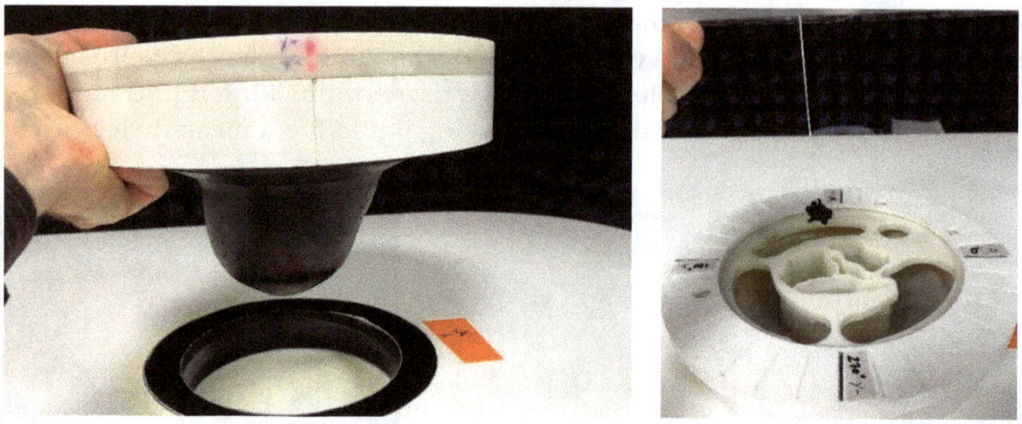

(a) (b)

Figure 6. Preparation of the breast phantom for the microwave breast imaging test: (**a**) Immersion of the breast in the circular opening of the examination table, filled with transition liquid; (**b**) Inclusion of the tumor phantom in the fibroglandular tissue-mimicking liquid.

2.4. The Imaging Algorithm

2.4.1. The Physical Considerations and Modeling

In order to properly design the data processing algorithms for such a device, it is fundamental to take into consideration the anatomy of the human female breast and translate it into an electromagnetic wave propagation problem to be resolved. As depicted in Figure 7, the breast skin layer, the fat, and the network of glandular tissue lobules and ducts of the human female breast have been considered to model the wave propagation path through the breast, before potentially reaching a tumor. As stated earlier, a network of sensors encircles a cylinder about which a vertical microwave imaging scan is performed.

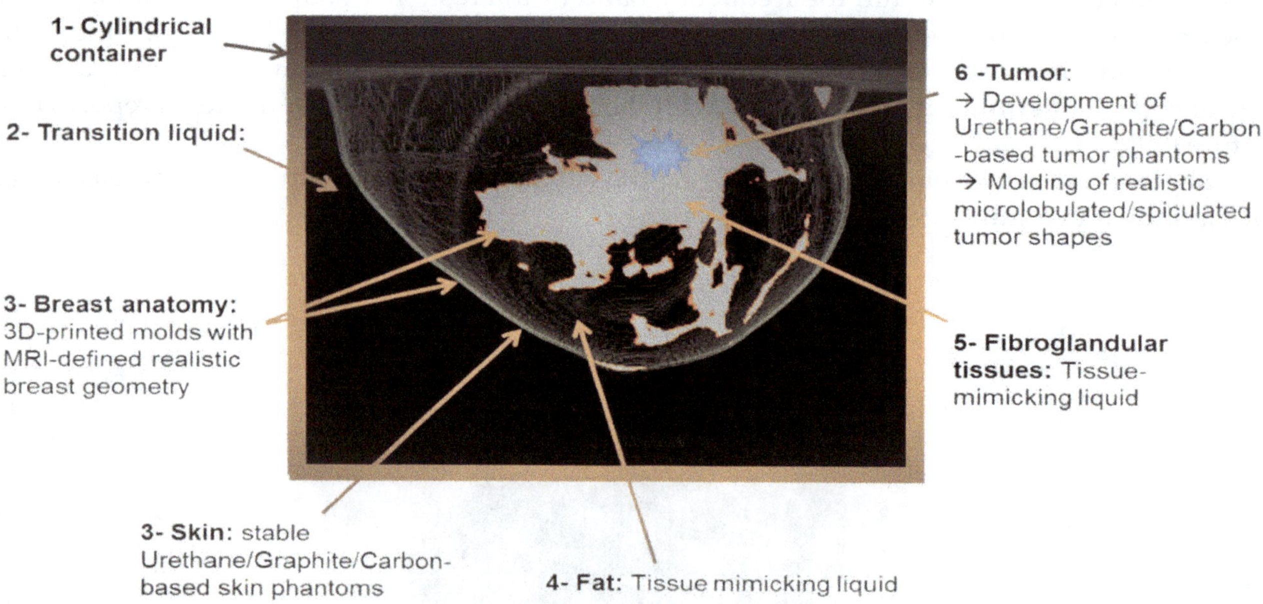

Figure 7. Realistic modeling of the near-field, non-planar, multi-layer, high permittivity transmission medium for electromagnetic wave penetration.

The cylinder is filled with coupling transition liquid into which the breast is immersed. The transition liquid allows for optimizing the transmission of the electromagnetic waves from the antennas into the breast (similar function as for the gel used in ultrasound echography for optimizing the transmission of the ultrasound waves from the probe to the interior of the body). Thus, the transition liquid has been designed to have real permittivity that well matches the permittivity of the human skin, as specified by Lazebnik et al. [28]. At the same time, the conductivity of the liquid has been designed to be such that it introduces non-negligible propagation losses, thus mitigating the strong multipath waves that propagate in the cylinder without ever entering the breast, as initially suggested in [36] by P. Meaney et al. The real permittivity of the transition liquid ranges between 25 and 30, and its conductivity ranges between 0.2 S/m and 1.2 S/m in the working frequency band F = [1–4] GHz. The liquid is based on organic oil and deionized water mixed at a given proportion such that the desired dielectric properties are achieved.

Given the above considerations, the data processing algorithms of such a device should be designed such that useful information for breast imaging is acquired if the electromagnetic wave that is emitted from a sensor is received by another sensor of the network in a bistatic configuration. This step comes after transition from the following chain of non-planar layers with distinct dielectric properties (real permittivity and conductivity), which are each:

Transmitting antenna → Cylinder → Transition liquid → Skin → Fat → Glandular tissue → Tumor
Receiving antenna ← Cylinder ← Transition liquid ← Skin ← Fat ← Glandular tissue ← Tumor

The contrast in terms of the dielectric properties of the consecutive layers is responsible for the intensity of the echoes that are generated due to the transition of the electromagnetic wave via the respective layers. Thus, a significant tumor echo would be evoked that is conditioned on sufficient dielectric contrast between the normal glandular tissue and the cancerous tissue.

In addition, both the breast tissue and the transition liquid are materials of non-negligible conductivity that introduce noticeable radar wave propagation losses. This means that even if sufficient dielectric contrast exists to evoke significant reflection from tumors, the propagation losses along the path between the sensors and the tumor will lead to reflected signals of weak intensity compared to the unwanted reflections originating closer to the sensors. Namely, it is the interaction (coupling) between the antennas themselves, as well as the reflections that are generated by the skin layer once the electromagnetic wave impinges on the external surface of the breast, which represent signals that are several orders of magnitude larger in intensity than the weak reflections originating from the interior breast tissues.

Given the above principles, which are related to the physical nature of the problem, an imaging algorithm that is carefully customized for the application has been designed.

2.4.2. The Data Pre-Processing Steps

Several pre-processing steps are applied to the data measured by each couple of transmitting/receiving antennas, before this data can be efficiently used for imaging. The objective of the pre-processing steps is to mitigate the strong coupling between the antennas and the strong interference originating from the skin and other interwall reflections close to the breast surface. In the actual experimental setup, the effective employment of the data pre-processing steps reveals useful radar target echoes 30–40 dB below the raw measured data power level. However, the data pre-processing steps, being directly linked to the nature of the measured signal, are susceptible to evolving once the imaging system is employed in the clinical setting.

- Data calibration at the presence of the breast

As a first step, drift correction, with respect to a reference channel, is applied to the raw data measured by each couple of transmitting/receiving antennas; any time-varying drifts are thus eliminated before further processing of the signal.

The presence of the breast at a close vicinity to the sensor network significantly modifies the measured coupling between sensors. For this reason, a calibration process is employed to dynamically estimate the coupling signal based on a bunch of data from the scan that has been measured at similar conditions. The data-driven estimation is performed in the frequency domain at each vertical scan position and for each Tx/Rx couple in the network. The estimated coupling signal $\mathbf{DCal}_{\mathbf{Txi/Rxj,H_n}}(f)$, is further subtracted from the drift-corrected raw data $\mathbf{Dat}_{\mathbf{DriftCorr,Txi/Rxj,H_n}}(f)$.

A multiplicative compensation factor $\mathbf{PhCen}_{\mathbf{Corr,Txi/Rxj}}(f, e_{r,trans}(f))$ is then applied to the calibrated data in order to geometrically align the data. The phase-center compensation term is computed for each Tx/Rx couple in the network for each operating frequency point and is subject to the dielectric constant $\mathbf{e}_{\mathbf{r,trans}}(f)$ of the transition liquid, as a function of the frequency. Conditioned on temperature preservation in the operating limits of the device, such that the transition liquid dielectric properties are known, this term does not require dynamic data-driven estimation; it is a priori defined and stored during the system characterization at factory.

$$\mathbf{Dat}_{\mathbf{CAL,Txi/Rxj,H_n}}(f) = (\mathbf{Dat}_{\mathbf{DriftCorr,Txi/Rxj,H_n}}(f) - \mathbf{DCal}_{\mathbf{Txi/Rxj,H_n}}(f)) \cdot \mathbf{PhCen}_{\mathbf{Corr,Txi/Rxj}}(f, \mathbf{e}_{\mathbf{r,trans}}(f)) \quad (1)$$

- Reconstruction of the breast external envelope

This estimation module uses as input a reduced set of data from the microwave breast imaging system, which after calibration for removal of the strong antenna coupling, is used to reconstruct the external surface of the breast with limited accuracy. The calibrated data is used in conjunction with an active contour model to estimate a simple closed contour representing the skin return boundary, based on bistatic wave-front detection, at each vertical scan position. The algorithm has been presented in more detail in [37] by P. Lawrence et al.

- Independent Component Analysis, in the frequency domain

The independent component analysis (ICA) is a well-known method for finding underlying factors, or components, from multivariate statistical data [38,39]. The ICA method has been used extensively in various application domains, among which medical imaging is included, for feature extraction and selection, or even pathology identification [40,41].

What distinguishes ICA from other methods is that it looks for components that are both statistically independent and non-Gaussian. Given a set of observations of stochastic processes $x_1(t), x_2(t), \ldots, x_m(t)$, where t denotes the sample index, assume that they are generated as a linear mixture of independent components $y = W \cdot x$, where W is some unknown matrix. Independent component analysis consists of estimating the mixing matrix W, such that the non-Gaussianity of the components $y_i(t)$ is maximized. The kurtosis and the negentropy are two of the most commonly employed measures of non-Gaussianity for estimating the mixing matrix W [38].

In the case of radar signals, ICA can be performed either in the time domain, or in the frequency domain [42–45]. In our data processing chain, we have opted for the frequency-domain ICA, applied to the calibrated data $\mathbf{DCal}_{\mathbf{Txi/Rxj,H_n}}(f)$ per Tx/Rx couple at each vertical scan position H_n.

Segmentation of the data vector in frames of appropriate length, via application of a sliding window in frequency, is initially applied. Principal component analysis (PCA) is subsequently performed for data pre-whitening and dimensionality reduction [46], prior to input into the ICA algorithm. The selected sliding step in frequency is an important parameter that is directly linked to the spectral properties of the underlying signal and the principal modes to be preserved after pre-processing. The ICA operation is denoted in Equation (2), where $\mathbf{Dat}_{\mathbf{PCA-TAB,Txi/Rxj,H_n}}$, $(M \cdot N_f)$ is the block of M principal modes that is provided as input to the ICA algorithm, $\mathbf{Dat}_{\mathbf{ICA-TAB,Txi/Rxj,H_n}}$, $(M \cdot N_f)$ is the block of M ICs, as estimated by the algorithm, M corresponds to the number of sliding windows in the frequency that is initially selected, and N_f is the number of frequency samples in the measured data vector.

$$\mathbf{Dat}_{\mathbf{ICA\text{-}TAB,Txi/Rxj,H_n}} = W^H \cdot \mathbf{Dat}_{\mathbf{PCA-TAB,Txi/Rxj,H_n}}, \forall H_n \text{ and } Tx_i/Rx_i \quad (2)$$

- Data filtering: IC Selection with Appropriate Spectral and Geometry-based Features

The clear function of the ICA data pre-processing step is to classify/separate useful against interference (strong clutter components), based on:

- The distinct spectral properties of the various radar target echoes i.e., frequency dispersion is normally translated to higher kurtosis [47,48].
- The estimated location from which each IC radar echo originates: an inverse fast Fourier transform (IFFT) for transformation of the IC from the frequency domain to the time domain is applied for this purpose; the correspondence between time and distance is established using as input the prior estimate of the breast contour, the known dielectric properties of the transition liquid, and an assumption on the average dielectric properties in the interior of the breast (directly derived from an assumption on the percentage of fibro-glandular versus adipose tissue in the breast).

Given the above considerations, two filtering steps are sequentially applied to the data:

- Filtering-out ICs with spectral profile incompatible with radar target echoes originating from the breast tissues, given the expected level of frequency dispersion; in the future, additional pattern features may be identified and employed at this filtering step, based on measurements with real breast tissues.
- Filtering-out ICs that are associated with radar target echoes originating from either very short distances (residual coupling) or very long distances (multipath) with respect to the sensors; the ICs that are filtered out at this step cannot physically correspond to the breast tissues, in terms of geometry.

- Propagation Loss Compensation

In order for the imaging algorithm to work properly, it is important to compensate for the electromagnetic wave propagation losses, which vary significantly along the working frequency band in the case of the highly-dispersive breast tissues.

Given the estimate of the distance from which the radar target echo that is associated with each IC originates (as estimated for the purpose of the distance-based filtering), a multiplicative propagation loss compensation term that is both frequency and distance dependent is applied to each IC. A characterization of the propagation loss model, which is applicable to the specific near-field radar imaging setup, is required to perform a good compensation. For now, an estimate, which is planned to be further refined in the future, is applied which achieves partial compensation of the propagation losses.

The energy focusing level, which is retrieved on the images, is expected to be degraded in the case of target sources for which the propagation loss compensation has not been properly performed at this pre-processing step. The propagation loss compensation term being dependent on the distance between the sensors and the target location to which each IC is associated means that it is also dependent on an assumption of the percentage of fibroglandular tissue pc_{fib} present along the specific bistatic radar path.

Given all of the above considerations, a filtered version of $\mathbf{DCal}_{\mathbf{Txi/Rxj,H_n}}(f)$ is reconstructed using the ICs obtained from the two filtering stages. A multiplicative propagation loss compensation term is applied separately to each IC before concatenation.

$$\mathrm{DCal-Filt}_{\mathrm{Txi/Rxj,H_n}}(f) = \sum_{i\in\{IC_{rem}\}} \mathrm{Dat}_{\mathrm{ICA-TAB,Txi/Rxj,H_n}}(i,f).\ \mathrm{LossComp}\ (f, d_i, pc_{fib}), \forall H_n \text{ and } Tx_i/Rx_i \quad (3)$$

In Equation (3), IC_{rem} denotes the set of IC indices that have been maintained after the two-step filtering, while d_i denotes the bistatic radar distance of the target echo that has been associated with the ith IC.

2.4.3. The TR-MUSIC (Time-Reversal Multiple Signal Classification) Imaging Algorithm

After pre-processing the signals, as measured by various combinations of transmitting/receiving antennas—thus in various bistatic configurations—are combined in a multistatic radar imaging algorithm to generate an image of the interior breast tissues. The combination of multistatic radar paths in the same imaging algorithm enhances the angular diversity of the input information, thus making the algorithm more robust against clutter (unwanted distributed interference echoes from the interior of the breast) and enhancing the focusing of the image energy on small pronounced targets.

The imaging algorithm that is used is the time-reversal multiple signal classification (TR-MUSIC) algorithm, which was originally conceived for the detection of obscured radar targets in heavily cluttered environments, in the case of surveillance and tracking defense radars [49]. The original definition of the algorithm works optimally for a finite collection of point targets, as is the case when small targets are observed by a radar with limited spatial resolution, or when the first-order Born approximation is valid for the scattering mechanisms that dominate the imaging scene [50]. Further studies have been subsequently performed to generalize the algorithm in cases of multiple scattering phenomena [51] or extended targets, as is the case when a target is large relative to the size of the radar resolution cell [52]. More recently, the algorithm has been also proposed for breast cancer detection in dense breasts [53–58], albeit limited to simulations and no experimental data.

The main steps of our implementation of the algorithm are outlined as follows:

- A limited number of N_{fsel} frequency points is selected from the total of measured frequency points in the operating band.
- Sectorization is performed, such that multiple images are formed at each frequency and each vertical position of the sensor network, each time using a different sector of the circular network. The selected number of sensors in the sector is further denoted as N_S. The total number of sectors required to scan over the full 360° around the breast is denoted as N_{sect}.

Both the selection of specific frequency points, and the physical size and number of elements in the sub-arrays (sectors) used for the elementary image formation, can be critical to the achievable system performance in terms of unambiguous target (tumor) detection in the breast.

Monochromatic (single frequency) images are formed for each selected frequency point and each sector of sensors as follows:

- The multistatic frequency response matrix (MFRM) is formed using the calibrated and filtered data at the specific frequency:

$$\mathbf{S_{sect}}(f) = \begin{bmatrix} \mathbf{S}_{Tx_1/Rx_1} & \mathbf{S}_{Tx_1/Rx_2} & \cdots & \mathbf{S}_{Tx_1/Rx_{N_s}} \\ \mathbf{S}_{Tx_2/Rx_1} & \ddots & \ddots & \vdots \\ \vdots & \ddots & \ddots & \vdots \\ \mathbf{S}_{Tx_{N_s}/Rx_1} & \cdots & \cdots & \mathbf{S}_{Tx_{N_s}/Rx_{N_s}} \end{bmatrix}, \ f = 1 : N_{fsel} \quad (4)$$

where:

$$S_{Tx_i/Rx_j}(f) = DCal - Filt_{Txi/Rxj,H_n}(f), \ \forall H_n \text{ and } Tx_i/Rx_i \quad (5)$$

as defined in Equation (3).

- The time-reversal operator is subsequently formed as:

$$T_{sect}(f) = S_{sect}(f)^H \cdot S_{sect}(f) \quad (6)$$

with H denoting the Hermitian transpose.

- Eigenvalue decomposition is performed on $T_{sect}(f)$, and an appropriate model order selection criterion is used to separate the resulting eigenspace into signal and noise subspaces [59]:

$$\{\text{Signal subspace}: \{\lambda_s, Q_s\} = \{\lambda_i, Q_i\}_{i=1}^{M_{ord}}, \text{ Noise subspace}: \{\lambda_N, Q_N\} = \{\lambda_i, Q_i\}_{i=M_{ord}+1}^{N_s}\} \tag{7}$$

where M_{ord} is the selected model order. The separation can be a challenging task, if in the imaging scene there are multiple interacting non-point targets, as is typically the case for breast imaging. The effective separability between the signal and noise subspace has a significant direct impact on the final imaging result, given that the principle for the formation of this type of image is the orthogonality between the two subspaces.

$$\mathbf{Q}_S^H \cdot \mathbf{Q}_N = 0 \tag{8}$$

- The image, or the so-called TR-MUSIC pseudospectrum at the pixel p and the frequency f, when using the sector of sensors sect at the vertical scan position h_j, is formed as:

$$Im_{sect,h_j}(p,f) = \frac{1}{\|(Q_N{}^H \cdot G_{sect}(p,f))^H \cdot (Q_N{}^H \cdot G_{sect}(p,f))\|} \tag{9}$$

where:

$$\mathbf{G}_{\mathbf{sect}}(p,f) = \left[\ \mathbf{g}_0\left(p_{TRx_{sect,1}}, p, f\right)\ \ \mathbf{g}_0\left(p_{TRx_{sect,2}}, p, f\right)\ \ \cdots\ \ \mathbf{g}_0\left(p_{TRx_{sect,N_s}}, p, f\right)\ \right]^T \tag{10}$$

is the illumination vector of the sector sensor array sect at the frequency f and the pixel location p in the imaging zone.

In Equation (10), $\mathbf{g}_0\left(p_{TRx_{sect,i}}, p, f\right)$ denotes the elementary Green function (i.e., the impulse response function of the propagation path) from the individual antenna at position $p_{TRx_{sect,i}}$ to the arbitrary point p in the scanning region at the frequency f, while T denotes the matrix transpose.

The TR-MUSIC pseudospectrum in Equation (9) gets maximized, thus highlighting a target presence, at the pixel location p, at which the orthogonality constraint between the sensor array illumination vector and the signal noise subspace is better met.

This arises from the assumption that a linear decomposition of the illumination vector $\mathbf{G}_{sect}(p,f)$ in the signal subspace Q_s exists such that:

$$\mathbf{G}_{\mathbf{sect}}(p,f) = Q_s \cdot B^{(m)}, \text{ with } B^{(m)} = \left[\ b_1^m\ \ b_2^m \cdots b_{M_{ord}}^m\ \right]^T \text{ a set of linear coefficients} \tag{11}$$

and the orthogonality constraint in Equation (8).

2.4.4. The Composite Image Formation

The monochromatic (single-frequency) image, as defined in Equation (9), may be difficult to be exploited as such for unambiguous and comprehensive interpretation of the imaging scene, due to inevitable corruption of the signal by residual noise and interference, even after pre-processing. Frequency diversity is commonly employed to mitigate the presence of frequency-dependent clutter (unwanted interference) radar echoes. The multi-frequency TR-MUSIC image at the sector sect and the vertical scan position h_j is defined in Equation (12):

$$Im_{sect,h_j}(p) = \sum_{f=1}^{N_{f_{sel}}} \frac{1}{\|(Q_N{}^H \cdot G_{sect}(p,f))^H \cdot (Q_N{}^H \cdot G_{sect}(p,f))\|} \tag{12}$$

In order to assure visibility of the breast over the full azimuth domain of 360°, integration is performed on multiple partial images, computed per sectors of sensors all around the breast.

The composite image that is formed using all the N_{sect} elementary multi-frequency images at a given vertical position of the sensor network is defined in Equation (13):

$$Im_{TOT,h_j}(p) = \frac{1}{N_{sect}} \cdot \sum_{i=1}^{N_{sect}} Im_{sect,h_j}(p) \quad (13)$$

The composite image of Equation (13) is the first type of image that is used for the validation of the imaging system using a well-controlled breast phantom, imaged at a single vertical position of the sensor network, in the vicinity of the tumor phantom.

Integration of multiple partial images of the complete imaging scene, computed all along the vertical scan of the sensor network, is further applied to form the full 3D image of the breast.

The composite image using data from multiple vertical scan positions of the sensor network is defined in Equation (14):

$$Im_{TOT,MultiH}(p) = \frac{1}{N_h} \cdot \sum_{j=1}^{N_h} Im_{TOT,h_j}(p) \quad (14)$$

where N_h is the number of vertical scan positions of the sensor network that are used to form the full 3D image.

2.4.5. The Focusing Metrics, as a Means of Adjustment of the Breast Mean Permittivity

In order to map the multistatic radar echoes to the imaging grid under investigation, a model for the electromagnetic wave propagation modes is employed, as defined in Equations (9) and (10).

In the actual version of the microwave imaging device, propagation in two homogeneous lossless media is considered in the model. Lossless media are justified, given that loss compensation has been applied to the pre-processed signals before entering the imaging algorithm, as defined in Section 2.4.2.

Separation of the space in two media is assumed, given that the heterogeneous distribution of the tissues in the interior of the breast is unknown and sought to be estimated by the imaging algorithm. Thus, the two media that are provided as a priori to the imaging algorithm are: the transition liquid between the antennas and the exterior breast surface, and then the interior of the breast associated with an "average" dielectric permittivity, which remains homogeneous per coronal slice of the breast. The breast external surface has been estimated prior, using a subset of the calibrated data, as mentioned briefly in Section 2.4.2; this information is exploited here to define the border between the two distinct media of propagation.

The elementary Green function $\mathbf{g_0}\left(p_{TRx_{sect,i}}, p, f\right)$ involved in Equation (10) is further defined as:

$$\mathbf{g_0}\left(p_{TRx_{sect,i}}, p, f\right) = j \cdot \mathbf{H}_0^{(1)}\left(\mathbf{k_{bg}}(f) \cdot \|p - p_{TRx_{sect,i}}\| + \mathbf{D\hat{k}_{breast}}(f) \cdot \hat{d}_{InBreast,i,p}\right) \quad (15)$$

where:

- $\mathbf{H}_0^{(1)}$ is the Hankel function of first kind and zero order: $\mathbf{H}_m^{(1)}(x) = (-j)^{m+1} \cdot \frac{e^{j \cdot x}}{x}$, with $m = 0$,
- $\mathbf{k_{bg}}(f) = \frac{2\pi f}{c_0} \cdot \sqrt{\mathbf{e_{r,trans}}(f)}$ is the wavenumber for propagation in the transition liquid,
- $\mathbf{D\hat{k}_{breast}}(f) = \frac{2\pi f}{c_0} \cdot \left(\sqrt{\mathbf{\hat{e}_{r,InBreast}}(f)} - \sqrt{\mathbf{e_{r,trans}}(f)}\right)$ is an 'average' differential wavenumber for propagation in the breast,
- c_0 is the speed of light in vacuum,
- $\mathbf{e_{r,trans}}(f)$ is the known dielectric constant of the transition liquid,
- $\mathbf{\hat{e}_{r,InBreast}}(f)$ is an estimate of the average equivalent dielectric constant of the breast, and
- $\hat{d}_{InBreast,i,p}$ is an estimate of the propagation path in the breast, in the case of a wave propagating from the sensor $TRx_{sect,i}$ to the pixel p, knowing the wavefront corresponding to the external surface of the breast.

The "average" equivalent dielectric constant of the breast is defined in Equation (16) as a function of the dielectric constant of the adipose and fibroglandular tissue, mixed at proportion pc_{fib}.

$$\hat{\mathbf{e}}_{\mathbf{r,InBreast}}(f) = (pc_{fib} \cdot \hat{\mathbf{e}}_{\mathbf{r,fibroglandular}}(f) + (1 - pc_{fib}) \cdot \hat{\mathbf{e}}_{\mathbf{r,adipose}}(f)) \cdot 10^{-2} \quad (16)$$

$\hat{\mathbf{e}}_{\mathbf{r,InBreast}}(f)$ is plotted in Figure 8 for various assumptions pc_{fib}, while considering for the adipose and fibroglandular tissue dielectric properties the ones of the corresponding tissue-mimicking liquids used to fill the breast phantom molds of the Wavelia microwave breast imaging system, as defined in Section 2.3.

Parametric images are generated under varying assumptions of percentage of fibroglandular tissue pc_{fib} along the propagation path from a given transmitting antenna, to the breast and back to a given receiving antenna. The parameter pc_{fib} impacts on both the estimate of the lossless elementary Green function $\mathbf{g_0}\left(p_{TRx_{sect,i}}, p, f\right)$, as defined in Equation (15), but also on the computation of the propagation loss compensation term LossComp (f, d_i, pc_{fib}), in Equation (3) of the data pre-processing chain.

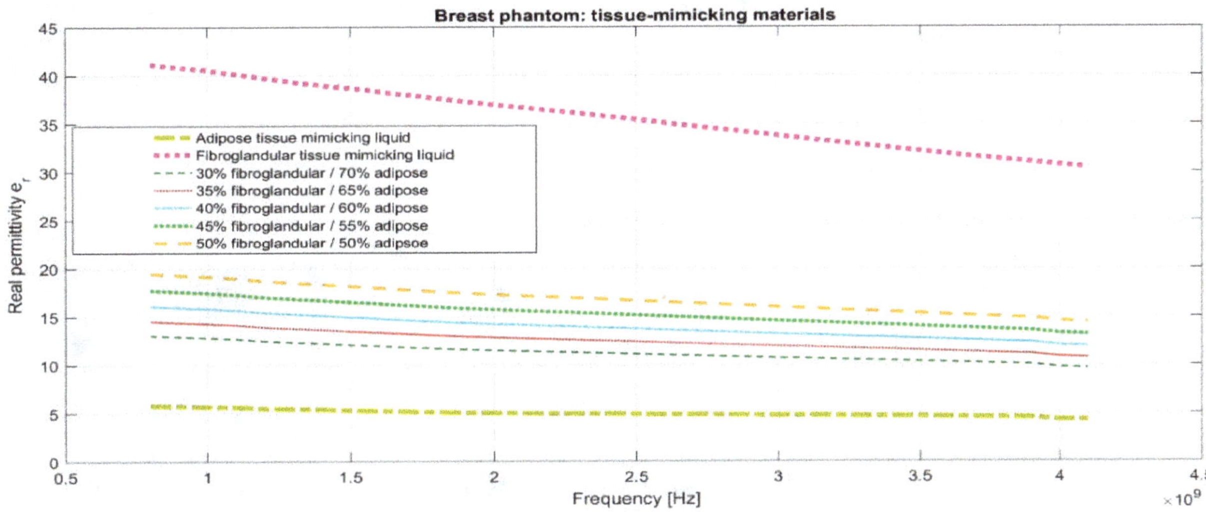

Figure 8. "Average" equivalent dielectric constant along a bistatic path through the breast, under various assumptions on the percentage of fibroglandular tissue pc_{fib}. Applicability to the breast phantoms used for the design validation of the microwave breast imaging system.

The generated set of parametric images is further evaluated in terms of focusing, using appropriate image focusing measures [60–62]. The optimal pc_{fib} assumption is automatically selected based on maximization of the focusing capability of the imaging algorithm, under the specific pc_{fib} assumption. Given the varying consistency of the heterogeneous breast along the vertical scan, the focusing operation is performed per vertical position of the sensor network, thus on the image type defined in Equation (13).

For the analysis presented in this paper and used for the on-site validation of the Wavelia imaging system before its pilot clinical test, the image curvature, as defined in [60] by S. Pertuz et al., is used as the focusing metric (FM) for the parametric images. The intensity of the TR-MUSIC pseudospectrum of Equation (13) is interpolated by means of a quadratic surface $f(x, y) = c0 \cdot x + c1 \cdot y + c2 \cdot x^2 + c3 \cdot y^2$, where the vector of coefficients C = [c0 c1 c2 c3]^T is computed through least squares by applying two convolution masks, as defined in [60] by S. Pertuz et al. The curvature of the quadratic surface is used as the focusing metric (FM) for the image:

$$FM = |c0| + |c1| + |c2| + |c3| \quad (17)$$

The quadratic surface fitting and FM computation is actually performed per regions of interest (ROIs) of limited size on the image. The selected ROI size is related to the image resolution, as well as the size of detectable scattering objects in the radar imaging scene. The maximal image curvature (FM) over all of the ROIs is computed per parametric image. The pc_{fib} associated with the image with overall maximal curvature is selected as optimal at a given vertical section of the breast (coronal breast size) in front of the sensor network. The composite multi-height image, as defined in Equation (14), is automatically formed via concatenation of all the coronal slices with maximal curvature (FM).

At the current stage of system development, the image formation is performed offline. It may take a few hours for the focusing algorithm to run the multiparametric (multi pc_{fib}) multi-sector images for all the vertical (coronal) slices of the breast. The total duration for the composite image formation will depend on the size of each breast (= i.e., number of coronal slices to be processed) and the number of assumptions on the background breast permittivity under test (=size of the parameter set pc_{fib}).

The actual implementation is valid, as such, in the case of a single dominant target (tumor) in each coronal slice of the breast. Both the breast phantoms and the clinical setting for the pilot first-in-human testing of the device are compliant with such a physical assumption. Appropriate complexification of the algorithm is planned for the near future in order to properly handle the realistic case of multiple lesions being present, sought to be detected, and accurately localized per coronal slice of the breast.

An example of the computed FM for a set of five pc_{fib}-parameterized images, as well as the result of optimal pc_{fib} selection, is shown in Figure 9. The FM values are appropriately rescaled by the algorithm, such that the resulting values are comparable among various coronal cross-sections of the breast. The depicted images are normalized to maximum intensity.

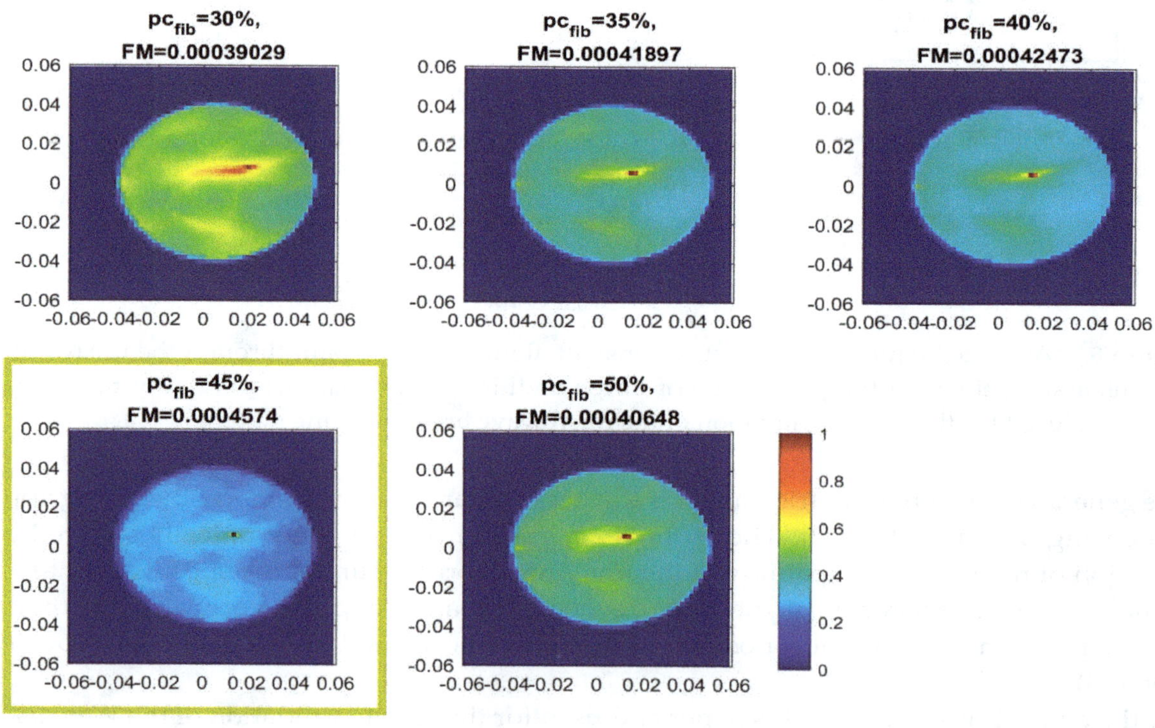

Figure 9. Example of focusing evaluation on a coronal breast slice. Parametric images generated for five assumptions in terms of percentage of fibroglandular tissue in the breast. Optimal pc_{fib} = 45%, automatically selected based on maximization of the focusing metric (FM). Single tumor (dominant scatterer) detected on the specific breast coronal slice.

2.5. The Optical Breast Scan and Metrology

As mentioned in Section 2.1, the Wavelia medical device consists of two subsystems, both performing a non-invasive examination: the microwave breast imaging subsystem, which is the main part of the system, and the optical breast contour detection subsystem, which plays an auxiliary role. The objective of the optical subsystem is triple:

- Compute the volume of the patient's breast, thus indirectly deriving the required volume of transition liquid such that the container of the microwave breast imaging subsystem is optimally filled after immersion of the breast;
- Compute the vertical extent of the pendulous breast, in order to optimally dimension the vertical scan of the microwave breast imaging system;
- Reconstruct fully the external envelope of the breast, with high precision; such information will further serve to control the potential level of deformation of the breast due to immersion in the transition liquid during the microwave imaging scan. It may also serve as an intermediate step when registering the 3D microwave image with reference to the 2D mammographic projections of the patient's breast, for comparison and validation of the microwave breast imaging modality.

The optical scan of the breast will be performed just before the microwave imaging scan, during the clinical testing of the Wavelia system. In order for the optically reconstructed breast envelope to be useful a priori information for the microwave imaging system, it is important that the patient is lying in the same prone position during both examinations. Thus, an identical examination table as the one used for the microwave imaging and shown in Figure 1, is integrated with the optical breast contour detection subsystem as well.

The patient is lying on the examination table, with her breast under examination inserted in the circular opening of the examination table. For this examination, there is no coupling liquid, as shown in Figure 2 for the microwave imaging system. The breast is in the air, hanging below the examination table. A 3D infrared camera is placed below the examination table at a distance of several tens of centimeters below the breast. A motorization system enables the azimuthal motion of the camera in one single horizontal plane. The azimuthal scan of the 3D camera permits reconstructing the external envelope of the breast with sub-millimetric precision.

In Figure 10, the reconstructed outer surface for the breast phantom that has been specified in detail in Section 2.3 and is used for the validation of the Wavelia imaging system on site is shown. Both a side view and a bottom view are indicatively shown, as provided to the system user for acceptance of the scan.

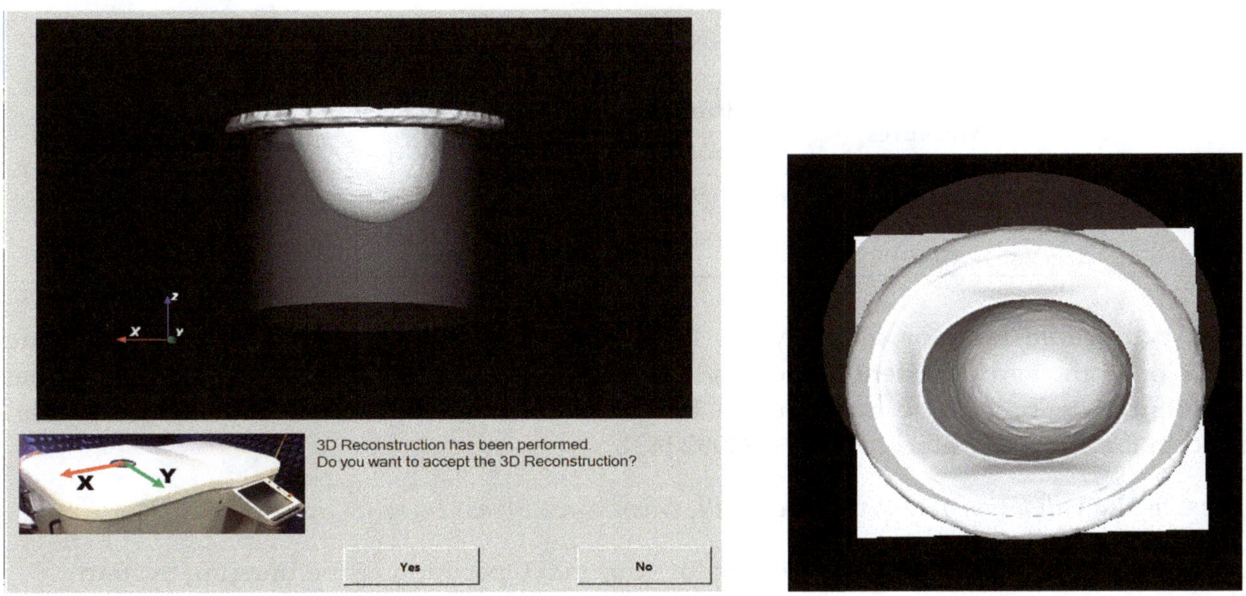

(a) (b)

Figure 10. Reconstructed outer surface of the breast phantom #1 (**a**) Screen capture from the Wavelia Optical Breast Contour Detection subsystem, as provided to the user, (**b**) Zoomed bottom view of the reconstructed outer surface of the breast.

In Figure 11, the reconstructed outer surface of a second breast phantom of different shape and a significantly bigger size is illustrated.

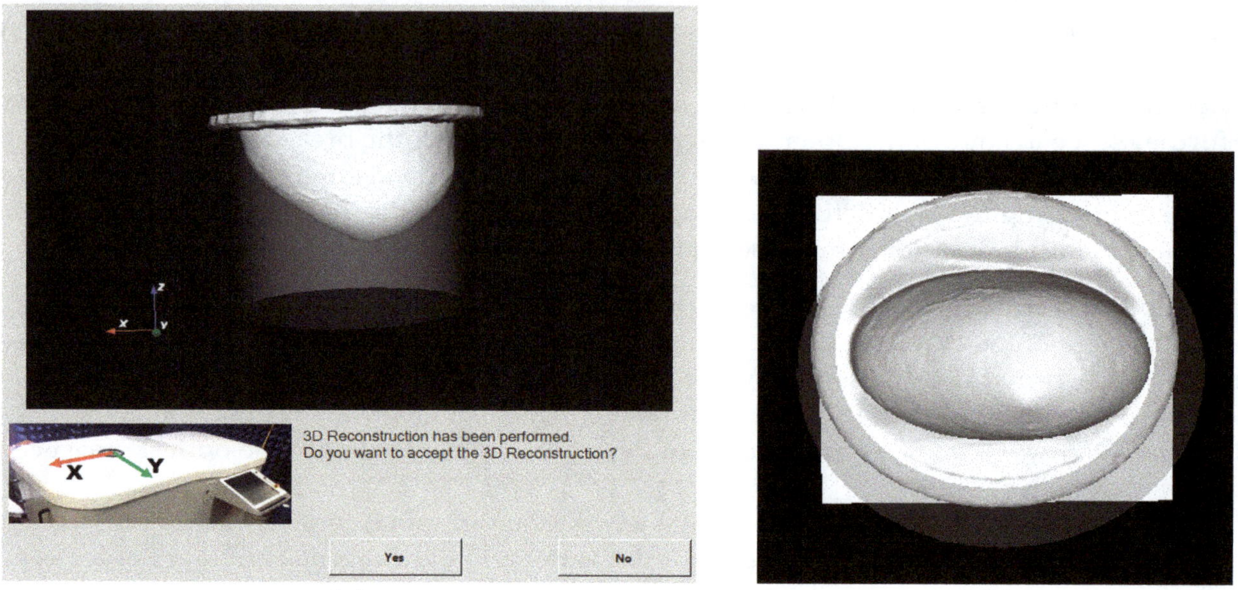

(a) (b)

Figure 11. Reconstructed outer surface of a second breast phantom #2, of significantly bigger size, (**a**) Screen capture from the Wavelia Optical Breast Contour Detection subsystem, as provided to the user, (**b**) Zoomed bottom view of the reconstructed outer surface of the breast.

In Table 1, the measurement results for both breast phantoms are given, for one optical scan performed at factory and another scan performed after the installation of the system on site. Reproducible results have been achieved with very good accuracy; these results served for the site acceptance of the optical system at the hospital.

Table 1. Breast Phantom Metrology, Based on the Optical Scan.

Measures	Breast Phantom #1		Breast Phantom #2	
	Site	Factory	Site	Factory
Breast Volume (mL)	698	696	1099	1097
Breast Vertical Extent (mm)	85	84	108	108

The achievable level of accuracy for both the computation of the breast volume and the computation of the vertical extent of the pendulous breast is compatible with the expected values and independent of the breast size and shape, as long as the breast is within the limits of acceptable sizes specified in the clinical protocol NCT03475992 [63].

2.6. The On-Site Validation Test Procedure for the Microwave Breast Imaging System

2.6.1. Controlled Environmental Conditions for Nominal Operation of the Imaging System

At this stage of prototype development, the imaging system is required to operate in a controlled environment, for the nominal system performance to be assured. The examination room temperature should range between 20–25 °C during the full examination, which takes approximately 1 h, including: the optical and microwave scan of both breasts of the patient, all the intermediate system preparation steps, the transition liquid preparation steps, and the system quality checks.

In order to assure compliance with these temperature limits during the examination, it is recommended that the room temperature does not exceed 21–22 °C at the beginning of the examination.

For the system on-site validation tests with breast phantoms, the temperature is monitored both at the beginning and at the end of each test. The monitoring is performed at the following control points:

- container filled with transition liquid: measurement at the center and close to the borders of the container
- breast mold compartments filled with fibroglandular tissue-mimicking liquid: measurement at three different points, or compartments

In Table 2, the temperature monitoring data for an on-site system validation test, which has been marked as compliant with the nominal operating conditions, is indicatively provided.

Table 2. Temperature Measurement Conditions: Breast Phantom Validation Test.

Transition Liquid		Fibroglandular Tissue	
Before the Scan	**After the Scan**	**Before the Scan**	**After the Scan**
22.7 °C–23.3 °C	23.0 °C–24.1 °C	20.6 °C	21.2 °C

2.6.2. System Stability Verification

A series of systematic tests are regularly performed at system installation in order to assess the repeatability of the measuring capability of the system. The assessment of the repeatability before performing a RF scan is fundamental to assure that a reliable and exploitable measurement can be performed.

A procedure for quantitative assessment of the system reliability has been developed. A reduced version of this is also performed automatically by the system before the examination of each patient. It consists of repeating a dummy (no breast immersion) measurement several times and performing three tests to quantify the level of variability of the complex measurements, both in terms of amplitude and phase.

- Verify that the amplitude envelope of the raw measured data keeps consistent with the lower and upper-level masks, as predefined at factory;
- Perform first and second-order statistics on raw measured data after drift correction: evaluate the stability, both in amplitude and phase, of the reference channel
- Perform first and second-order statistics on calibrated data: evaluate the multi-run stability, both in amplitude and phase, on a limited set of T*x*/R*x* couples.

2.6.3. Imaging Test with Complex Breast Phantom at Two Azimuthal Rotational Positions

For the on-site validation of the system imaging performance after installation, a controlled test with a complex breast phantom is performed. A tumor phantom is included at a given known position in the breast. Quantitative evaluation of a series of metrics is performed for the quality assessment and validation of the scan. For this reason, it is important that repeated testing with the exact breast and tumor location configuration has been prior performed and thoroughly characterized at the factory. The breast and tumor phantoms that are used for the on-site system validation have been defined in Section 2.3.

The scan is repeated for two distinct azimuthal rotations of the phantom (azimuthal rotation of both the breast and tumor by 180°, such that the relative location of the tumorous inclusion in the breast remains constant). The purpose of the breast rotation is to identify and characterize any "non-symmetries" in the system imaging performance, due to residual uncalibrated imperfections of the system circular network. For the definite on-site validation of the system after installation, a follow-up of the system imaging performance, as evaluated on the two azimuthal rotations of the breast phantom, is performed over several days.

After the system acceptance on site, and while the pilot clinical test is running on patients, the scan of the two breast phantom positions is recommended to be repeated and evaluated at regular intervals in time (e.g., regular monthly, or bi-monthly, interventions by the device manufacturer on site for control and maintenance). It is important to put into place such a regular follow-up in order to better assure the pilot clinical trial data quality, using a system at the prototype level of development.

In Figure 12, a top view of the Wavelia examination table, after installation of the breast phantom for the regular validation test, is shown. The breast phantom is maintained at the known position, using a supporting ring structure. The tumor is inserted at the predefined 3D location, using a rigid string of known length, inserted via a hole at a precisely known (x, y) position on the phantom support structure. A photo of the two azimuthal rotation positions of the phantom, as used for system validation, is shown in Figure 12a,b.

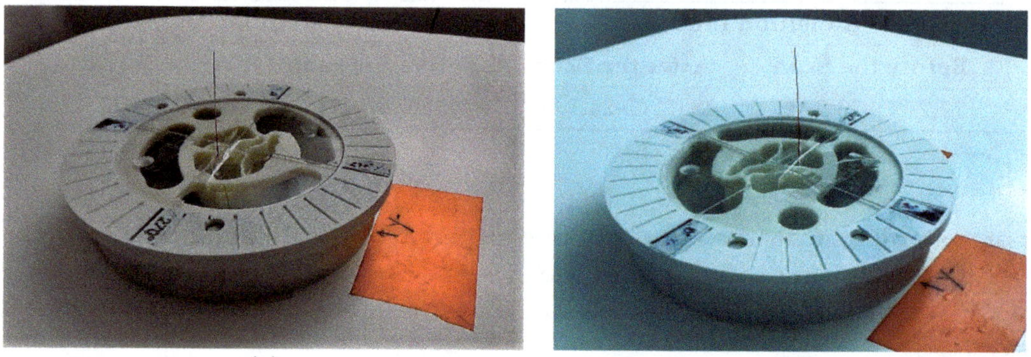

(**a**) (**b**)

Figure 12. Breast phantom ready for the microwave imaging test: examination table top view (**a**) Breast phantom rotational position #1; (**b**) Breast phantom rotational position #2.

2.6.4. Centering Assessment of the Reconstructed Breast Outer Surface

The breast-centering quality test is performed each time on a single breast contour that is associated with a single vertical scan position of the sensor network predefined by the user. A coronal slice close to the middle vertical extent of the pendulous breast is normally selected for the evaluation of the centering of the breast with respect to the imaging zone.

Given the breast contour estimate gc chosen for the breast-centering assessment, at each point X along this test contour, the minimum bistatic distance $r_{gc}(x)$ between this point and any pair of RF sensors (among the reduced set of pairs preselected for use with this estimation module) that can "see" that point, is computed.

In order to assess the centering quality of the estimated contour, an ideally centered reference contour is derived by translating the estimated contour by a varying amount x_T around the 2D region of interest until it yields the largest value of $\oint_{gc_T} r_{gc_T}(gc_T(s))ds$, where $gc_T = gc + x_T$ is the translated contour and $r_{gc_T}(x)$ denotes the minimum bistatic distance to a point x on this translated contour. For this ideal centered reference contour, the minimum bistatic distances, associated to each point x of this curve, denoted by $r_c(x)$, are similarly calculated as for the estimated contour.

For brevity, the notation x is used in the sequel of this section to refer to a given point along the estimated breast contour, and also to refer to the corresponding point $x + x_T$ on the ideally centered reference contour.

The centering assessment is then performed by comparing the bistatic ratio:

$$b_r := \max_{x \in gc}\left(\frac{|r_c(x) - r_{gc}(x)|}{r_c(x)}\right) \quad (18)$$

to the threshold value $B_r \cdot p_{dist\_thresh}$ where B_r is the largest bistatic ratio of any possible translation of the estimated contour, and p_{dist_thresh} is a user-defined parameter, which is by default set to 0.85 for the system validation test.

If b_r exceeds $B_r \cdot p_{dist\_thresh}$, then the estimated breast contour is marked as remarkably off-centered, and the breast centering confidence level P is set to a minimal value that is preset via the parameter $perc_{at\_max\_dis\,tan\,ce}$. Otherwise, the ratio $b_r/(B_r \cdot p_{dist\_thresh})$ is used to compute the breast centering confidence level, as defined in Equation (19):

$$p = \begin{cases} 100 \cdot perc_{at\_max\_distance}, & \text{if } b_r > B_r \cdot p_{dist\_thresh} \\ 100 - 100(1 - perc_{at\_max\_distance}) \frac{b_r}{B_r \cdot p_{dist\_thresh}}, & \text{otherwise} \end{cases} \quad (19)$$

To this extent, the centering assessment will have a confidence level percentage ranging between a maximum of 100 (if the test contour is coincident with the ideal centered contour) and a minimum of $100 \cdot perc_{at\_max\_distance}$. For the on-site validation tests, the minimal value 50% has been used for all of the centering assessment tests.

In Figure 13a,c the breast surface contour estimate chosen for the breast centering assessment (depicted in blue) and the associated ideally centered contour (depicted in cyan) are shown for the tests at the breast rotational position #1, on Test Date 1 and Test Date 2, correspondingly. The red dots depict the location of the sensors, while the black circle represents the inner wall of the transition liquid container.

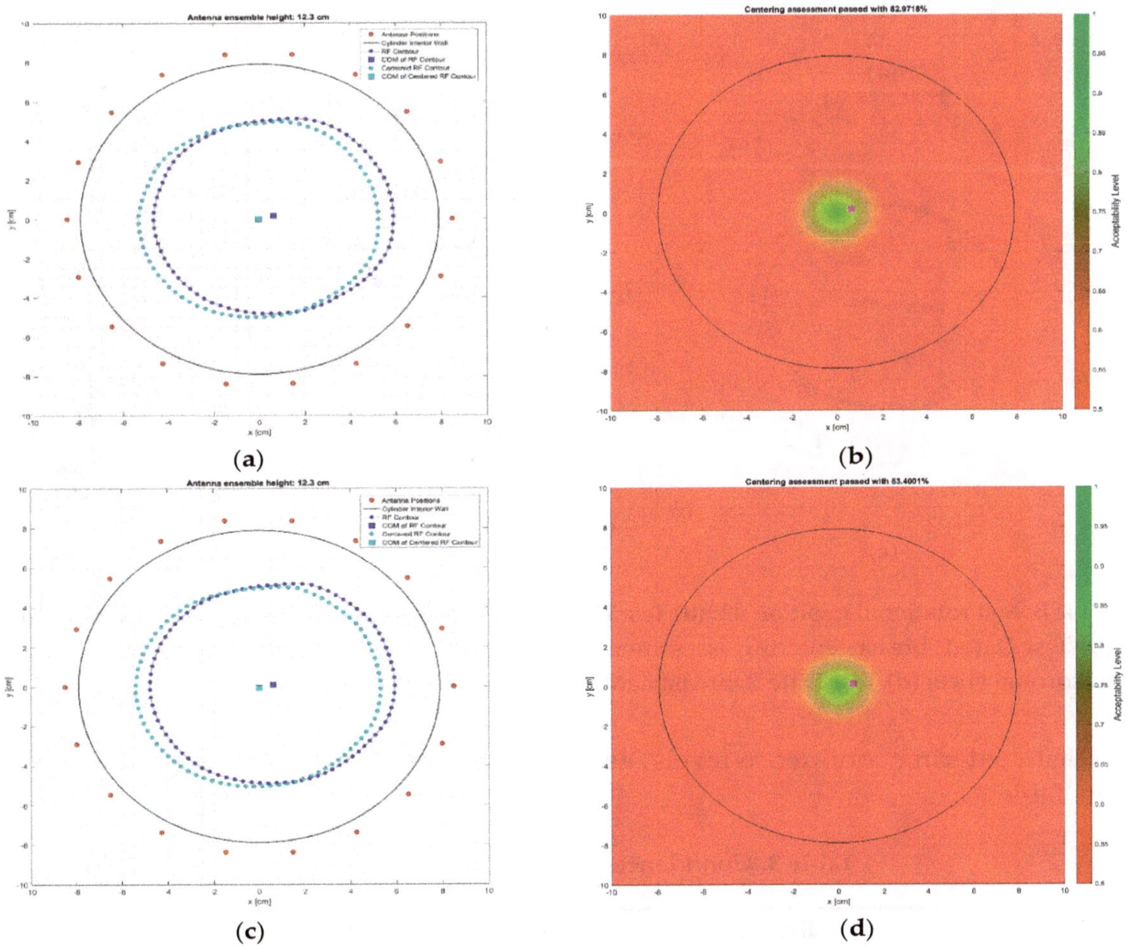

Figure 13. Breast rotational position #1: (**a**) Test Date 1, estimated outer breast surface at a given coronal slice; (**b**) Test Date 1, breast centering assessment map; (**c**) Test Date 2, estimated outer breast surface at a given coronal slice; (**d**) Test Date 2, breast centering assessment map.

The associated spatial map of breast-centering assessment is shown in Figure 13b,d for the two test dates of the breast rotational position #1, correspondingly.

In either figure, the purple square represents the location of the center of mass of the breast surface contour estimate that was used for the breast-centering assessment; the resulting breast-centering confidence level is marked on the title of each figure. The black circle depicts the inner wall of the transition liquid container.

The results for the breast rotational position #2 are given in Figure 14a,b for the data recorded on Test Date 1, and in Figure 14c,d for Test Date 2. All of the notations are consistent with the definitions provided earlier as explanation to Figure 13.

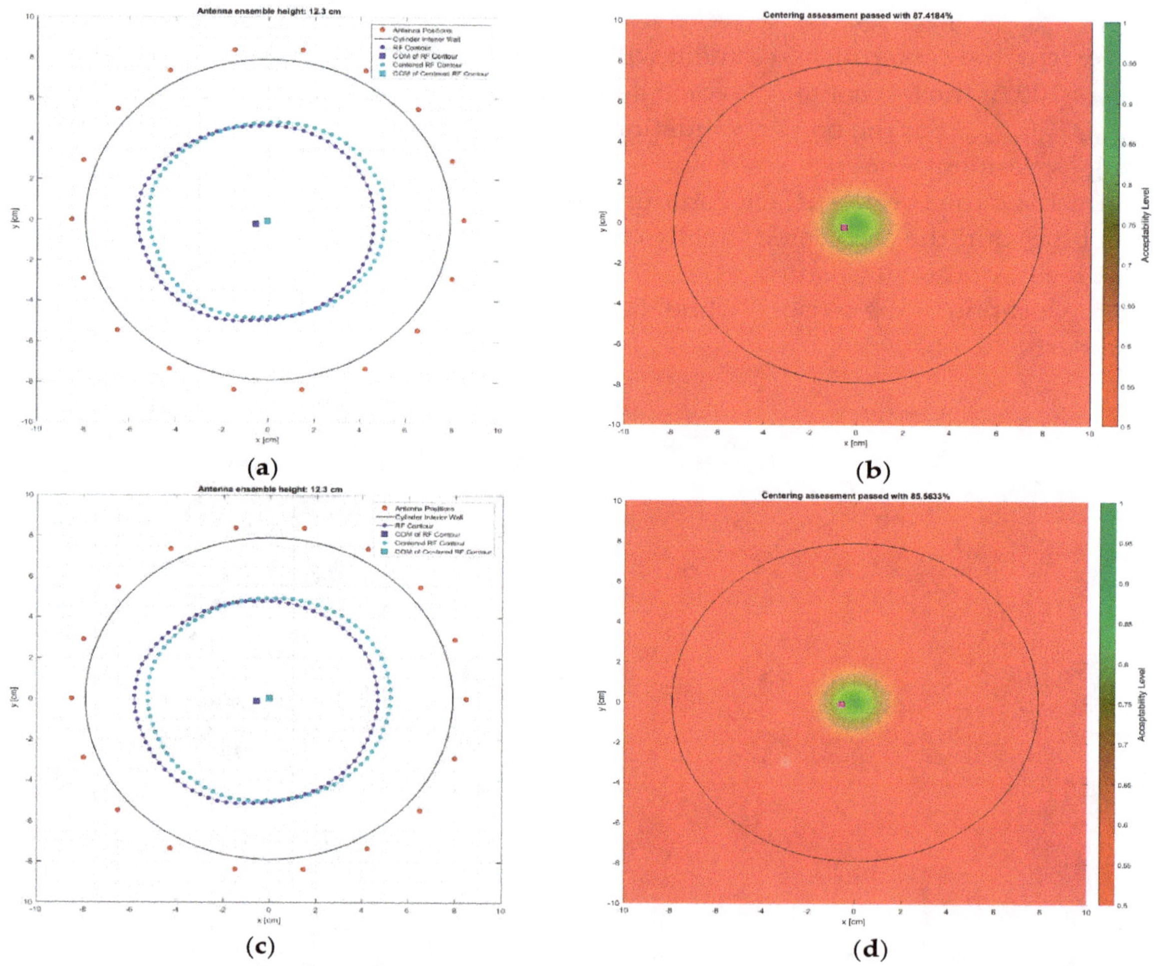

Figure 14. Breast rotational position #2: (**a**) Test Date 1, estimated outer breast surface at a given coronal slice; (**b**) Test Date 1, breast centering assessment map; (**c**) Test Date 2, estimated outer breast surface at a given coronal slice; (**d**) Test Date 2, breast centering assessment map.

The breast-centering confidence levels, as computed for all four test cases, are comparatively presented in Table 3.

Table 3. Confidence Level for Breast Centering.

Breast	Test Date 1	Test Date 2
Rotational position #1	82.97%	83.40%
Rotational position #2	87.42%	85.86%

It is shown that the natural off-centering of the breast phantom at the selected coronal slice is repeatedly identified with a fair level of accuracy, associated with centering confidence levels varying between 83–87.4%. It is worth noting that a slight offset is repeatedly identified between the estimates for the two distinct rotational positions of the breast phantom. This is an indication of a slight non-symmetry in the reconstructed geometry, introduced either by the sensor network itself, or possibly due to a non-homogeneous thermal distribution in the interior of the examination table.

2.6.5. Image Quality Assessment (QA) Metrics for System Performance Acceptance

The microwave breast imaging system evaluation and acceptance is performed based on a series of quality metrics which are computed on multistatic radar images of the breast phantoms, as defined in Equations (13) and (14).

- QA Metric 1: Focusing Metric (FM) evaluated on the composite image formed at single vertical position of the sensor network (as per Equation (13)), in front of the tumor:

The FM is evaluated on a series of images, parameterized by the assumed percentage of fibroglandular tissue pc_{fib} in the breast.

- ○ Acceptance Criterion (AC) #1: The optimal pc_{fib} value, for which the focusing measure is maximized, should remain constant at every repetition of the controlled imaging test, and for every rotational position of the breast phantom (testing with pc_{fib} intervals equal to 5%).
- ○ AC#2: the value of the focusing measure, for the optimal pc_{fib}, should exceed a preset threshold value thr_{QA_1}.

- QA Metric 2: Intensity of the TR-MUSIC pseudospectrum at the tumor location (Im_{max}), evaluated on the composite image formed at a single vertical position of the sensor network (as per Equation (13)), in front of the tumor:

The Im_{max} is evaluated for a series of images parameterized by the assumed percentage of fibroglandular tissue pc_{fib} in the breast:

- ○ AC#3: The optimal pc_{fib} value for which Im_{max} is maximized should remain constant at every repetition of the controlled imaging test, and for every rotational position of the breast phantom (testing with pc_{fib} intervals equal to 5%).
- ○ AC#4: The value of Im_{max}, for the optimal pc_{fib} value, should exceed a preset threshold value thr_{QA_2}.
- ○ AC#5: The two patterns $FM(pc_{fib})$ and $Im_{max}(pc_{fib})$ should be consistent with each other, meaning that maximization and identical slope(s) are observed for the same pc_{fib} values on both patterns.

- QA Metric 3: Variation of the maximal achievable focusing FM over the height, evaluated for images formed using various vertical scan positions of the sensor network (as per Equation (14)):

- ○ AC#6: The maximal FM should be observed at the same height: the one closer to the tumor, at every repetition of the controlled imaging test, and for every rotational position of the breast phantom.
- ○ AC#7: The contrast between the maximal FM and the FM achievable at all of the other heights should exceed a given threshold thr_{QA_3}.

- QA Metric 4: Ratio between the average image intensity at the exterior of the breast and the Im_{max} in the interior of the breast: Evaluation on the composite image formed using data from multiple vertical scan positions of the sensor network (as per Equation (14)):

The multi-height image is formed via concatenation of the single-height images with pc_{fib} automatically selected to allow optimal image focusing independently per height.

- ○ AC#8: The ratio should not exceed a preset upper-limit value UL_{QA_4}.

3. Results

In this section, indicative results are presented from the test campaign that has been recently carried out for the site acceptance of the Wavelia microwave breast imaging system after its installation at the Galway University Hospital for a pilot first-in-human clinical test [63]. The series of image quality assessment (QA) metrics, as defined in Section 2.6.5, have been evaluated on four scans of a realistically complex breast phantom, as detailed in Section 2.6.3.

3.1. QA Metrics 1 and 2: Images Formed at Single Vertical Position of the Sensor Network

3.1.1. Breast Rotational Position #1

In Figure 15, the experimental setup for the tests at the rotational position #1 of the breast phantom is illustrated. For these tests, the microlobulated tumor of average size (14 mm) has been immersed in the fibroglandular tissue-mimicking liquid, at the location $(x, y, z) = (20, 0, 110)$ mm (=center of the tumorous lesion).

The test has been repeated on two distinct dates. Imaging results from the two identical tests are presented and compared in this section.

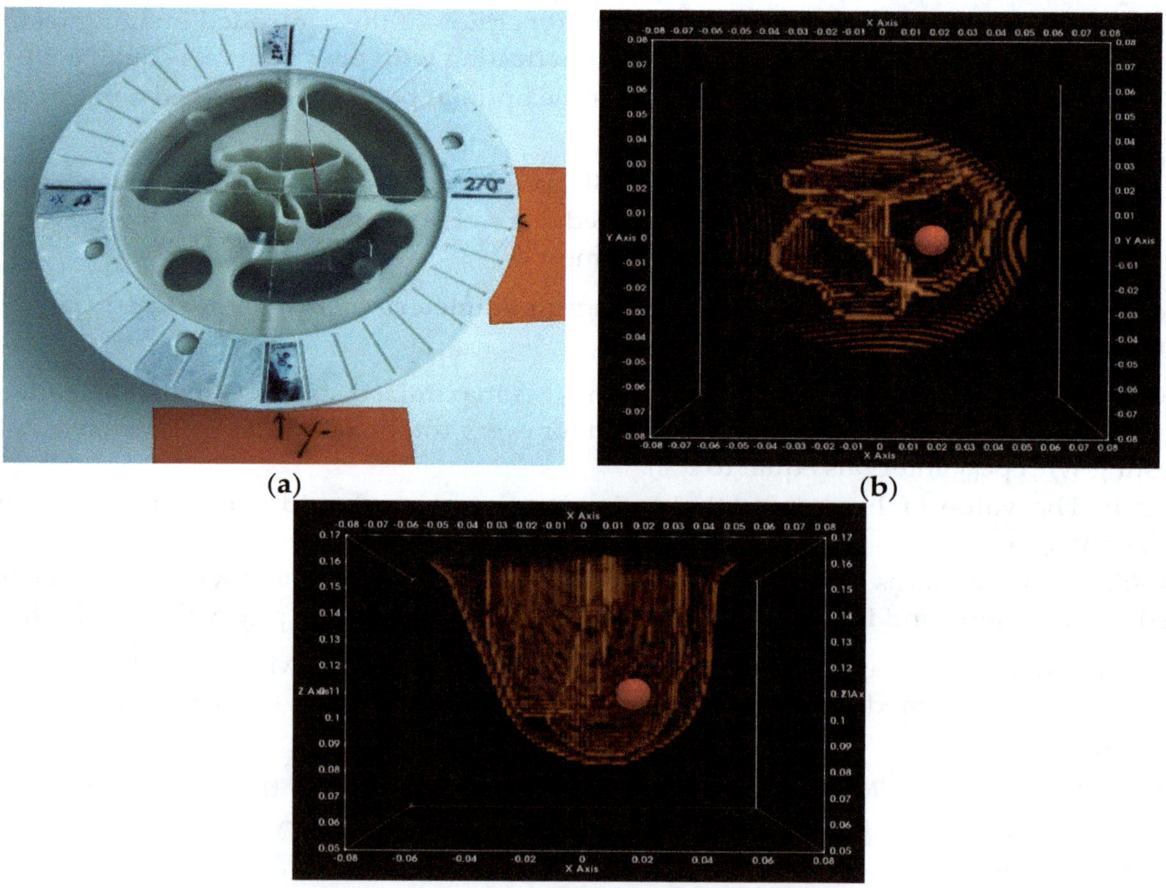

(a) (b) (c)

Figure 15. Experimental setup for the breast rotational position #1: (**a**) Photo—Top view of the breast phantom, installed on the examination table; (**b**) Schematic definition of the tumor location (red sphere with a 14-mm diameter, equal to the average diameter of the microlobulated tumor phantom), in the fibroglandular tissue of the breast (the outer surface of both the fibroglandular mold and the outer breast surface mold are depicted with orange color)—Top View; (**c**) Schematic definition of the tumor location in the fibroglandular tissue of the breast—Side View.

In Figure 16, the composite TR-MUSIC pseudospectra, as formed using Equation (13) and data from a single vertical scan position of the sensor network, are depicted for the two data snapshots recorded on two different dates. The full imaging domain, both in the interior and the exterior of the breast phantom, is evaluated. The objective of such a visualization is to highlight the absence of any significant artifact radar echoes at the exterior of the breast, in the case of both measurements.

These composite images have been formed with the integration of monochromatic (single-frequency) TR-MUSIC pseudospectra, computed as per Equations (9)–(13), using:

- a given number Nfreq of frequency points, uniformly spanning the working frequency band,
- a given number Nsec of sectors of antenna sub-arrays spanning the full 360° azimuth domain around the breast.

The images that have been formed under the assumption pc_{fib} that resulted in maximized focusing are here depicted. The optimal pc_{fib} has been automatically selected with the method that has been defined in Section 2.4.5.

The applied data processing chain is meant to result, ideally, in the formation of very spiked images indicating the probability of the target presence on each pixel of the imaging domain. The unambiguously detected and accurately localized targets are expected to be associated with constellations of very small bright spots, highlighting the target position in an overall dark spatial map. In Figure 16a,b, a clear and pronounced peak of the TR-MUSIC pseudospectrum is visible on both images in the vicinity of the ground truth location of the tumor.

It is noticeable that the intensity of the TR-MUSIC pseudospectrum is slightly higher on the first Test Date 1, as compared to Test Date 2. In addition, two secondary radar echoes (of significantly lower intensity compared to the dominant echo, which is clearly attributed to the tumor) are present on the image of Test Date 1. These secondary echoes can be attributed to a "cavity" of adipose tissue that is formed in between the three compartments of the mold filled with fibroglandular tissue-mimicking liquid in the breast phantom. This adipose 'cavity', which has significant negative dielectric contrast with respect to the surrounding fibroglandular tissue, is visible in Figure 17a, and can be spatially correlated with the secondary radar echoes seen in Figure 16a.

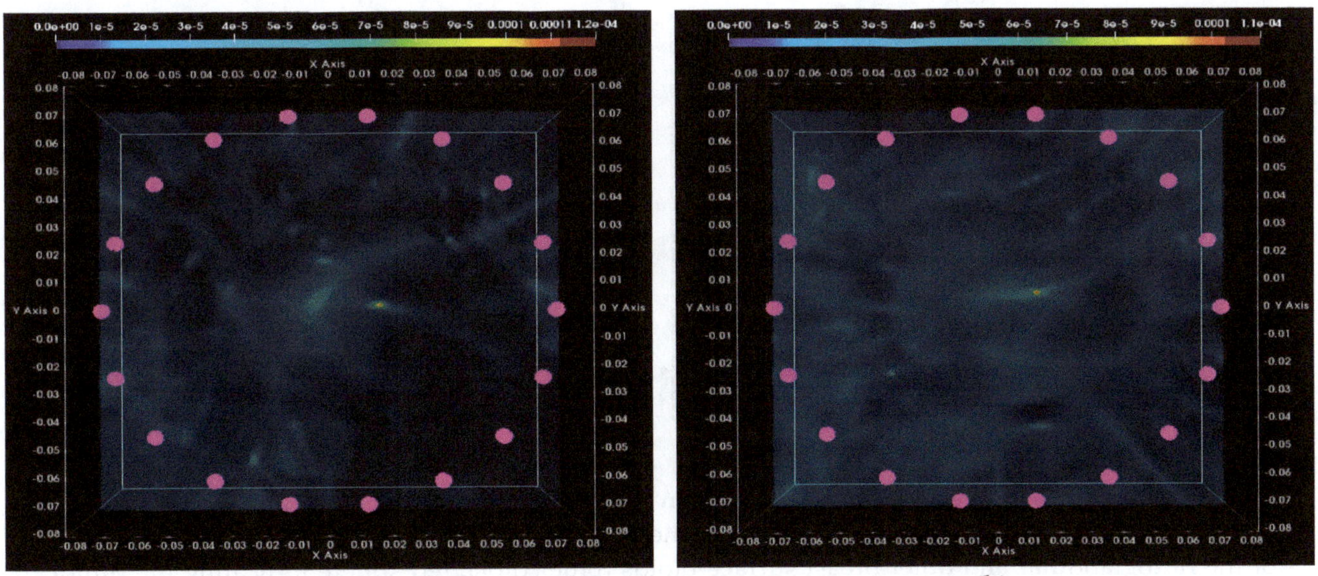

(a) (b)

Figure 16. Breast rotational position #1—image formed at a single vertical position of the sensor network, in front of the tumor; top XY view of the full imaging domain (the antennae center positions are depicted with purple dots): (**a**) Test Date 1; (**b**) Test Date 2.

In Figure 17a,b, the same images as Figure 16a,b are shown, but after having filtered out the parts corresponding to the exterior of the breast phantom. The breast external contour has been a priori extracted from the data as defined in Section 2.4.2, and is used here for spatial filtering in order for the image to be easier interpretable from a physical point of view. The borders of the fibroglandular tissue-mimicking molds, which are a priori known, and a red sphere with diameter equal to the average size of the microlobulated tumor, have also been superimposed on the images in Figure 17a,b. The objective of this second visualization is a straightforward linking of the bright spots on the images of Figure 16a,b and the experimental setup.

In Figure 17c,d, an alternative viewpoint is provided for the same images of the breast interior. The selected viewpoint would correspond to a front-side view of the breast, while the patient is in the standing position. The borders of the fibroglandular tissue mimicking molds have not been superimposed with the images in this third visualization.

Clean images that can be clearly associated with unambiguous detection of the tumor have been retrieved on both tests of the rotational position 1 of the breast phantom.

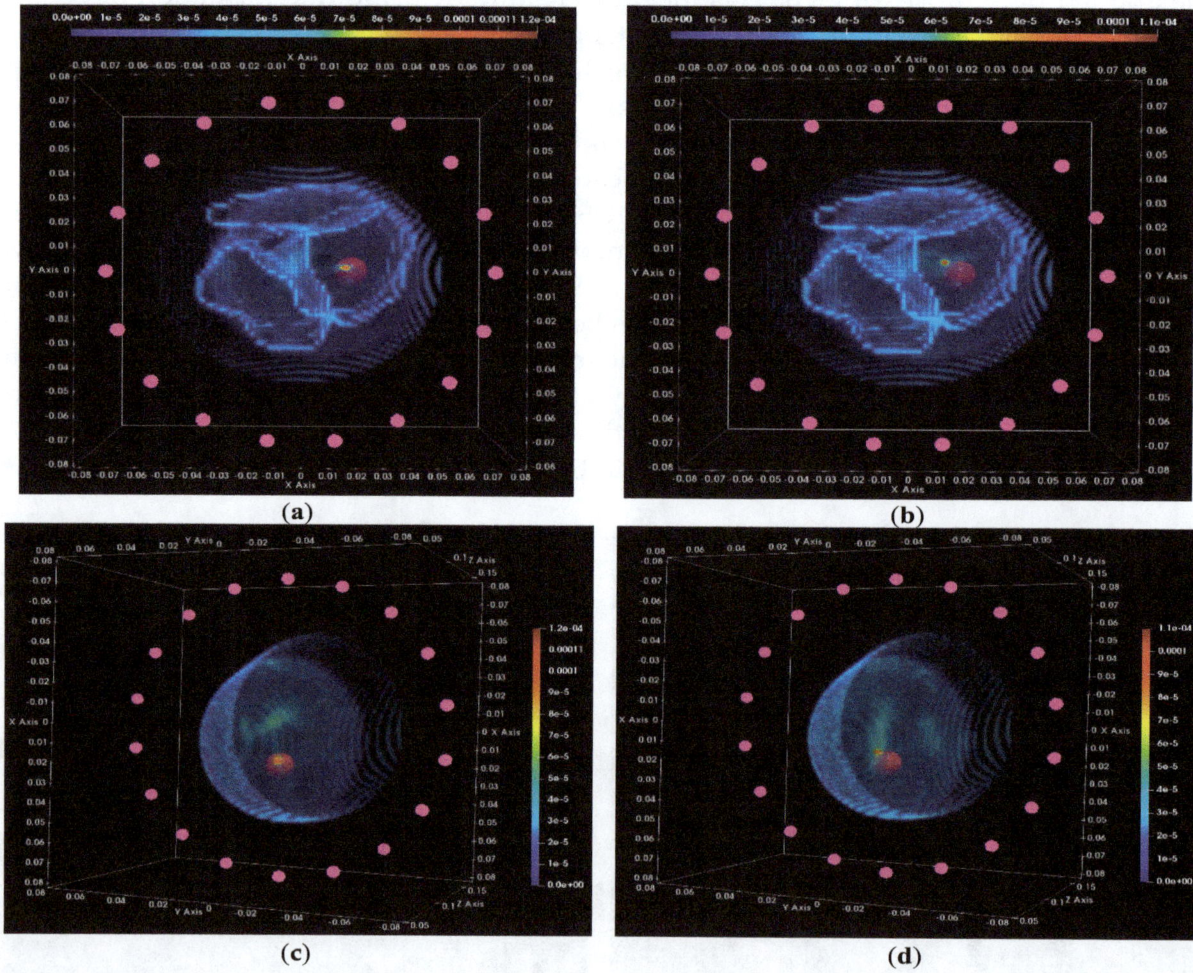

Figure 17. Breast rotational position #1—image in the interior of the breast only, formed at a single vertical position of the sensor network, in front of the tumor: (**a**) Test Date 1, top XY view, superposition of the fibroglandular and outer breast surface molds (blue color), red sphere indicating the tumor location; (**b**) Test Date 2, top XY view, superposition of the fibroglandular and outer breast surface molds (blue color), red sphere indicating the tumor location; (**c**) Test Date 1, 3D view, superposition of the outer breast surface mold (blue color), red sphere indicating the tumor location; (**d**) Test Date 2, 3D view, superposition of the outer breast surface mold (blue color), red sphere indicating the tumor location.

The evaluation of the QA metric 1 is shown in Figure 18a,b for the two images, formed on Test Date 1 and Test Date 2 correspondingly. It can be observed that maximal focusing is achieved for pc_{fib} = 40% on Test Date 1, while on Test Date 2, the optimal pc_{fib} value is 45%.

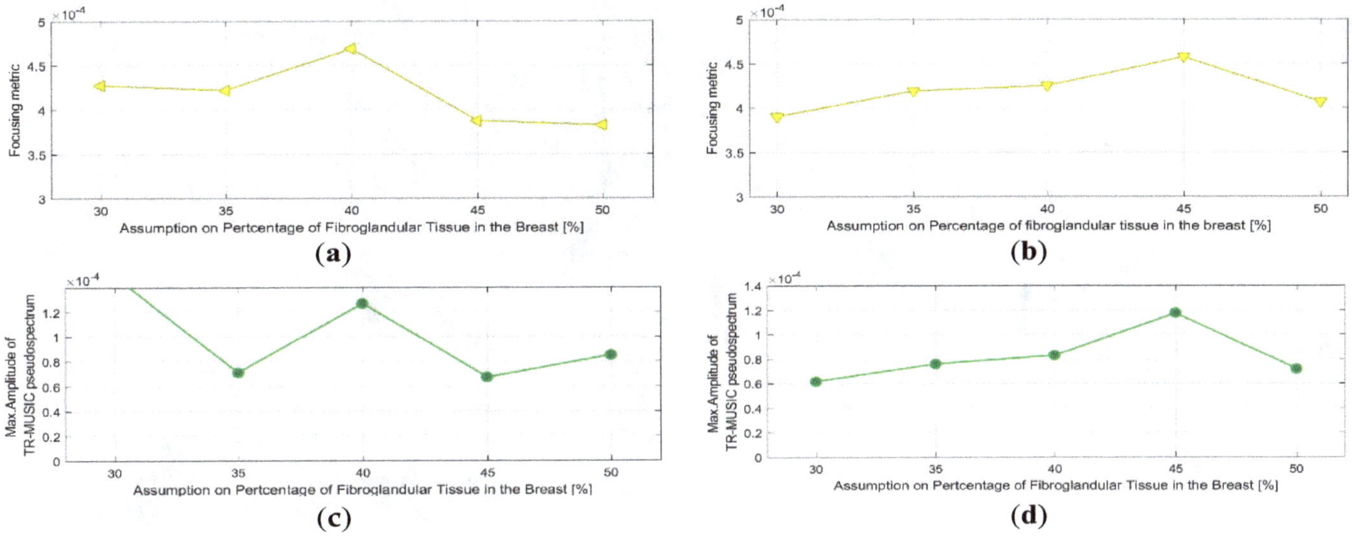

Figure 18. Breast rotational position #1: (**a**) Test Date 1, image quality assessment (QA) metric 1; (**b**) Test Date 2, image QA metric 1; (**c**) Test Date 1, image QA metric 2; (**d**) Test Date 2, image QA metric 2.

The acceptance test (AC) #1 would strictly fail in such a case. However, given the proximity of the 'average' breast tissue dielectric properties that are associated with the two pc_{fib} values, as depicted in Figure 8, and also considering the constrained and yet non-optimized stability and robustness of both the imaging system and the transition liquid itself against slight variations in the nominal environmental operating conditions (e.g., slight temperature variations), such a variation in the optimal pc_{fib} value, in terms of focusing, is still considered acceptable for the on-site validation tests of the actual version of the imaging system prototype.

The threshold value for the optimal focusing metric (FM) per image has been set to $thr_{QA\_1} = 0.0004$. This is valid for the specific experimental setup, which has been reproduced both at factory and after system installation on-site. This is the threshold value that is used with acceptance test #2 all along the on-site validation of the imaging system. Both tests at the rotational position 1 of the breast are thus validated in terms of AC #2.

The evaluation of the QA metric 2 is shown in Figure 18c,d for the two images, formed on Test Date 1 and Test Date 2, correspondingly. It can be observed that the maximal intensity Im_{max} of the TR-MUSIC pseudospectra is maximized for the same pc_{fib} values as the FM. Concerning acceptance test #3, the same considerations hold as for AC#1. In terms of acceptance test #4, the threshold value for the image intensity at the target (tumor) position has been set to $thr_{QA\_2} = 0.0001$, while performing tests with the same experimental setup as at the factory. This is the threshold value that is used with the AC #4 all along the on-site validation of the imaging system. Both tests at the rotational position 1 of the breast are thus validated in terms of AC #4. Finally, the two patterns FM (pc_{fib}) and Im_{max} (pc_{fib}) remain consistent between each other, as far as the dependence on pc_{fib} is concerned, with the exception of the outlier point: Im_{max} (pc_{fib}), pc_{fib} = 30%. Acceptance test #5 is validated in such a case of similarity between the two patterns at the given prototype state of the imaging system.

3.1.2. Breast Rotational Position #2

In this section, the same QA metrics 1 and 2 are evaluated for the two imaging tests that have been performed at the rotational position 2 of the same breast phantom on two distinct dates: Test Date 1 and Test Date 2. The breast phantom is rotated by 180°, with respect to the two first tests, which have been thoroughly evaluated and validated in terms of QA 1 and QA 2 in the previous section. In Figure 19, the experimental setup for the tests at the rotational position #2 of the breast phantom is illustrated.

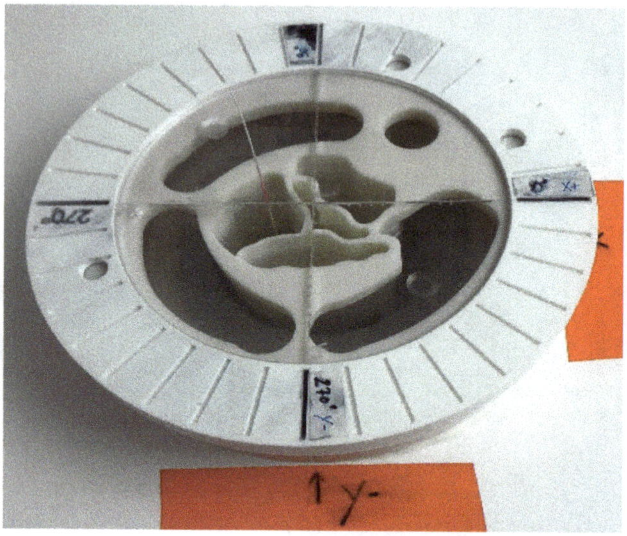

(a)

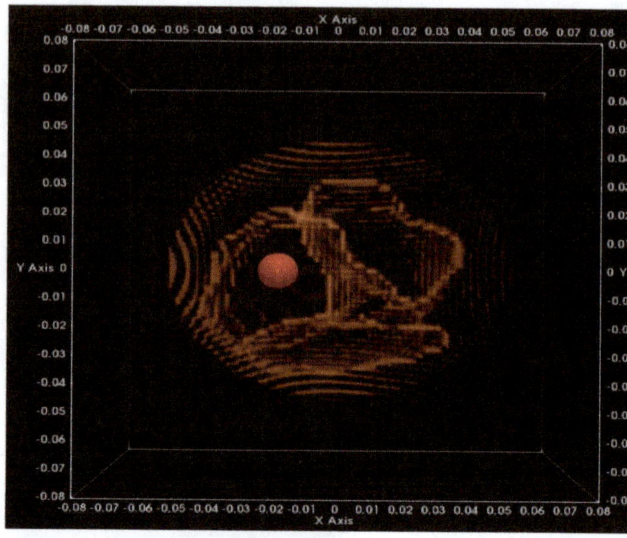

(b)

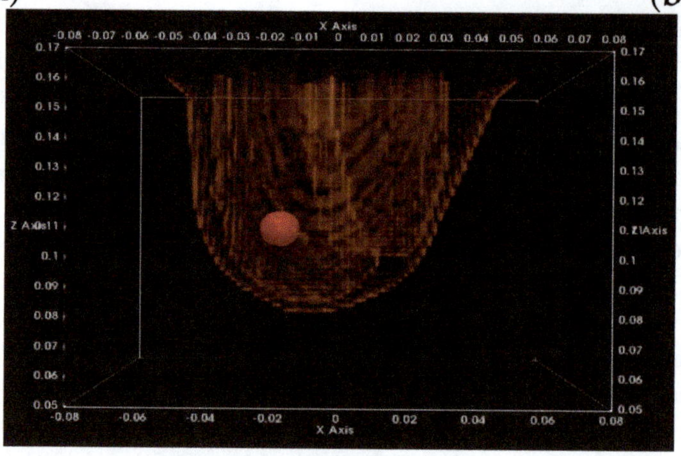

(c)

Figure 19. Experimental setup for the breast rotational position #2: (**a**) Photo—Top view of the breast phantom, installed on the examination table; (**b**) Schematic definition of the tumor location (red sphere of diameter 14 mm, equal to the average diameter of the microlobulated tumor phantom) in the fibroglandular tissue of the breast (the outer surface of both the fibroglandular mold and the outer breast surface mold are depicted with orange color)—Top View; (**c**) Schematic definition of the tumor location in the fibroglandular tissue of the breast—Side View.

For these tests, a microlobulated tumor of average size (14 mm) has been immersed in the fibroglandular tissue-mimicking liquid at the location $(x, y, z) = (-20, 0, 110)$ mm (=center of the tumorous lesion).

In Figure 20, the composite TR-MUSIC pseudospectra, as formed using the Equation (13), and data from a single vertical scan position of the sensor network are depicted for the two data snapshots recorded on two different dates.

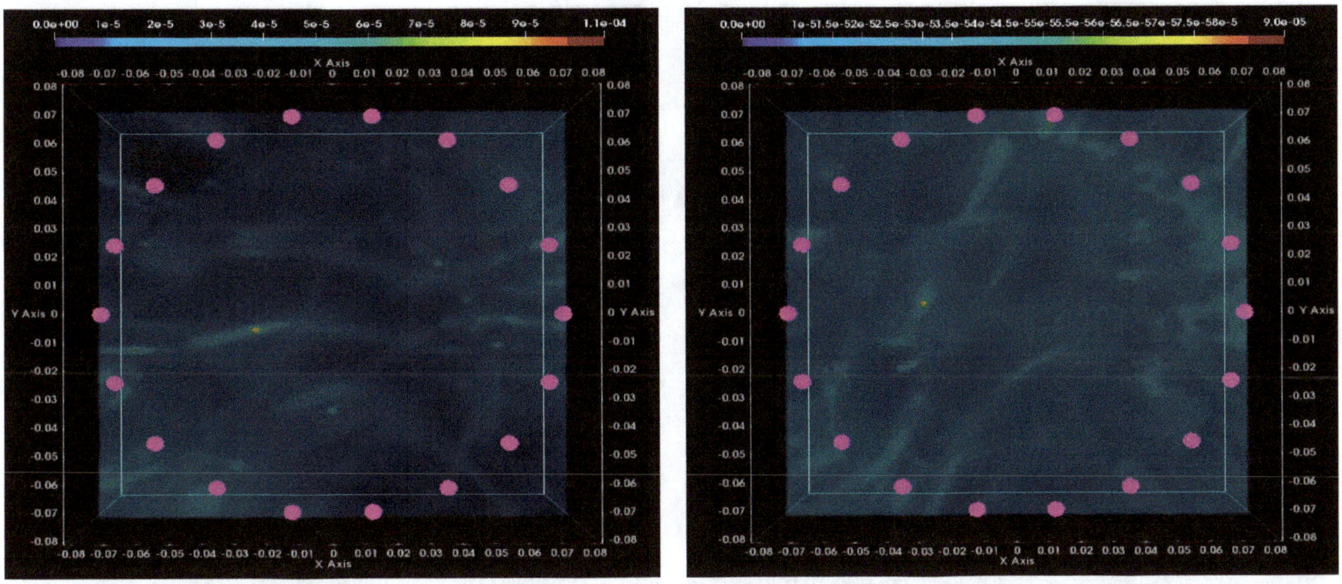

(a) (b)

Figure 20. Breast rotational position #2—image formed at a single vertical position of the sensor network, in front of the tumor, top XY view of the full imaging domain (the antennae center positions are depicted with purple spots): (**a**) Test Date 1; (**b**) Test Date 2.

These images have been formed in exactly the same way, as detailed in Section 3.1.1 for the images in Figure 16. A clear and pronounced peak of the TR-MUSIC pseudospectrum is visible on both images in the vicinity of the ground truth location of the tumor. However, when comparing these images with the ones in Figure 16, it is noticeable that the maximal intensity of the TR-MUSIC pseudospectrum in Figure 20b is lower than the maximal intensity in the three other images. The dominant peak that is unambiguously associated with the tumor multistatic radar echo is also slightly misplaced with respect to the ground truth location of the tumor. The observed shift can be better seen in Figure 21b. The four images in Figure 21 have been formed in exactly the same way as the corresponding images in Figure 17 in Section 3.1.1.

Clean images that can be clearly associated with unambiguous detection of the tumor have been retrieved from both tests at rotational position 2 of the breast phantom. The imaging performance is slightly degraded on Test Date 2; however, such a level of degradation lies within the limits of acceptable variability in the system performance at this stage of development. All four datasets presented in the article are thus examples of test data that have served the on-site validation of the imaging system. The quantified evaluation of the system performance, in terms of the QA metrics 1 and 2, is shown in Figure 22 for the two tests at rotational position 2 of the breast phantom.

The result representation in Figure 22 is identical to the one in Figure 18 for the two tests at rotational position 1 of the breast phantom, which has been detailed in Section 3.1.1.

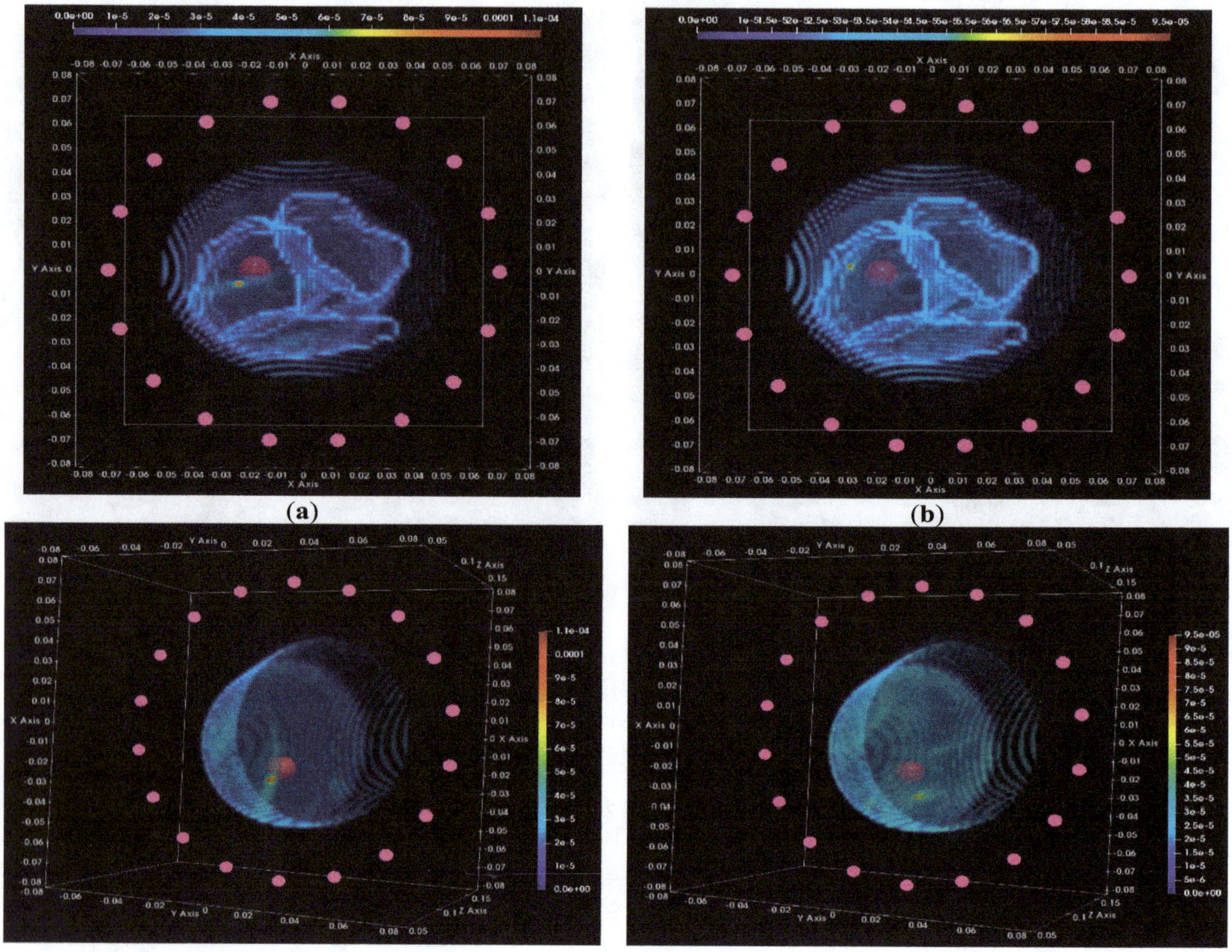

(c) (d)

Figure 21. Breast rotational position #2—image in the interior of the breast only, formed at a single vertical position of the sensor network, in front of the tumor: (**a**) Test Date 1, top XY view, superposition of the fibroglandular and outer breast surface molds (blue color), red sphere indicating the tumor location; (**b**) Test Date 2, top XY view, superposition of the fibroglandular and outer breast surface molds (blue color), red sphere indicating the tumor location; (**c**) Test Date 1, 3D view, superposition of the outer breast surface mold (blue color), red sphere indicating the tumor location; (**d**) Test Date 2, 3D view, superposition of the outer breast surface mold (blue color), red sphere indicating the tumor location.

It can be observed in Figure 22a,b that maximal focusing is achieved for pc_{fib} = 35% on both test dates. The optimal pc_{fib} value remains constant between the two test dates, as required by acceptance test #1; however, this value is lower than the optimal value identified for rotational position 1 of the breast phantom. This phenomenon of slightly shifted optimal pc_{fib}, depending on the orientation of the breast phantom with respect to the sensor network, has been consistently observed on more validation test datasets of the imaging system, and could be attributed to the slight inhomogeneity in the temperature spatial distribution in the interior of the device, at its actual version. This is accepted as such, and validated for the clinical pilot testing of the system; a thermoregulation of the device interior is planned to be put in place when upgrading the device design in the future, such that this type of inhomogeneity can be avoided. The 'average' breast tissue dielectric properties that are associated with each pc_{fib} value are defined in Figure 8.

Considering the threshold value $thr_{QA\_1} = 0.0004$ for the optimal focusing metric (FM) per image, as defined in Section 3.1.1, acceptance test #2 is clearly validated on Test Date 1, but it is hardly reached on Test Date 2, as can be observed in Figure 22a,b.

The evaluation of the QA metric 2 is shown in Figure 22c,d. It is shown that the maximal intensity Im_{max} of the TR-MUSIC pseudospectra is maximized for the same pc_{fib} values as the FM, such that AC #3 is validated on both test dates. Given the threshold value for the image intensity at the target (tumor) position, $thr_{QA\_2} = 0.0001$, as specified in Section 3.1.1, AC #4 is clearly validated on Test Date 1 and just met on the Test Date 2.

The two patterns: FM (pc_{fib}) and Im_{max} (pc_{fib}) remain consistent between each other, as far as the dependence on pc_{fib} is concerned; acceptance test #5 is validated on both test dates.

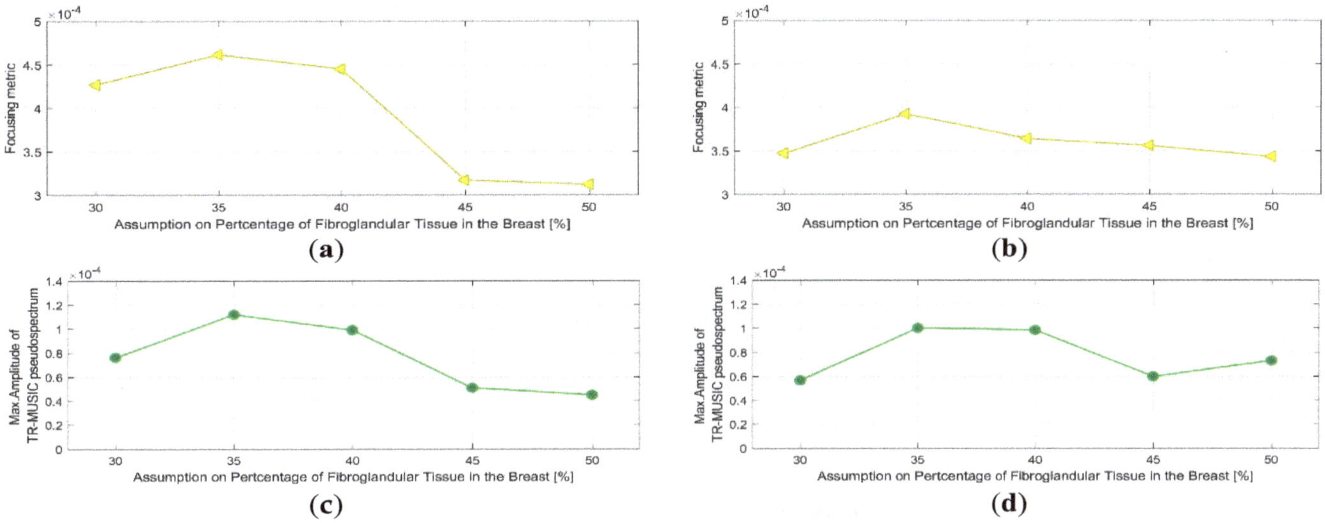

Figure 22. Breast rotational position #2: (**a**) Test Date 1, image QA metric 1; (**b**) Test Date 2, image QA metric 1; (**c**) Test Date 1, image QA metric 2; (**d**) Test Date 2, image QA metric 2.

3.2. QA Metrics 3 and 4: Images Formed at Multiple Vertical Positions of the Sensor Network

In Figure 23, the maximal focusing metric (FM), as extracted from Figure 18a,b and Figure 22a,b for the four test datasets at single H = 118 mm (sensor network in front of the tumor), is plotted as evaluated on images that have been formed using six different vertical scan positions of the sensor network (vertical sampling rate = 5 mm). The result, which is QA metric 3 as defined in Section 2.6.5, is plotted in Figure 23a,b for the breast rotational position 1, Test Date 1, and Test Date 2, correspondingly. In Figure 23c,d, QA metric 3 is plotted for the breast rotational position 2, Test Date 1, and Test Date 2, accordingly. The maximal FM is observed at the same height, H = 118 mm, for both rotational positions of the breast phantom, and for both repetitions of either of the two controlled imaging tests. AC #6 is validated based on the results presented for the four test datasets, as shown in Figure 23.

Ideally, an overall contrast between the maximal FM (at H = 118 mm, coronal slice of the breast on which the tumor is better 'seen' by the sensor network) and the FM that is achievable at any other coronal breast slice should exceed a given threshold $thr_{QA\_3} = 1.2$, as is the case in Figure 23b for breast rotational position 1 on Test Date 2. While such a case represents the goal in terms of unambiguous retrieval of the tumor echo along the vertical scan of the heterogeneous breast, AC #7 is validated also in the case of Figure 23a,c, where the contrast in terms of FM exceeds the value $thr_{QA\_3} = 1.1$. In the case of Figure 23d, the computed contrast is 1.08. It has been concluded in the course of the on-site validation of the imaging system that the three first test datasets are validated in terms of AC #7, while the fourth test dataset hardly meets the set threshold value. It is interesting to notice that the breast rotational position 2—Test Date 2 scan is the only one that has been marked as invalid (or potentially critically valid) by the total of three quantitative evaluation tests: AC#2, AC#4, and AC#7.

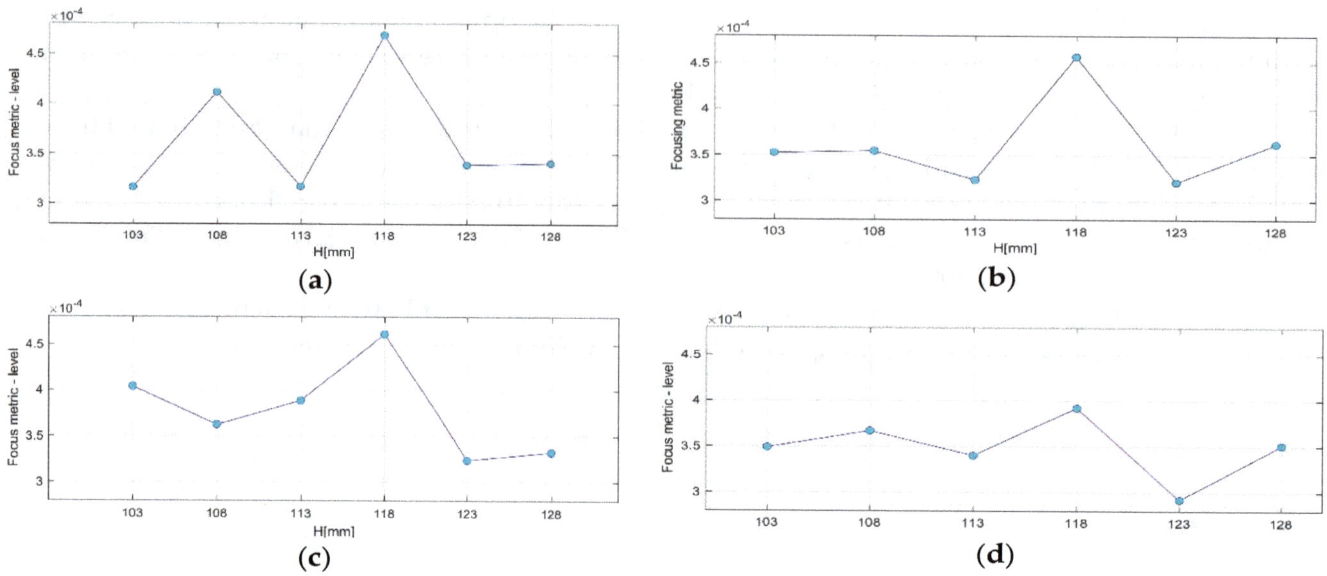

Figure 23. Imaging focusing analysis on 3D multi-H data: (**a**) Rotational position #1—Test Date 1; (**b**) Rotational position #1—Test Date 2; (**c**) Rotational position #2—Test Date 1; (**d**) Rotational position #2—Test Date 2.

In Figure 24, a top and side view of the composite image formed using the data from the six vertical scan positions of the sensor network (as per Equation (14)) are shown for breast rotation position 1 on Test Date 1. The ground truth location of the tumor phantom is illustrated with a spherical inclusion with a diameter of 14 mm, which is equal to the average size of the microlobulated tumor that is superimposed on the images. This type of multi-height composite image has been formed via concatenation of the single-height images with automatically selected pc_{fib}, to allow optimal image focusing independently per height, as explained in Section 2.4.5. The sensor positions, as mapped on the inner wall of the container filled with transition liquid, are illustrated with the purple dots that are overlaid on the images. Overlapping zones exist in the 3D imaging domain among the elementary images formed from data at a single vertical scan position of the sensor network. Intensity normalization operations are also involved in the concatenation of the elementary images for formation of the composite multi-height image; this is the reason why the scaling of the intensity is different for the single-height (formed as per Equation (13)) and the multi-height images (formed as per Equation (14)). The difference in scaling depends on the number of integrated vertical scan positions and the amount of overlap among the elementary images. These parameters are not detailed any further in this paper.

In Figure 25, a top and side view of the composite image formed using the data from the six vertical scan positions of the sensor network (as per Equation (14)) are shown for breast rotation position 1 on Test Date 2.

By comparing the imaging results in Figures 24 and 25, it is clear that while unambiguous detectability of the tumor in the breast interior is assured all along the six vertical scan positions, the maximal intensity of the composite TR-MUSIC pseudospectrum in the breast (tumor constellation of echoes) is lower in Figure 25 as compared to Figure 24. Few spots of unfiltered clutter/interference close to the sensor network are also visible in the images in Figure 25. It is well seen on the side view in Figure 25b that the unfiltered interferers appear a bit higher than the tumor (=closer to the examination table).

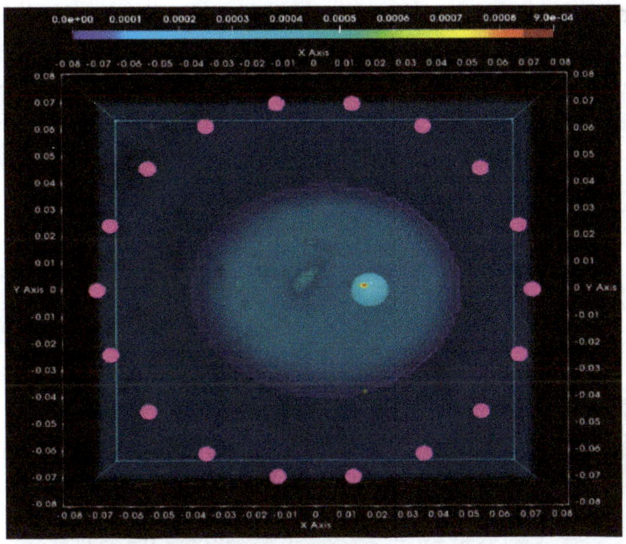

(a)

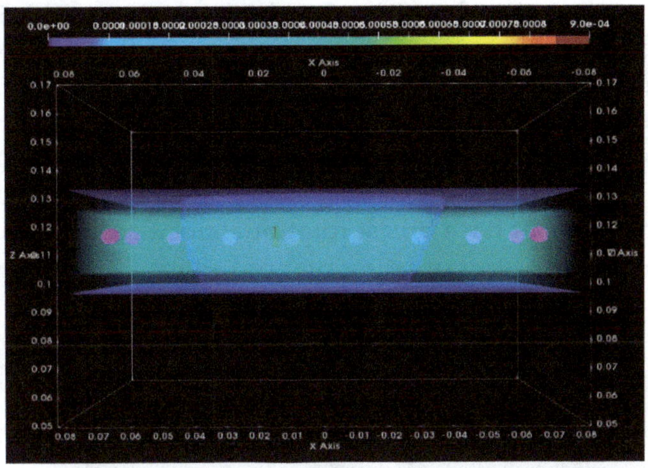

(b)

Figure 24. Breast rotational position #1—Test Date 1—image formed using six vertical positions of the sensor network in the vicinity of the tumor—image in the interior of the breast superimposed with the image of the full imaging domain: (**a**) top XY view; (**b**) side XZ view.

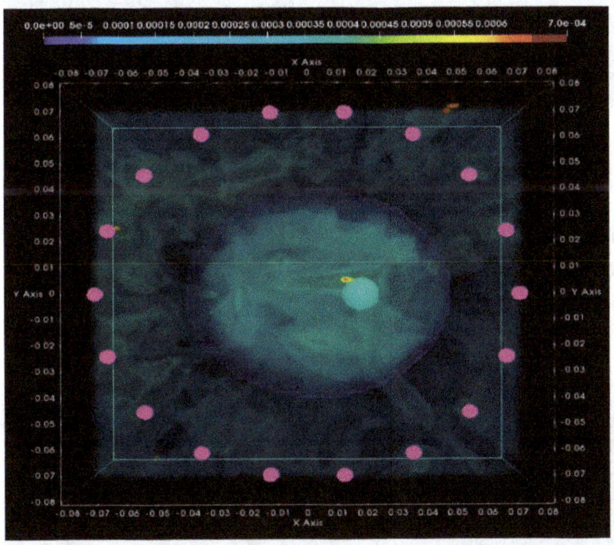

(a)

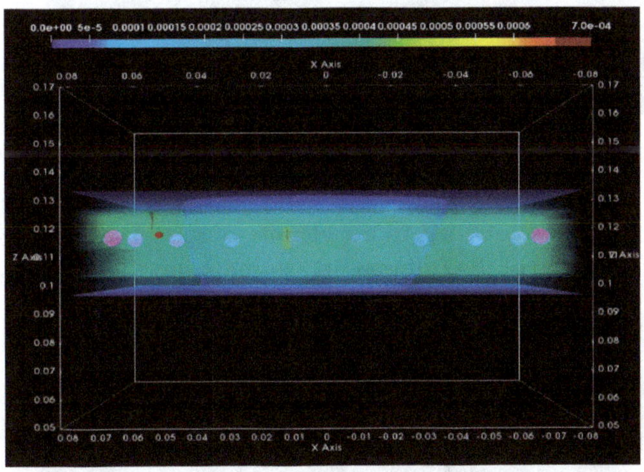

(b)

Figure 25. Breast rotational position #1—Test Date 2—image formed using six vertical positions of the sensor network, in the vicinity of the tumor—image in the interior of the breast superimposed with the image of the full imaging domain: (**a**) top XY view; (**b**) side XZ view.

In Figures 26 and 27, a top and side view of the composite images formed using the data from the same six vertical scan positions of the sensor network (as per Equation (14)) are shown for breast rotation position 2, on Test Date 1 and Test Date 2, correspondingly. The image intensity associated with the constellation of tumor radar echoes is a bit lower on both test dates, as compared to the images in Figure 24. The constellation of more than a single peaked spot is associated with the tumor on the TR-MUSIC pseudospectra of Figure 26. This is acceptable, given the size and irregular shape of the target, as seen in Figure 5.

In both Figures 26 and 27, a slightly higher level of overall intensity in the exterior of the breast phantom (level of residual interferer echoes) is observed, as compared to the images in Figures 23 and 24. This is an indicator of the slightly degraded imaging performance of the system in the case of breast rotational position 2 on both test dates. This is quantifiable by means of QA metric 4, i.e., the ratio between the average image intensity in the non-focused image in the exterior of the breast versus the maximal image intensity in the focused image in the interior of the breast (clearly associated with the tumor radar echo on all the presented images). The values of QA metric 4 are given in Table 4 for all four composite images in Figures 24–27. Ideally, QA metric 4 should not exceed the upper limit value $UL_{QA\_4} = 10\%$ for on-site acceptance of a test scan using the specific controlled imaging scenario. The scans of both breast rotational positions on Test Date 2 (this is not the same date for both scans) are thus at the limit of being marked as incompatible in terms of AC #8.

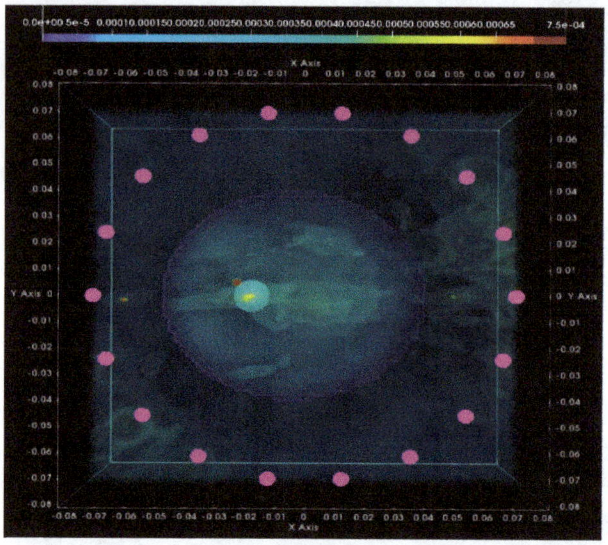

(a)

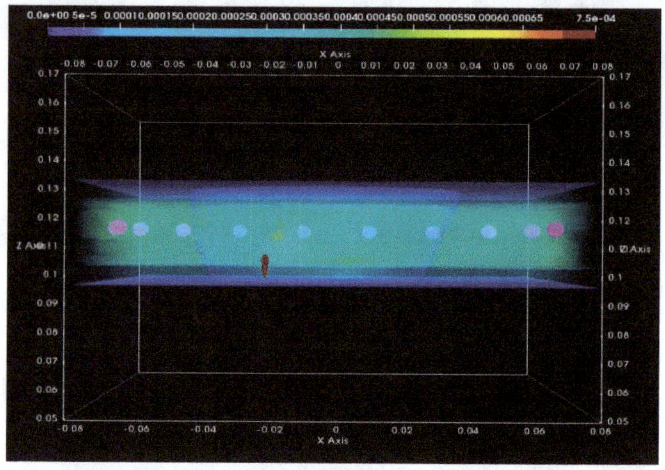

(b)

Figure 26. Breast rotational position #2—Test Date 1—image formed using six vertical positions of the sensor network, in the vicinity of the tumor—image in the interior of the breast superimposed with the image of the full imaging domain: (**a**) top XY view; (**b**) side XZ view.

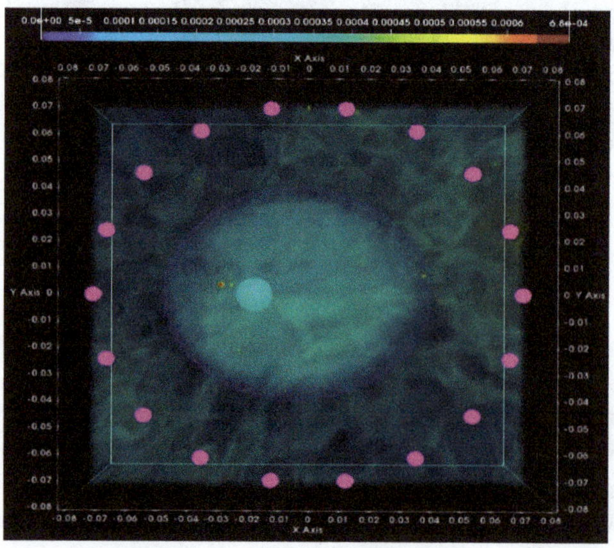

(a)

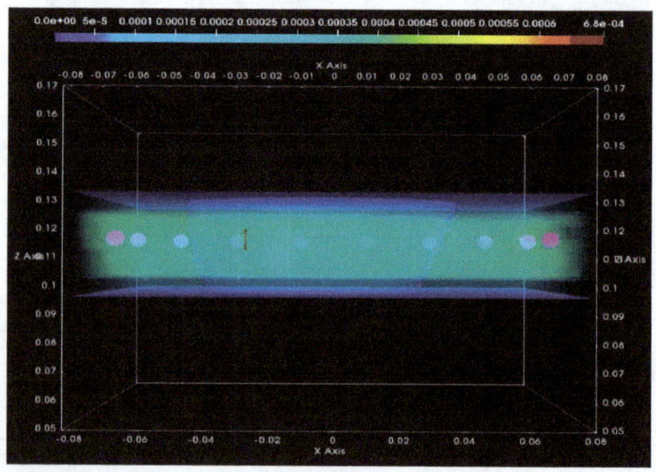

(b)

Figure 27. Breast rotational position #2—Test Date 1—image formed using six vertical positions of the sensor network, in the vicinity of the tumor—image in the interior of the breast superimposed with the image of the full imaging domain: (**a**) top XY view; (**b**) side XZ view.

Table 4. QA Metric 4, Evaluated for the Four Analyzed Test Datasets.

Breast	Test Date 1	Test Date 2
Rotational position #1	7.41%	10.38%
Rotational position #2	4.68%	11.42%

4. Discussion and Conclusions

In Table 5, a summary of the acceptance test results is reported for the four breast phantom scans, which have been thoroughly analyzed in Section 3.

Site acceptance of the imaging system is suggested, if more than $N_{test}/2$ valid tests are consistently reported, at every scan repetition, during a one-week test validation period ($N_{test} = 8$ is the total number of acceptance tests performed and evaluated after each scan, as defined in Section 2.6.5).

Table 5. Summary of Acceptance Test Results.

Acceptance Test (AC)	Rotational Position #1		Rotational Position #2	
	Test Date 1	Test Date 2	Test Date 1	Test Date 2
#1	-	-	-	-
#2	+	+	+	×
#3	-	-	-	-
#4	+	+	+	-
#5	-	+	+	+
#6	+	+	+	+
#7	-	+	-	×
#8	+	-	+	-

+, Valid; -, Critically Valid; ×, Invalid.

This summarized result presentation makes clear the degradation that has been observed for the scan at breast rotational position #2, on Test Date 2, when compared to the other three scans, in terms of the defined QA metrics. This is indicative of the expected and acceptable level of variability in the performance of the imaging system prototype.

At this stage of system development, and toward pilot clinical testing, all the "critically valid" AC test results in Table 5 have been considered acceptable. On-site acceptance of the imaging system is validated with such results, provided that such a performance is consistently achieved along the total duration of the one-week validation period.

In the case of the breast phantom defined in Section 2.3 and used for the validation tests of the system, even if a single tumor model is inserted in the breast phantom under test, the complex geometry of the plastic molds, filled with either adipose or fibroglandular tissue-mimicking liquid, may result in unfiltered radar echoes originating from the corners on the mold surface, which may be erroneously seen as "scattering objects of interest". This complexity renders the test scenario, which is used for system validation, particularly challenging (from a radar point of view), and does not necessarily correspond to a physical complexity that is expected to be found in the real breast; less discontinuous transitions and a less structured multi-layered configuration is naturally expected to be found in the real breast, but cannot be easily reproduced in a phantom.

On the other hand, it is clear that any perturbation that may be introduced in the microwave breast scan due to either an intentional motion of the patient or unintentional 'micromotions' of living body cells during the scan, has not been considered so far, and its impact will be investigated based on clinical data only. Interference due to blood flow in the breast, or due to the interface between the examination table and the patient's chest wall have not been investigated either. The inherent interpatient anatomical variability and its impact on the pre-processing modules for sensor coupling and breast skin echo suppression will also need to be carefully investigated during the pilot clinical test. Finally, the interpatient variability in terms of: normal and cancerous breast tissue dielectric properties and associated contrasts, breast density, and skin texture depending on age, are all examples of physical phenomena that have not been modeled by the phantoms used for the system design and validation.

Given the above considerations on potential sources of mismodeling of the breast with the available phantoms, it is inevitable that some adjustments of both the hardware and software modules of the system architecture may need to be performed as a conclusion of the planned pilot clinical testing. Such adjustments may be required such that the intended imaging performance, as validated with the indicative results presented in this paper, is assured and validated when processing the clinical data from patient breast scans as well.

Author Contributions: A.F. designed the radar signal processing algorithms for microwave breast image formation and tumor detection, conceived the QA metrics for on-site system validation, processed and evaluated the experimental data, wrote the original draft of the paper; L.D. supervised the installation of the imaging system at the Galway University Hospital, inspected and validated all the hardware system components after installation, performed all the experiments, reviewed and edited the draft paper; J.D.G.C. conceived and developed the calibration method for the optical sub-system, conceived and developed the breast surface reconstruction method for the optical sub-system, developed the piloting software of the Wavelia system including Graphical User Interface (GUI) appropriate for the clinical setting; P.L. conceived and developed the breast surface reconstruction method for the microwave imaging system, developed the breast centering assessment module for quality check of the microwave breast scan; G.R. designed the advanced mechanical support of the probe array of the RF subsystem, the mechanical architecture of the optical subsystem and contributed to the installation of the system at the hospital. J.-G.B. participated to the design of the electrical architecture of both RF and optical subsystems and contributed to the installation of the system at the hospital.

References

1. Fear, E.C.; Stuchly, M.A. Microwave detection of breast cancer. *IEEE Trans. Microw. Theory Tech.* **2000**, *48*, 1854–1863. [CrossRef]
2. Fear, E.C.; Hagness, S.C.; Meaney, P.M.; Okoniewski, M.; Stuchly, M.A. Enhancing breast tumor detection with near-field imaging. *IEEE Microw. Mag.* **2002**, *3*, 48–56. [CrossRef]
3. Fear, E.C.; Meaney, P.M.; Stuchly, M.A. Microwaves for Breast Cancer Detection? *IEEE Potentials* **2003**, *22*, 12–18. [CrossRef]
4. Klemm, M.; Craddock, I.; Leendertz, J.; Preece, A.; Benjamin, R. Experimental and clinical results of breast cancer detection using UWB microwave radar. In Proceedings of the 2008 IEEE Antennas and Propagation Society International Symposium, San Diego, CA, USA, 5–11 July 2008. [CrossRef]
5. Porter, E.; Santorelli, A.; Coates, M.; Popovic, M. An experimental system for time-domain microwave breast imaging. In Proceedings of the 5th European Conference on Antennas and Propagation (EUCAP), Rome, Italy, 11–15 April 2011.
6. Meaney, P.M.; Fanning, M.W.; Li, D.; Poplack, S.P.; Paulsen, K.D. A clinical prototype for active microwave imaging of the breast. *IEEE Trans. Microw. Theory Tech.* **2000**, *48*, 1841–1853. [CrossRef]
7. Meaney, P.M.; Fanning, M.W.; Zhou, T.; Golnabi, A.; Geimer, S.D.; Paulsen, K.D. Clinical microwave breast imaging—2D results and the evolution to 3D. In Proceedings of the 2009 International Conference on Electromagnetics in Advanced Applications, Torino, Italy, 14–18 September 2009. [CrossRef]
8. Meaney, P.M.; Kaufman, P.A.; Muffly, L.S.; Click, M.; Poplack, S.P.; Wells, W.A.; Schwartz, G.N.; di Florio-Alexander, R.M.; Tosteson, T.D.; Li, Z.; et al. Microwave imaging for neoadjuvant chemotherapy monitoring: Initial clinical experience. *Breast Cancer Res.* **2013**, *15*, 35. [CrossRef] [PubMed]
9. Shere, M.; Preece, A.; Craddock, I.; Leendertz, J.; Klemm, M. Multistatic radar: First trials of a new breast imaging modality. *Breast Cancer Res.* **2009**, *11* (Suppl. S2), O5. [CrossRef]
10. Fear, E.C.; Bourqui, J.; Curtis, C.; Mew, D.; Docktor, B.; Romano, C. Microwave breast imaging with a monostatic radar-based system: A study of application to patients. *IEEE Trans. Microw. Theory Tech.* **2013**, *61*, 2119–2128. [CrossRef]

11. Porter, E.; Coates, M.; Popovic, M. An Early Clinical Study of Time-Domain Microwave Radar for Breast Health Monitoring. *IEEE Trans. Biomed. Eng.* **2016**, *63*, 530–539. [CrossRef] [PubMed]
12. Kwon, S.; Lee, S. Recent Advances in Microwave Imaging for Breast Cancer Detection. *Int. J. Biomed. Imaging* **2016**, *2016*, 5054912. [CrossRef] [PubMed]
13. O'Loughlin, D.; O'Halloran, M.J.; Moloney, B.M.; Glavin, M.; Jones, E.; Elahi, M.A. Microwave Breast Imaging: Clinical Advances and Remaining Challenges. *IEEE Trans. Biomed. Eng.* **2018**. [CrossRef] [PubMed]
14. Conceição, R.; Mohr, J.; O'Halloran, M. *An Introduction to Microwave Imaging for Breast Cancer Detection*; Springer: Berlin, Germany, 2016. [CrossRef]
15. Hadjiiski, L.; Sahiner, B.; Chan, H.-P. Advances in computer-aided diagnosis for breast cancer. *Curr. Opin. Obstet. Gynecol.* **2006**, *18*, 64–70. [CrossRef] [PubMed]
16. Tang, J.; Rangayyan, R.M.; Xu, J.; el Naqa, I.; Yang, Y. Computer-aided detection and diagnosis of breast cancer with mammography: Recent advances. *IEEE Trans. Inf. Technol. Biomed.* **2009**, *13*, 236–251. [CrossRef] [PubMed]
17. Li, Q.; Nishikawa, R.M. *Computer-Aided Detection and Diagnosis in Medical Imaging*; Taylor & Francis: Thames, UK, 2010.
18. Joines, W.T.; Zhang, Y.; Li, C.; Jirtle, R.L. The measured electrical properties of normal and malignant human tissues from 50 to 900 MHz. *Med. Phys.* **1994**, *21*, 547–550. [CrossRef] [PubMed]
19. Gabriel, C. *Compilation of the Dielectric Properties of Body Tissues at RF and Microwave Frequencies*; Report N.AL/OE-TR-1996-0037; King's College London: London, UK, 1996.
20. Campbell, A.M.; Land, D.V. Dielectric properties of female human breast tissue measured in vitro at 3.2 GHz. *Phys. Med. Biol.* **1992**, *37*, 193. [CrossRef] [PubMed]
21. Chen, Y.; Gunawan, E.; Low, K.S.; Wang, S.C.; Soh, C.B.; Putti, T.C. Effect of lesion morphology on microwave signature in 2-D ultra-wideband breast imaging. *IEEE Trans. Biomed. Eng.* **2008**, *55*, 2011–2021. [CrossRef] [PubMed]
22. Davis, S.K.; van Veen, B.D.; Hagness, S.C.; Kelcz, F. Breast tumor characterization based on ultrawideband microwave backscatter. *IEEE Trans. Biomed. Eng.* **2008**, *55*, 237–246. [CrossRef] [PubMed]
23. Conceicao, R.C.; O'Halloran, M.; Capote, R.M.; Ferreira, C.S.; Matela, N.; Ferreira, H.A.; Glavin, M.; Jones, E.; Almeida, P. Development of breast and tumour models for simulation of novel multimodal PEM-UWB technique for detection and classification of breast tumours. In Proceedings of the 2012 IEEE Nuclear Science Symposium and Medical Imaging Conference Record (NSS/MIC), Anaheim, CA, USA, 27 October–3 November 2012. [CrossRef]
24. Cherniakov, M. *Bistatic Radar: Emerging Technology*; John Wiley & Sons: Hoboken, NJ, USA, 2008. [CrossRef]
25. Skolnik, M.I. *Radar Handbook*; McGraw-Hill Education–Europe: London, UK, 2008.
26. Lazebnik, M.; Popovic, D.; McCartney, L.; Watkins, C.B.; Lindstrom, M.J.; Harter, J.; Sewall, S.; Ogilvie, T.; Magliocco, A.; Breslin, T.M.; et al. A large-scale study of the ultrawideband microwave dielectric properties of normal, benign and malignant breast tissues obtained from cancer surgeries. *Phys. Med. Biol.* **2007**, *52*, 6093. [CrossRef] [PubMed]
27. Zastrow, E.; Davis, S.K.; Lazebnik, M.; Kelcz, F.; van Veen, B.D.; Hagness, S.C. Development of anatomically realistic numerical breast phantoms with accurate dielectric properties for modeling microwave interactions with the human breast. *IEEE Trans. Biomed. Eng.* **2008**, *55*, 2792–2800. [CrossRef] [PubMed]
28. Lazebnik, M.; McCartney, L.; Popovic, D.; Watkins, C.B.; Lindstrom, M.J.; Harter, J.; Sewall, S.; Magliocco, A.; Booske, J.H.; Okoniewski, M.; et al. A large-scale study of the ultrawideband microwave dielectric properties of normal breast tissue obtained from reduction surgeries. *Phys. Med. Biol.* **2007**, *52*, 2637. [CrossRef] [PubMed]
29. Sugitani, T.; Kubota, S.I.; Kuroki, S.I.; Sogo, K.; Arihiro, K.; Okada, M.; Kadoya, T.; Hide, M.; Oda, M.; Kikkawa, T. Complex permittivities of breast tumor tissues obtained from cancer surgeries. *Appl. Phys. Lett.* **2014**, *104*, 253702. [CrossRef]
30. Martellosio, A.; Pasian, M.; Bozzi, M.; Perregrini, L.; Mazzanti, A.; Svelto, F.; Summers, P.E.; Renne, G.; Preda, L.; Bellomi, M. Dielectric Properties Characterization From 0.5 to 50 GHz of Breast Cancer Tissues. *IEEE Trans. Microw. Theory Tech.* **2016**, *65*, 998–1011. [CrossRef]
31. Conceição, R.C.; O'Halloran, M.; Glavin, M.; Jones, E. Numerical modelling for ultra wideband radar breast cancer detection and classification. *Prog. Electromagn. Res. B* **2011**, *34*, 145–171. [CrossRef]

32. Fasoula, A.; Bernard, J.; Robin, G.; Duchesne, L. Elaborated breast phantoms and experimental benchmarking of a microwave breast imaging system before first clinical studyTitle. In Proceedings of the 12th European Conference on Antennas and Propagation 2018, London, UK, 9–13 April 2018.
33. Fasoula, A.; Anwar, S.; Toutain, Y.; Duchesne, L. Microwave vision: From RF safety to medical imaging. In Proceedings of the 11th European Conference on Antennas and Propagation, Paris, France, 19–24 March 2017. [CrossRef]
34. Joachimowicz, N.; Conessa, C.; Henriksson, T.; Duchêne, B. Breast phantoms for microwave imaging. *IEEE Antennas Wirel. Propag. Lett.* **2014**, *13*, 1333–1336. [CrossRef]
35. Garrett, J.; Fear, E. A New Breast Phantom with a Durable Skin Layer for Microwave Breast Imaging. *IEEE Trans. Antennas Propag.* **2015**, *63*, 1693–1700. [CrossRef]
36. Meaney, P.M.; Shubitidze, F.; Fanning, M.W.; Kmiec, M.; Epstein, N.R.; Paulsen, K.D. Surface wave multipath signals in near-field microwave imaging. *Int. J. Biomed. Imaging* **2012**, *2012*, 697253. [CrossRef] [PubMed]
37. Lawrence, P.; Fasoula, A.; Duchesne, L. RF-based Breast Surface Estimation—Registration with Reference Imaging Modality. In Proceedings of the IEEE International Symposium on Antennas and Propagation and USNC-URSI Radio Science Meeting, Boston, MA, USA, 8–13 July 2018.
38. Hyvärinen, A.; Oja, E. Independent Component Analysis: Algorithms and Applications. *Neural Netw.* **2000**, *13*, 411–430. [CrossRef]
39. Karhunen, J.; Oja, E. Applications of ICA. Feature Extraction by ICA. *Indep. Compon. Anal.* **2001**, *1*, 391–405.
40. Eguizabal, A.; Laughney, A.M.; García-Allende, P.B.; Krishnaswamy, V.; Wells, W.A.; Paulsen, K.D.; Pogue, B.W.; Lopez-Higuera, J.M.; Conde, O.M. Direct identification of breast cancer pathologies using blind separation of label-free localized reflectance measurements. *Biomed. Opt. Express* **2013**, *4*, 1104–1118. [CrossRef] [PubMed]
41. Laughney, A.M.; Krishnaswamy, V.; Rizzo, E.J.; Schwab, M.C.; Barth, R.J.; Cuccia, D.J.; Tromberg, B.J.; Paulsen, K.D.; Pogue, B.W.; Wells, W.A. Spectral discrimination of breast pathologies in situ using spatial frequency domain imaging. *Breast Cancer Res.* **2013**, *15*, R61. [CrossRef] [PubMed]
42. Chaumette, E.; Comon, P.; Muller, D. ICA-based technique for radiating sources estimation: Application to airport surveillance. *IEE Proc. Part F Radar Signal Process.* **1993**, *140*, 395–401. [CrossRef]
43. Gaikwad, A.N.; Singh, D.; Nigam, M.J. Application of clutter reduction techniques for detection of metallic and low dielectric target behind the brick wall by stepped frequency continuous wave radar in ultra-wideband range. *IET Radar Sonar Navig.* **2011**, *5*, 416–425. [CrossRef]
44. Zakrzewski, M.; Vanhala, J. Separating respiration artifact in microwave Doppler radar heart monitoring by independent component analysis. In Proceedings of the 2010 IEEE Sensors, Kona, HI, USA, 1–4 November 2010. [CrossRef]
45. Zarzoso, V.; Comon, P. Automated Extraction of Atrial Fibrillation Activity from the Surface ECG Using Independent Component Analysis in the Frequency Domain. In Proceedings of the Medical Physics and Biomedical Engineering World Congress, Munchen, Germany, 7–12 September 2009.
46. Stoica, P.; Moses, R.L.; Hall, P. *Introduction to Spectral Analysis*; Prentice Hall: Upper Saddle River, NJ, USA, 2005. [CrossRef]
47. DeCarlo, L.T. On the Meaning and Use of Kurtosis. *Psychol. Methods* **1997**, *2*, 292–307. [CrossRef]
48. Aly, O.A.M.; Omar, A.S. Detection and localization of RF radar pulses in noise environments using wavelet packet transforn and higher order statistics. *Prog. Electromagn. Res.* **2006**, *58*, 301–317. [CrossRef]
49. Devaney, A.J. Super-Resolution Processing of Multi-Static Data Using Time Reversal and MUSIC, Northeastern University Report. Available online: http://www.ece.neu.edu/faculty/devaney/ajd/preprints.htm (accessed on 23 March 2018).
50. Born, M.; Wolf, E. *Principles of Optics: Electromagnetic Theory of Propagation, Interference and Diffraction of Light*; Elsevier: New York, NY, USA, 1994. [CrossRef]
51. Gruber, F.K.; Marengo, E.A.; Devaney, A.J. Time-reversal imaging with multiple signal classification considering multiple scattering between the targets. *J. Acoust. Soc. Am.* **2004**, *115*, 3042–3047. [CrossRef]
52. Marengo, E.A.; Gruber, F.K.; Simonetti, F. Time-reversal MUSIC imaging of extended targets. *IEEE Trans. Image Process.* **2007**, *16*, 1967–1984. [CrossRef] [PubMed]
53. Kosmas, P.; Rappaport, C.M. Time reversal with the FDTD method for microwave breast cancer detection. *IEEE Trans. Microw. Theory Tech.* **2005**, *53*, 2317–2323. [CrossRef]

54. Kosmas, P.; Rappaport, C.M. A matched-filter FDTD-based time reversal approach for microwave breast cancer detection. *IEEE Trans. Antennas Propag.* **2006**, *54*, 1257–1264. [CrossRef]
55. Kosmas, P. Application of the DORT technique to FDTD-Based time reversal for microwave breast cancer detection. In Proceedings of the 37th European Microwave Conference, Munich, Germany, 9–12 October 2007. [CrossRef]
56. Kosmas, P.; Laranjeira, S.; Dixon, J.H.; Li, X.; Chen, Y. Time reversal microwave breast imaging for contrast-enhanced tumor classification. In Proceedings of the 2010 Annual International Conference of the IEEE Engineering in Medicine and Biology, Buenos Aires, Argentina, 31 August–4 September 2010. [CrossRef]
57. Hossain, M.D.; Mohan, A.S.; Abedin, M.J. Beamspace Time-Reversal Microwave Imaging for Breast Cancer Detection. *IEEE Antennas Wirel. Propag. Lett.* **2013**, *12*, 241–244. [CrossRef]
58. Hossain, M.D.; Mohan, A.S. Cancer Detection in Highly Dense Breasts Using Coherently Focused Time-Reversal Microwave Imaging. *IEEE Trans. Comput. Imaging* **2017**, *3*, 928–939. [CrossRef]
59. Stoica, P.; Selen, Y. Model-order selection. *IEEE Signal Process. Mag.* **2004**, *21*, 36–47. [CrossRef]
60. Pertuz, S.; Puig, D.; Garcia, M.A. Analysis of focus measure operators for shape-from-focus. *Pattern Recognit.* **2013**, *46*, 1415–1432. [CrossRef]
61. O'Loughlin, D.; Krewer, F.; Glavin, M.; Jones, E.; O'Halloran, M. Estimating average dielectric properties for microwave breast imaging using focal quality metrics. In Proceedings of the 2016 10th European Conference on Antennas and Propagation, Davos, Switzerland, 10–15 April 2016. [CrossRef]
62. O'loughlin, D.; Krewer, F.; Glavin, M.; Jones, E.; O'halloran, M. Focal quality metrics for the objective evaluation of confocal microwave images. *Int. J. Microw. Wirel. Technol.* **2017**, *9*, 1365–1372. [CrossRef]
63. Registered Cinical Trial Protocol. Available online: https://clinicaltrials.gov/ct2/show/NCT03475992 (accessed on 23 March 2018).

12

Characteristics of a Surgical Snare Using Microwave Energy

Masashi Sugiyama [1,*] and Kazuyuki Saito [2]

1 Graduate School of Science and Engineering, Chiba University, Chiba 263-8522, Japan
2 Center for Frontier Medical Engineering, Chiba University, Chiba 263-8522, Japan; saito@faculty.chiba-u.jp
* Correspondence: m-sugiyama@chiba-u.jp

Abstract: Currently, minimally invasive treatments that insert various treatment devices into an endoscope are actively being performed. A high-frequency (HF) snare is commonly used as an energy device inserted into an endoscope. However, using a high-frequency snare, problems usually occur, such as the obstruction of the visual field caused by smoke. On the other hand, microwave heating produces less smoke and provides a better visual field. In this study, a snare using microwave energy inserted into an endoscope is proposed, and its characteristics are evaluated.

Keywords: microwave; EMR; snare; numerical calculation

---

1. Introduction

In recent years, electromagnetic field techniques have been widely used in medical applications. Examples of these applications are microwave hyperthermia [1], microwave coagulation therapy used for liver cancer [2,3], cardiac catheter ablation for ventricular arrhythmia [4], and hyperthermia treatment for benign prostatic hyperplasia. These technologies are used to simulate the thermal effect of living tissue by the electromagnetic field.

One of the applications of the thermal effect is endoscopic mucosal resection (EMR) [5]. A schematic diagram of EMR is shown in Figure 1. EMR is mainly used for lesions of the stomach and the esophagus. The medical doctor inserts the endoscope into the mouth of the patient, and a snare is inserted into the forceps channel of the endoscope. The snare diameter can be changed to a certain extent. The doctor can put the snare on the location of the lesion and then squeeze and heat the lesion with the snare. An image of the surgery being performed can be viewed from a video monitor. The doctor can remove the lesion areas while stopping bleeding. EMR is performed at various medical institutions, and many cases have been reported [6,7]. However, as the current snare works at high-frequency (HF) currents (300 kHz to 5 MHz), the tissue will be carbonized, and smoke will be generated because of the excessively high temperature. The occurrence of perforations is also reported [8]. In addition, to the best of the author's knowledge, there are no studies on snare development.

In this study, we designed an EMR snare using microwave energy. Microwave heating is derived from the vibration of water molecules. There are three advantages of using microwave energy. First, it has high tissue coagulation ability. Second, it does not generate smoke at the time of surgery because of mild heating. Third, tissue coagulation can be performed even under liquid conditions. With the use of HF currents, such currents are dispersed in the liquid, so the heating capability is lowered. By contrast, microwave energy does not have these limitations. For these reasons, microwave snares are considered to improve the quality of treatment.

In this study, the heating characteristics of a high frequency snare and a microwave snare are examined by numerical analysis and in vivo experiments.

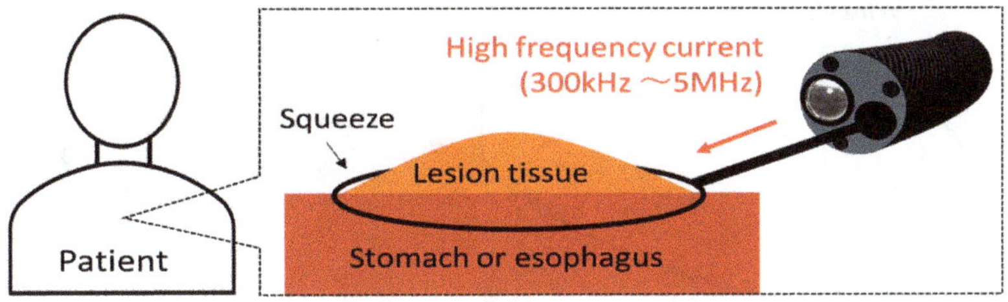

Figure 1. Schematic diagram of endoscopic mucosal resection (EMR).

2. Materials and Methods

2.1. Device Structure

Figure 2 shows the schematic diagram of the proposed microwave snare. It consists of a coaxial cable and a connecting wire. The inner and outer conductors are connected, and the connecting wire configures the main body of the snare. The coaxial cable is covered with a movable heath. This device operates like a loop antenna by exciting microwave energy from the end of the coaxial cable. The target part is grabbed and heated. Then, the snare is tightened while heating, and the target part can be removed. Figure 3 shows a schematic diagram of a commercially available snare. This snare consists of a wire electrode and a sheath electrode. The HF current runs between these two electrodes and causes Joule heating to be generated in the target tissue.

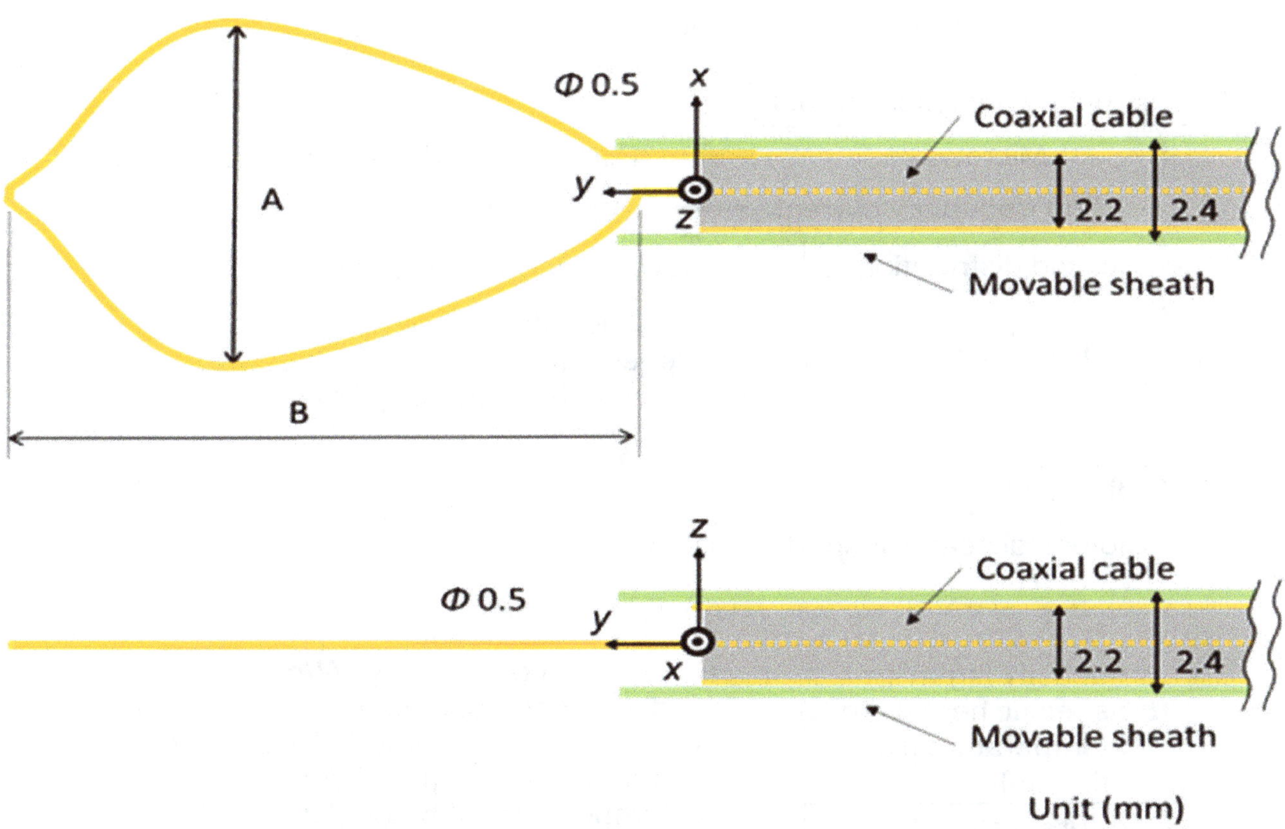

Figure 2. Schematic diagram of the proposed microwave snare.

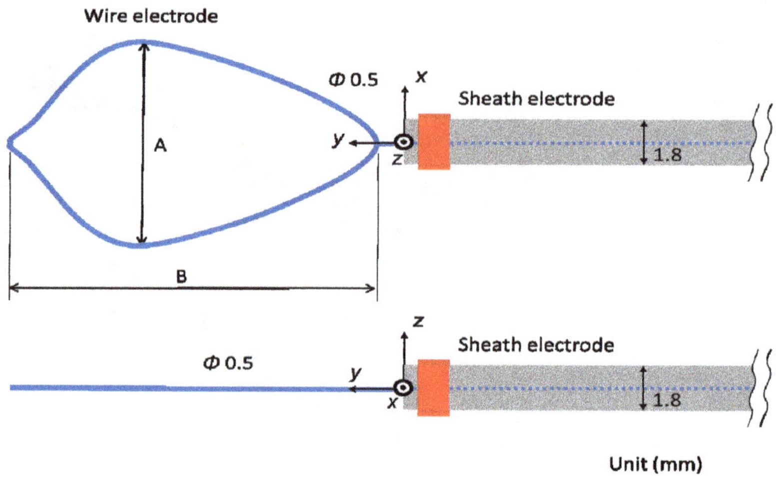

Figure 3. Schematic diagram of a commercially available snare.

2.2. Electromagnetic Field Analysis

The numerical analysis is shown in Figure 4. Analysis of the snare using microwave energy was performed with a self-developed program by utilizing the finite difference time domain (FDTD) method [9]. In addition, the HF current was analyzed with the finite element method (FEM) of CST (Computer Simulation Technology) EM Studio 2018. As FEM performs analysis in the frequency domain, this calculation takes time in the HF region. However, FEM is better than the FDTD method in the low-frequency region because it takes time for the signal to decay in the FDTD method. The electric field distribution near the device is first calculated.

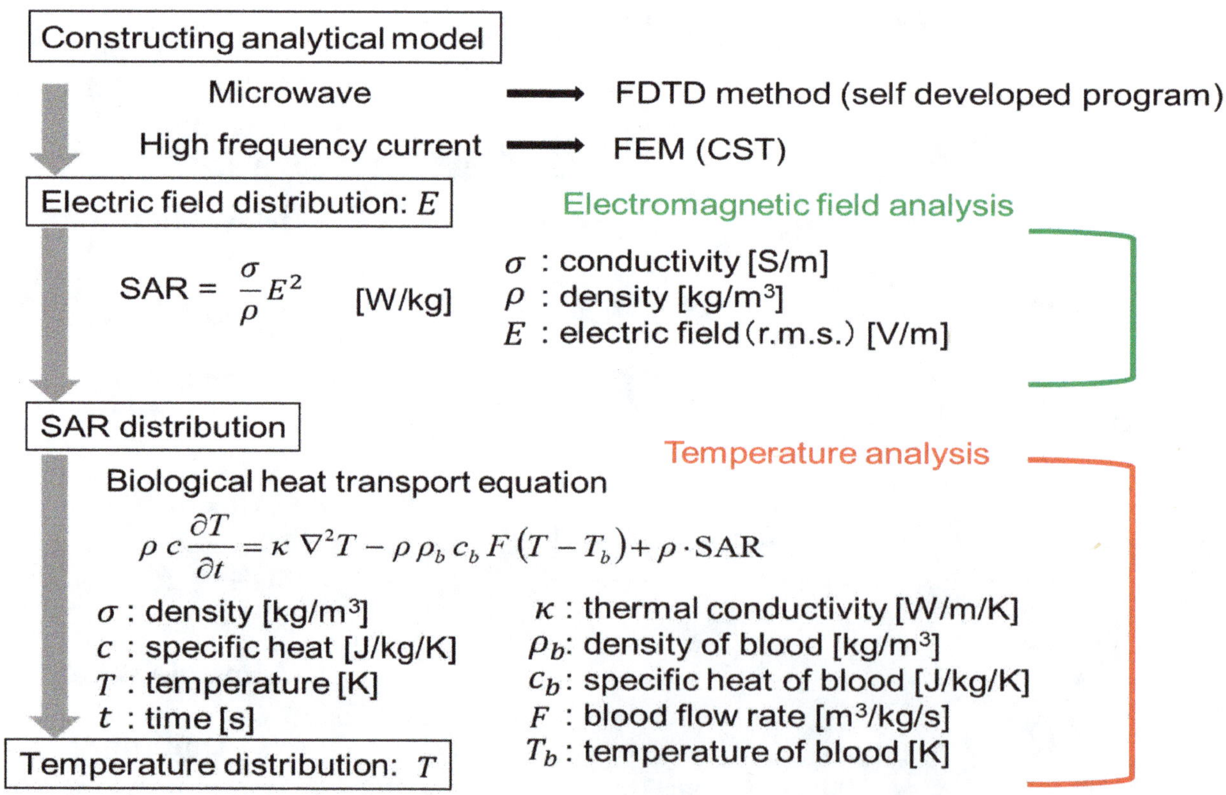

Figure 4. Numerical analysis procedure. FE—finite element.

Then, the specific absorption rate (SAR) in the biological tissue is determined. The SAR can be calculated by Equation (1):

$$\mathrm{SAR} = \frac{\sigma}{\rho}E^2 \quad (1)$$

In this equation, σ is the conductivity (S/m), ρ is the density (kg/m^3), and E is the electric field (V/m) (r.m.s). Using this calculated SAR distribution as the heat source, the temperature distribution can be determined by solving the bioheat transfer equation [10]. The analytical parameters are shown in Table 1. The values in Table 1 are set considering realistic use at each energy. Therefore, the powers and the time of the "microwave" and the "HF" are not the same. In the HF snare, electric current flows directly to the living tissue, so its power is smaller than that of the microwave snare.

Table 1. Analytical parameters.

Parameters	Microwave Snare	High Frequency Snare
Calculation method	FDTD	FEM
Power (W)	60	30
Heating time (s)	10	3

The analytical model is assumed to be used in EMR, and the situation is simulated, where the snare is used in stomach tissue on air. To simulate the grasping process of stomach tissue with the snare, a grasped stomach tissue is protruded. Three patterns of the length of the exposed snare are calculated to consider the squeezing process.

For each model, the electric field is obtained by inputting a voltage of 2.45 GHz for the microwave and 500 kHz for the HF voltage from the end of the cable to calculate the SAR distributions. Other electrical parameters are shown in Table 2 [11].

Table 2. Electrical constants.

Electrical Constants	Frequency	Stomach
Relative permittivity	500 kHz	2060
	2.45 GHz	43.0
Conductivity (S/m)	500 kHz	0.55
	2.45 GHz	1.69

2.3. Temperature Analysis

The bioheat transfer equation used to obtain the temperature distribution of the living tissue is shown in Equation (2).

$$\rho c \frac{\partial T}{\partial t} = \kappa \nabla^2 T - \rho \rho_b c_b F(T - T_b) + \rho \cdot \mathrm{SAR} \quad (2)$$

T is the temperature and t is the time in the equation. ρ is the density (kg/m^3) of the tissue and ρ_b is the density of blood. c is the specific heat (J/kg/K) of the tissue and c_b is the specific heat of blood. κ is the thermal conductivity (W/m/K), and F is the blood flow rate (m^3/kg/s). The first term on the right side of this equation shows the diffusion of heat in the living body, the second term shows the dispersion of heat by blood flow, and the third term shows the heat generation source in the living body. The initial temperatures of the tissue, blood, and air are all 37 °C. Thermal constants are shown in Table 3 [11]. When the temperature reaches about 100 °C by microwave heating, moisture evaporates, so no further temperature increase occurs. Therefore, in the temperature analysis of microwave energy, the maximum temperature is limited to 100 °C. On the other hand, the temperature rises abruptly, and the tissue will be carbonized with the use of a HF current. An increase in temperature of 100 °C or more is considered. Therefore, the temperature was not limited.

Table 3. Thermal constants.

Thermal Constants	Objects	Values
Specific heat (J/kg/K)	Stomach Fluororesin Blood	3690 1000 3960
Thermal conductivity (W/m/K)	Stomach Fluororesin	0.53 0.23
Density (kg/m^3)	Stomach Fluororesin Blood	1088 2200 1050
Blood flow rate (m^3/kg/s)	Stomach	1.43×10^{-5}

3. Results

3.1. Calculated Results

The temperature distributions at the xy plane at $z = -0.3$ mm are shown in Figure 5 when the snare using a HF current is utilized. These are also shown in Figure 6 when the microwave snare is used. The observation surface in Figure 6 is set to be the same as that for a HF current. Regarding the exposed part's length, (a), (b), and (c) represent 1/2 λ, 3/8λ, and 1/4λ, respectively. λ represents a wavelength of 2.45 GHz microwave energy in stomach tissue. Table 4 shows the relationship between the total length and the size of the snare. The lengths A and B are shown in Figures 2 and 3, respectively. The white lines in Figures 5 and 6 indicate snare outlines. In addition, cross sections of $x = 0$ when the snare's exposed part length is 1/2λ are shown in Figures 7 and 8. The white lines in Figures 7 and 8 indicate the boundary between the stomach and air. In Figures 5–8, the device body is grayed out because this part is excluded from the temperature evaluation. In Figure 5, high temperatures are observed at the xy plane ($z = -0.3$ mm) at $x = y = 0$ in all cases. This is the root of the snare. It can be inferred that perforation is caused by this localized heating. Compared with the temperature distribution in Figure 5a–c), it can be estimated that most of the current is concentrated at the root of the snare, so there is no difference in temperature distribution for different snare lengths. On the other hand, in the microwave snare, the entire gripping part is heated in Figure 6. This is advantageous for tissue removal by the snare. From Figures 7 and 8, the maximum tissue coagulation depth over 60 °C, which is the tissue coagulation temperature, is 1.5 mm and 5.8 mm with the HF current and the microwave energy, respectively. Because microwave energy heats to a greater depth than the HF current does, caution may be required in clinical application. The SAR distribution of the microwave snare is shown in Figure 9. In this figure, a high SAR is observed at the vicinity and root of the snare. Therefore, the microwave snare can be heated regardless of the shape of the snare.

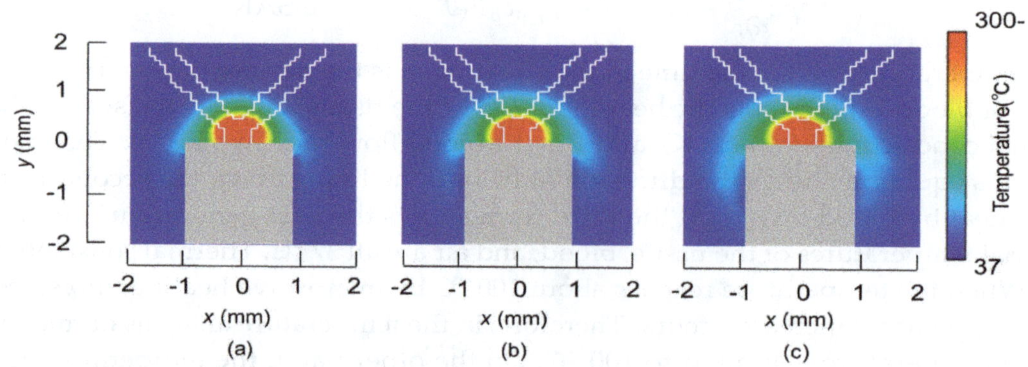

Figure 5. Temperature distributions of the high frequency snare at $z = -0.3$ mm.

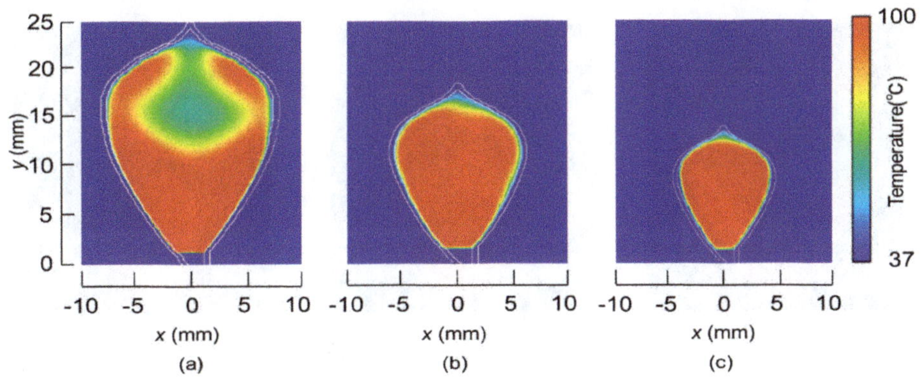

Figure 6. Temperature distributions of the microwave snare at $z = -0.3$ mm.

Table 4. Relationship between the total length and size of the snare.

Sizes	A (mm)	B (mm)
1/2λ	15	23
3/8λ	11	15
1/4λ	8	13

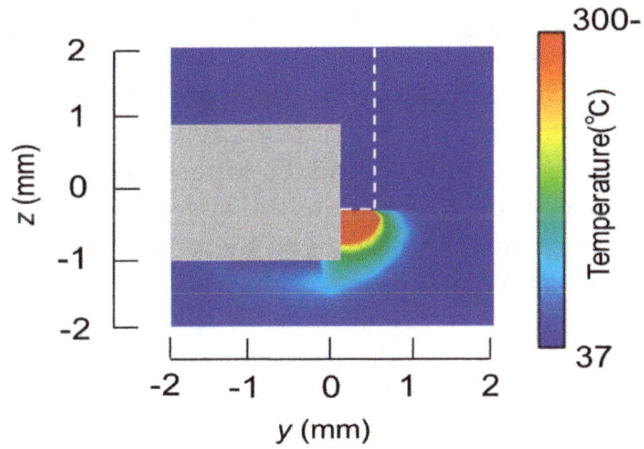

Figure 7. Temperature distributions of the high frequency snare at $x = 0$ mm.

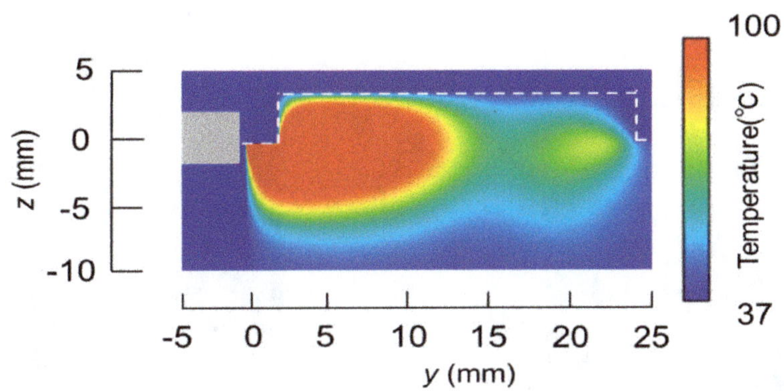

Figure 8. Temperature distribution of the microwave snare at $x = 0$ mm.

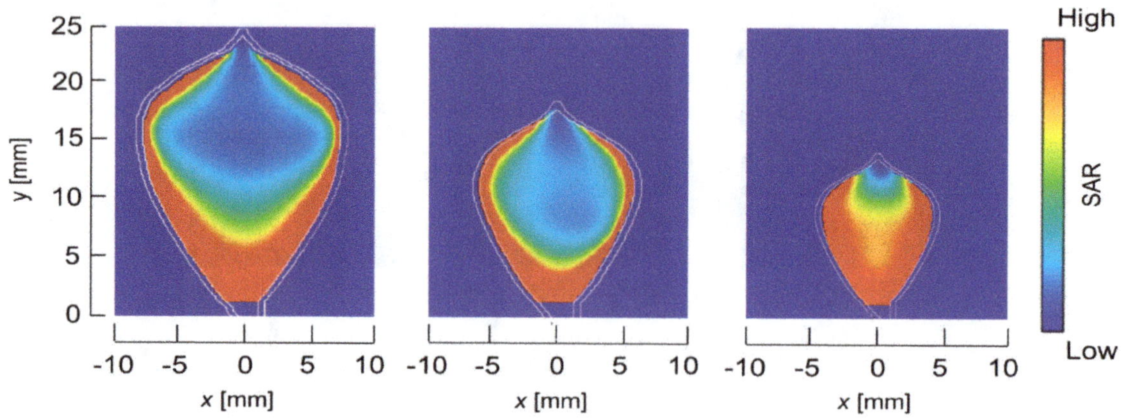

Figure 9. SAR distribution of the microwave snare at $z = -0.3$ mm.

3.2. Experimental Validation

Figure 10 shows an image of the prototype device. The dimensions of the device are the same as those of the numerical model. The snare is made of annealing copper. The device is connected to the experimental system, shown in Figure 11. The 2.45 GHz microwave energy is inputted from the microwave generator through the power reflection meter to the end of the prototype device. Porcine liver was used because it can be easily obtained in this experiment, and discoloration can be easily observed. The dielectric and thermal properties of porcine liver are similar to those of human liver, and there are no substantial differences in electrical properties between the stomach and the liver. The center of porcine liver is protruded to simulate the surgical condition of EMR. The protruding part is squeezed with a snare, coagulated, and removed by reducing the exposed diameter of the snare while heating. The input power is 58 W.

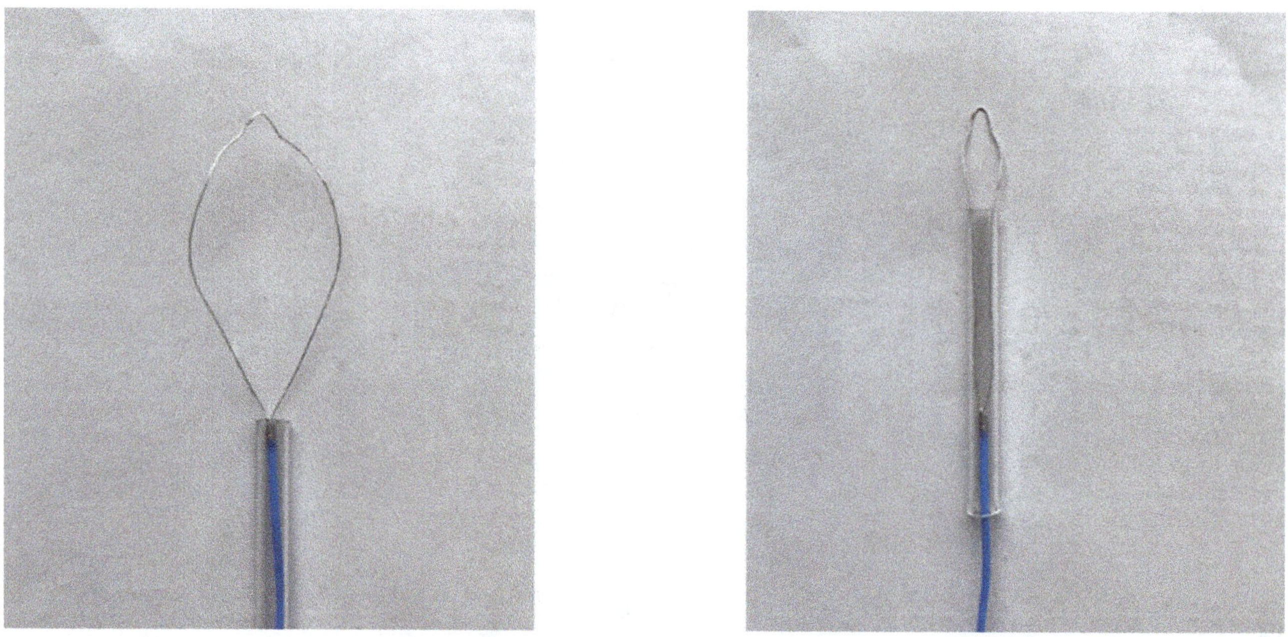

Figure 10. Prototype device.

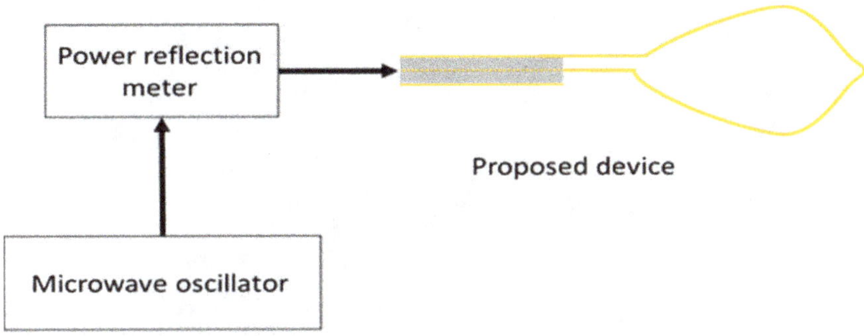

Figure 11. Experimental system.

The liver tissue surface after the experiment is shown in Figure 12a, and the removed tissue is shown in Figure 12b. It can be confirmed that discoloration occurs in the entire gripping part, even in the center part, which is the furthest part from the snare. In addition, there is no blackened part in the discolored portion of the tissue. It can be concluded that the entire gripping part can be heat coagulated by the device, and the tissue can be heated without charring by the device. Figures 13 and 14 show the overall view during the heating process. In Figure 13, during the HF current heating, smoke and sparks are observed. On the other hand, during the microwave heating, these are not observed (Figure 14).

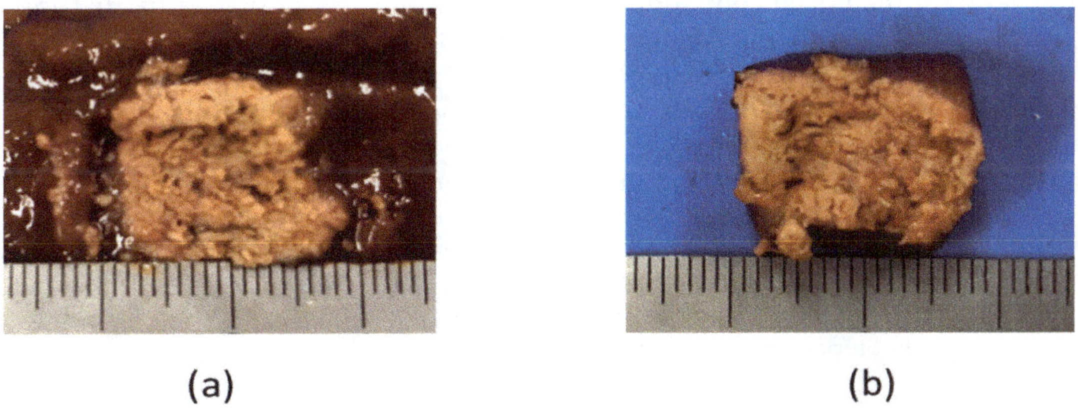

Figure 12. Liver tissue surface after the experiment.

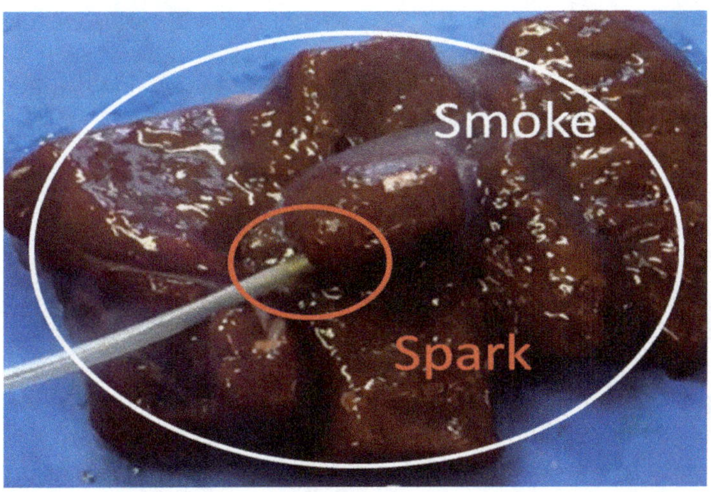

Figure 13. Heating with the high frequency current snare.

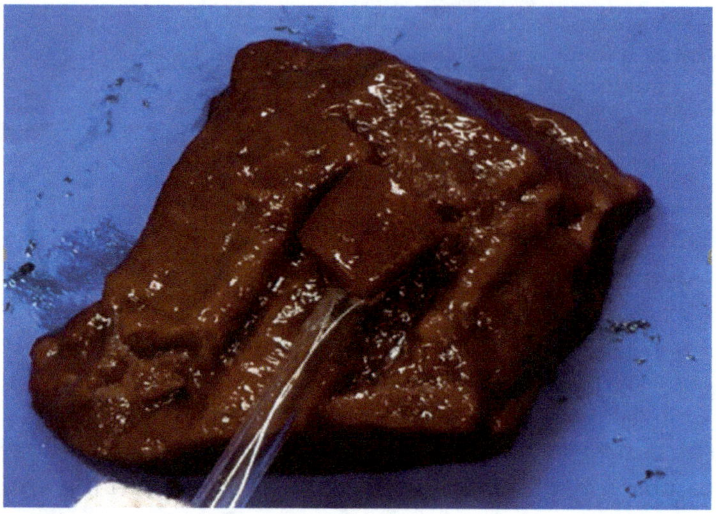

Figure 14. Heating with the microwave snare.

4. Discussion

In this study, we proposed a snare using microwave energy for EMR. The effectiveness of this snare was evaluated by numerical analysis and a heating experiment. In the numerical analysis, analytical models were made for the HF current and the microwave, and the temperature distributions of the target part were obtained for comparison and evaluation. The temperature distribution was calculated by using the bioheat transfer equation with SAR as the heat source. The results confirm that sufficient heating for tissue coagulation was possible with the proposed device. From the heating experiment of the prototype device, it was also confirmed that the entire gripping part could be coagulated without carburization. We plan to develop devices that can be used for animal experimentation.

Author Contributions: Calculations and experiments—M.S.; Conceptualization and supervise—K.S.

Acknowledgments: The authors would like to thank Aditya Rakhmadi and Yunxiao Peng for their generous support and cooperation in preparing this paper.

References

1. Converse, M.; Bond, E.J.; Hagness, S.C.; Van Veen, B.D. Ultrawide band microwave space-time beam-forming for hyperthermia treatment of brest cancer. *IEEE Trans. Microwave Theory Tech.* **2004**, *52*, 1876–1889. [CrossRef]
2. Seki, T.; Wakabayashi, M.; Nakagawa, T.; Itoh, T.; Shiro, T.; Kunieda, K.; Sato, M.; Uchiyama, S.; Inoue, K. Ultrasonically guided percutaneous microwave coagulation therapy for small carcinoma. *Cancer* **1995**, *74*, 817–825. [CrossRef]
3. Liang, P.; Dong, B.; Yu, X.; Chang, Z.; Su, L.; Peng, J.; Nan, Q.; Wang, H. Computer-aided dynamic simulation of microwave-induced thermal distribution in coagulation of liver cancer. *IEEE Trans. Biomed. Eng.* **2001**, *48*, 821–829. [CrossRef] [PubMed]
4. Nevels, R.D.; Arndt, G.D.; Raffoul, G.W.; Carl, J.R.; Pacifico, A. Microwave catheter design. *IEEE Trans. Biomed. Eng.* **1998**, *45*, 885–890. [CrossRef] [PubMed]
5. Soetikno, R.M.; Gotoda, T.; Nakanishi, Y.; Soehendra, N. Endoscopic mucosal resection. *Gastrointest. Endosc.* **2003**, *57*, 567–579. [CrossRef] [PubMed]
6. Ahlenstiel, G.; Hourigan, L.F.; Brown, G.; Zanati, S.; Williams, S.J.; Singh, R.; Moss, A.; Sonson, R.; Bourke, M.J.; The Australian Colonic Endoscopic Mucosal Resection (ACE) Study Group. Actual endoscopic versus predicted surgical mortality for treatment of advanced mucosal neoplasia of the colon. *Gastrointest. Endosc.* **2014**, *80*, 668–676. [CrossRef] [PubMed]

7. Heresbach, D.; Kornhauser, R.; Seyrig, J.A.; Coumaros, D.; Claviere, C.; Bury, A.; Cottereau, J.; Canard, J.M.; Chaussade, S.; Baudet, A.; et al. A national survey of endoscopic mucosal resection for superficial gastrointestinal neoplasia. *Endoscopy* **2010**, *42*, 806–813. [CrossRef] [PubMed]
8. Ahmad, N.A.; Kockman, M.L.; Long, W.B.; Fruth, E.E.; Ginsberg, G.G. Efficacy, safety, and clinical outcomes of endoscopic mucosal resection: A. study of 101 cases. *Gastrointest. Endosc.* **2002**, *57*, 567–579. [CrossRef] [PubMed]
9. Yee, K.S. Numerical Solution of Initial Boundary Value Problems Involving Maxwell's Equations in Isotropic Media. IEEE Trans. *Antennas Propagat.* **1966**, *14*, 302–307.
10. Pennes, H.H. Physical properties of Tissue. *J. Appl. Physiol.* **1948**, *1*, 93–122. [CrossRef] [PubMed]
11. IT'IS Foundation. Available online: https://itis.swiss/news-events/news/latest-news/ (accessed on 31 October 2018).

Permissions

All chapters in this book were first published by MDPI; hereby published with permission under the Creative Commons Attribution License or equivalent. Every chapter published in this book has been scrutinized by our experts. Their significance has been extensively debated. The topics covered herein carry significant findings which will fuel the growth of the discipline. They may even be implemented as practical applications or may be referred to as a beginning point for another development.

The contributors of this book come from diverse backgrounds, making this book a truly international effort. This book will bring forth new frontiers with its revolutionizing research information and detailed analysis of the nascent developments around the world.

We would like to thank all the contributing authors for lending their expertise to make the book truly unique. They have played a crucial role in the development of this book. Without their invaluable contributions this book wouldn't have been possible. They have made vital efforts to compile up to date information on the varied aspects of this subject to make this book a valuable addition to the collection of many professionals and students.

This book was conceptualized with the vision of imparting up-to-date information and advanced data in this field. To ensure the same, a matchless editorial board was set up. Every individual on the board went through rigorous rounds of assessment to prove their worth. After which they invested a large part of their time researching and compiling the most relevant data for our readers.

The editorial board has been involved in producing this book since its inception. They have spent rigorous hours researching and exploring the diverse topics which have resulted in the successful publishing of this book. They have passed on their knowledge of decades through this book. To expedite this challenging task, the publisher supported the team at every step. A small team of assistant editors was also appointed to further simplify the editing procedure and attain best results for the readers.

Apart from the editorial board, the designing team has also invested a significant amount of their time in understanding the subject and creating the most relevant covers. They scrutinized every image to scout for the most suitable representation of the subject and create an appropriate cover for the book.

The publishing team has been an ardent support to the editorial, designing and production team. Their endless efforts to recruit the best for this project, has resulted in the accomplishment of this book. They are a veteran in the field of academics and their pool of knowledge is as vast as their experience in printing. Their expertise and guidance has proved useful at every step. Their uncompromising quality standards have made this book an exceptional effort. Their encouragement from time to time has been an inspiration for everyone.

The publisher and the editorial board hope that this book will prove to be a valuable piece of knowledge for researchers, students, practitioners and scholars across the globe.

List of Contributors

Yanjun Liu
College of Information Science and Engineering, Northeastern University, Shenyang 110819, China
Institute of Electrical Engineering Chinese Academy of Sciences, Beijing 100190, China

Guoqiang Liu
Institute of Electrical Engineering Chinese Academy of Sciences, Beijing 100190, China
School of Electronics, Electrical and Communication Engineering, University of Chinese Academy of Sciences, Beijing 100190, China

Dan Yang
College of Information Science and Engineering, Northeastern University, Shenyang 110819, China
Key Laboratory of Data Analytics and Optimization for Smart Industry MOE, Northeastern University, Shenyang 110819, China
Liaoning Province Key Laboratory of Infrared Optoelectric Materials and Micro-Nano Devices, Northeastern University, Shenyang 110819, China

Bin Xu
College of Computer Science and Engineering, Northeastern University, Shenyang 110819, China

Brian M. Moloney
Department of Diagnostic Radiology, Galway University Hospitals, Galway H91 YR71, Ireland
Discipline of Surgery, Lambe Institute for Translational Research, School of Medicine, National University of Ireland Galway, Galway H91 YR71, Ireland

Sami Abd Elwahab and Michael J. Kerin
Discipline of Surgery, Lambe Institute for Translational Research, School of Medicine, National University of Ireland Galway, Galway H91 YR71, Ireland

Ilja Merunka
Department of Electromagnetic Field, Czech Technical University in Prague, 166 27 Prague, Czech Republic

Tyson Reimer
Department of Physics and Astronomy, University of Manitoba, Winnipeg, MB R3T 2N2, Canada

Stephen Pistorius
Department of Physics and Astronomy, University of Manitoba, Winnipeg, MB R3T 2N2, Canada
Research Institute in Oncology and Hematology, University of Manitoba, Winnipeg, MB R3E 0V9, Canada

Mario Solis-Nepote
Research Institute in Oncology and Hematology, University of Manitoba, Winnipeg, MB R3E 0V9, Canada

Lesya Anishchenko
Remote Sensing Laboratory, Bauman Moscow State Technical University, Moscow 105005, Russia

Bárbara L. Oliveira, Martin Glavin and Edward Jones
Electrical and Electronic Engineering, National University of Ireland Galway, H91 TK33 Galway, Ireland

Daniela Godinho and Raquel C. Conceição
Instituto de Biofísica e Engenharia Biomédica, Faculdade de Ciencias da Universidade de Lisboa, Campo Grande, 1749-016 Lisboa, Portugal

Martin O'Halloran
Translational Medical Device Lab, National University of Ireland Galway, H91 TK33 Galway, Ireland

Alessandra La Gioia, Emily Porter, Atif Shahzad, Saqib Salahuddin and Marggie Jones
Department of Electrical and Electronic Engineering, National University of Ireland Galway, Galway, Ireland

Declan O'Loughlin
Electrical and Electronic Engineering, National University of Ireland Galway, Galway H91 CF50, Ireland

Zhenzhuang Miao, Panagiotis Kosmas and Syed Ahsan
Faculty of Natural and Mathematical Sciences, King's College London, Strand, London WC2R 2LS, UK

Tuba Yilmaz
Department of Electronics and Communication Engineering, Istanbul Technical University, 34469 Istanbul, Turkey

Robert Foster
Department of Electronic, Electrical and Systems Engineering, University of Birmingham, Birmingham B15 2TT, UK

Yang Hao
School of Electronic Engineering and Computer Science, Queen Mary University of London, London E1 4NS, UK

Nadine Joachimowicz, Christophe Conessa and Olivier Meyer
Group of Electrical Engineering, Paris (GeePs: CNRS—CentraleSupélec—Université Paris-Sud—Sorbonne Université), 91190 Gif-sur-Yvette, France

Bernard Duchêne
Laboratoire des Signaux et Systemes (L2S, UMR 8506: CNRS—CentraleSupélec—Université Paris-Sud), 91190 Gif-sur-Yvette, France

Rosa Scapaticci and Lorenzo Crocco
National Research Council of Italy—Institute for the Electromagnetic Sensing of the Environment, 80124 Napoli, Italy

Vanni Lopresto and Rosanna Pinto
Italian National Agency for New Technologies, Energy and Sustainable Economic Development, Division of Health Protection Technologies, Casaccia Research Center, 00123 Rome, Italy

Marta Cavagnaro
Department of Information Engineering, Electronics and Telecommunications, Sapienza University of Rome, 00184 Rome, Italy

Angie Fasoula, Luc Duchesne, Julio Daniel Gil Cano, Peter Lawrence, Guillaume Robin and Jean-Gael Bernard
MVG Industries, 91140 Villebon sur Yvette, France

Masashi Sugiyama
Graduate School of Science and Engineering, Chiba University, Chiba 263-8522, Japan

Kazuyuki Saito
Center for Frontier Medical Engineering, Chiba University, Chiba 263-8522, Japan

Index